POLITICS IN HEALING

Suppression and Manipulation in American Medicine

POLITICS IN HEALING
Suppression and Manipulation in American Medicine

Daniel Haley

POTOMAC VALLEY PRESS
Washington, DC

POLITICS IN HEALING
Suppression and Manipulation in American Medicine

© Copyright 2000 by Daniel Haley
First Printing - September 2000
Second Printing - May 2001
Third Printing - September 2002

Disclaimer

This book is for informational purposes only. It is not intended to diagnose, prevent, or treat any disease and should not be considered as a substitute for consultation with a licensed health care professional.

Cover by Mike Loyd, Houston, Texas

ISBN# 0-9701150-0-8
LCN 00-091629

POTOMAC VALLEY PRESS
Washington, DC

Printed in the United States of America

DEDICATION:

For Berk and Elinor Bedell, who helped make this book possible, and for Dan and Tracey Kirsch, who suggested it, and for Isabel, Ferda, Adam, and Luka, my posterity.

ACKNOWLEDGEMENTS

I am particularly indebted to former Congressman Berkley Bedell and his wife, Elinor, and to writer and former journalist Ruth Montgomery for their continuous encouragement, reading, editing, and commenting on each chapter as the book progressed. Also to Dr. Julian Whitaker for much help and for writing the Introduction. Also to Attorney James Turner, Chairman of the Board of Citizens for Health, for early and continuing encouragement, and for briefing on legal and political matters.

I am deeply indebted to many who supplied information for this book. Chapter by Chapter:

On the Hoxsey Story: vital to this chapter was the help of the late Mildred Nelson, and her sister, Mrs. Liz Jonas.

On Dr. Koch: the late Larry Thatcher, who gave me total access to his files; the late Dr. Spencer Way, the last of the Koch doctors; Paul Koch, Esq., Dr. Koch's son; Claudia Koch, Dr. Koch's granddaughter, Dr. Lawrence Reilly, and also a close friend of Dr. Koch's who prefers to remain - Anonymous.

On the Rife Story: writer and scholar Barry Lynes helped me greatly, and also Bud Curtis.

On Krebiozen: Barry Lynes helped, here too, and put me in touch with Mrs. Margaret Fuhro, who was at the Krebiozen demonstrations in Washington in the 1960's. She provided articles and pictures about them, and helped to edit the chapter. Robert Ivy, Dr. Ivy's son, also was helpful.

On DMSO: my thanks to Dr. Stanley Jacob, who went over the chapter to help me avoid mistakes. My appreciation to Pat McGrady Jr. for allowing the use of the name of his late father's book on DMSO as the title for my chapter.

On Colostrum: former Congressman Berkley Bedell brought

this story to me and all the people who figured in it.

On Gaston Naessens: this chapter could not have been written without the gracious help of Gaston and Jacinte Naessens.

On Electromedicine: my thanks to Dr. Robert Becker and to Dr. Daniel Kirsch for patiently explaining many intricate points.

On Hydrazine Sulfate: my thanks to Dr. Joseph Gold, who contributed a great deal to this chapter, and who corrected the manuscript more than once; to Jeff Kamen, for the use of his excellent articles in *Penthouse* magazine; to Col. Edward Heft, for supplying information from the Internet.

On the Fiercest Battle: my thanks for help with this chapter to Dr. Stanislaw Burzynski, his attorney, Rick Jaffe, and his patients, especially Mary Jo Siegel, and to Ric Schiff, to writer Tom Elias for the information in his book *Burzynski Breakthrough* and to Dr. William Regelson, who loaned me the Elias book. I am also indebted to Dr. Ralph Moss for permitting me to use the title of his Burzynski chapter (*Cancer Industry)* for my chapter.

Don and Karen Rott and Attorney Merrilie Maull were very helpful in editing the book, and I am grateful to Dan Kirsch and Richard Floyd for help in the final preparation.

I am deeply grateful to Alan Lummus for patiently coaxing me out of computer illiteracy into a slight knowledge of word processing, and for similar help, my thanks to John and June Dumas, to Delbra Anthony, Cristy Eversole, and Dusty Ansley.

In acquiring knowledge over the years which led to this book, I am deeply indebted to the late Stephen Fuqua, brilliant nutritionist, who taught me much, especially that the body has the ability to heal itself, if helped. I am similarly indebted to Dr. William Lee Cowden, and also to Professor Eleanor Macdonald, who in the 1930's started the first cancer registry anywhere, for her inexhaustible knowledge of cancer, and for her encouragement.

The cover was suggested by Phillip Schaeffer of Corporate Communications, Santa Barbara, CA, with some input from Charles Gumbiner, and executed by Mike Lloyd of Houston, TX.

POLITICS IN HEALING

TABLE OF CONTENTS

FOREWORD

It has been my good fortune to get to read the manuscript of a book written by former legislator Dan Haley documenting a serious problem that exists in our society. It points out documented facts that clearly illustrate the suppression of new medical treatments if those treatments come from other than conventional sources.

I have been tremendously impressed with this manuscript.

Such a book could only be written by a person such as Mr. Haley who has experience in the field of politics and a willingness to search out the facts. Thank God it is not written by a doctor giving you his or her beliefs, but rather by an investigative person reporting documented facts.

It is extremely important that the facts in this book be made available to the public. It points out how innovation in medicine is suppressed in our society by current laws, regulations and policies, and what has happened as a result.

I served for 12 years in the United States Congress. I found most members truly dedicated to trying to do the right thing. Unfortunately, too frequently we did not have sufficient facts to be able to make the right decisions. Few members of Congress are aware of the problem which the facts in this book clearly point out. It is only by getting these facts to the people and the politicians that we can hope to see the problem addressed and innovation and creativity encouraged and rewarded in medicine and health as it is in almost every other area of our society.

There is growing interest in alternative medicine. I would expect that many of those who read the book would recommend it to their friends, and furnish it to their legislators. I would expect it to be widely read in the alternative community, and I would hope in government circles as well.

Berkley Bedell
Former Member of U.S. Congress
Founder and President
National Foundation for
Alternative Medicine

NOTE: Former Congressman Bedell originated the idea for the Office of Alternative Medicine (OAM), and for the Access to Medical Treatment Act. The healing crises he survived via alternative medicine are described in Chapters 7 and 8.

INTRODUCTION

The struggle between good and evil is a common theme. In modern cinema evil has often claimed the souls of corporate or government leaders, while good is embodied in one or two individuals who "take on City Hall," trying to right a wrong or give voice to the truth. In the movies the good guys usually prevail, as it makes us all happy to see good triumph over evil. Very few cheer for evil over good.

When the movie ends and we return to the daylight of real life, a strange phenomenon occurs. We suspend belief in the struggles between good and evil. What was so real, so believable, so contemporary on the screen only moments ago inexplicably disappears as we walk to our cars. We delude ourselves with the comfortable notion that real life does not embody such stark differences between good and evil. We see only various shades of gray.

Why do we do this? Why do we deny the presence of good and evil when they are so clearly and believably expressed in art? Surely it is because acknowledgement of real-life evil is uncomfortable.

Daniel Haley has written a very important book about the medical profession, detailing the struggles between good and evil as no one ever has before.

Of course, others have been written about scientific discovery and the titanic struggles of ego and belief systems over the ages. We know about the travails of Galileo, how the Catholic Church threatened him with torture if he did not recant his thesis that the earth was round. Galileo recanted, publicly embracing the prevailing view that the earth was flat and was the center of the universe, and for the last eight years of his life was kept under house arrest by the Church. And Dr. Ignaz Semmelweis, who was ridiculed for his crusade to convince his colleagues that their failure to wash their hands before assisting women in childbirth was the cause of the infections that killed over half of the women giving birth during that time. He died in an insane asylum.

But was the Catholic Church, the reigning authority of Galileo's day, evil? Were the physicians of Semmelweis' era? Many would say they were, but I would not be so harsh in judgment. Virtually every scientific discovery over the ages has met a wall of resistance vested in the prevailing belief system and buttressed by rigid bias, dead set - often viciously so - against the innovation and the innovator.

On the other hand, the struggles chronicled in Daniel Haley's book are different. Here a common pattern emerges. The authority figures first recognize and thus acknowledge the value of the discovery. Next, they try to separate the innovator from his discovery, to essentially steal it, usually with a profit motive in mind. And finally, without fail, they pursue a no-holds-barred course to destroy the discoverer. This, ladies and gentlemen, is evil.

As you read this book, you may find some of the episodes Daniel Haley relates hard to believe. You may ask yourself could the author, in his zealousness to make his point, have massaged the data or fabricated these horrendous events?

The answer is no. Incredible as these stories may seem, they are true. This book is very well researched and extensively documented. The information comes from numerous newspaper accounts, court records, evidence presented at jury trials, and, in some cases, testimony from people who were helped by the therapies.

The test of the veracity of this book for me was how the author handled the case of Stanislaw Burzynski, M.D. I have very personal experience with the struggles of Dr. Burzynski, having visited his clinic five times, spoken with numerous patients who survived terminal cancer as a result of his therapy, and interviewed his major opponents in the FDA and academic medicine. I know that this account is accurate. If anything, it understates the energy and force that the government used in trying to destroy Dr. Burzynski. Only the evil will try to destroy a man and his medicine at the same time that they're trying to steal it from him.

For those who want stories to have a happy ending, this book is not an easy read, for evil often wins over good. Valuable therapies have been buried, sick people have been sacrificed, and the lives of innovative scientists and physicians have been shattered. However, this book does much more than tell tales that need to be told. First, it can put you on guard as to what the face of evil actually looks like. It identifies individuals and organizations such as the American Cancer Society that are not worthy of our trust and certainly not our money.

It can also be used as a blueprint for researching your options and protecting yourself should you become ill. All too often individuals with serious cancers who go the accepted route of chemotherapy and radiation suffer not only from cancer, but also from a lack of understanding as to how the medical profession functions and how it has turned its back on its mission.

Finally, this book can serve as a call for action. It makes you want to go out and start a crusade to change things and Haley, a one-time legislator, spells out specifically what needs to be changed. How long are we going to tolerate authority figures who at will, if not at whim, destroy innovation? I am convinced that the best protection against the evil that lurks among us - and make no mistake that it lurks among us - is information. Daniel Haley's contribution is as good a start as you're likely to find.

Julian Whitaker, M.D.
Whitaker Wellness Institute
Newport Beach, California

Author's Preface

Without the experience of six years (1970-76) as a member of the New York State Legislature, I might never have perceived the political patterns described in this book. During the Albany years, I learned to look under the tables and behind the doors to try to figure out what was really going on. It sometimes seemed that the main problems (not the penny ante stuff the press runs after) were occurring on such a large scale and at such a level that one couldn't even see them. That principle is applicable to the ten stories in this book, stories that should not have happened, stories about political harassment and suppression. This is not skullduggery by elected officials, whom the press will always go after, but by the appointed ones whom the press routinely ignores.

Over a period of 10 - 15 years, I kept hearing about effective, non-toxic therapies which saved many lives and would have saved many more but for political machinations and interference by the American Medical Association (AMA) and the U.S. Food and Drug Administration (FDA). "Why would they do such things?" I wondered. The Watergate scandal source known only as "Deep Throat" had the answer: "FOLLOW THE MONEY". Few institutions exercise more influence over government at all levels than the AMA, one of whose principal sources of income - if not its principal one - is advertising by pharmaceutical drug companies. As for the FDA, between 2/3 and 3/4 of its employees take jobs in the pharmaceutical companies (the very sector they were regulating) upon retiring from the government.

Involvement of government means politics - and politics is a field I know something about. As I learned more about these matters, it occurred to me that maybe someday I could be helpful.

This is not an encyclopedia of everything that's out there in alternative medicine. It is not even about medicine, but rather about political intrusion in medicine and healing.

I have written these ten stories as a reporter telling the tragic truth about politics in healing and cancer. Each story stands alone and can be read independently of the others. Together, they tell a much bigger story of the existence behind the scenes of a solidly entrenched policy of manipulation and suppression that has been - and is - profoundly dangerous to American health.

Not a doctor, I advocate no specific therapy but rather a <u>free market where non-toxic therapies can compete freely and openly with the toxic therapies</u> currently accepted by the medical establishment, <u>and the freedom for doctors and patients to use them</u>. This book is not intended and should not be understood to offer any medical advice. Instead, it reports on things which, sadly, actually happened, and, even more sadly, are still happening.

The August 26, 2002 issue of *Business Week* stated: "The performance we get for what we invest in health care is probably the biggest business failure in American history." This is predictable in classic economic theory, which holds that the most regulated parts of an economy will perform the worst, and the American health system is the most overregulated and most expensive in the world. The FDA and the AMA have prohibited in healthcare the "creative destruction" that lets breakthrough technologies push aside obsolete ones, starting with the horse and buggy. If IBM had had an FDA to protect them, as the drug companies do, we'd probably still be using punch cards. Every therapy in this book is or was nontoxic. Most are not available, not because they didn't work, but for political reasons, generally aimed at keeping off the market products that might compete too strongly with pharmaceutical drugs. We do not need to pay bureaucrats to protect us from things that can't hurt us. Therefore, I believe that the FDA should have no authority to regulate NON-toxic or harmless therapies. If this were American law, costs of prescription drugs would plummet from the competition of a free market.

Daniel Haley

WHAT'S WRONG WITH AMERICA'S HEALTHCARE SYSTEM?

Politics and healing might be thought of as a contradiction in terms. Surely there can't be politics in cancer and healing; surely when breakthroughs are made, the medical profession puts them to use. That's the way it is, isn't it? It would be nice if it were that simple.

In most fields, competition usually arranges for the best product to prevail - not always, but usually. In ten stories, *Politics in Healing* shows that a free market in health products does not exist in the U.S. Effective and non-toxic products (many for cancer) have been shoved aside during most of the 20th century. Pushed forward in their stead have been "approved" therapies, usually extremely toxic, which did not win their spurs in the open competition of a free market. Instead, approval was dictated and administered from the top down by "Official Medicine". Official Medicine consists of the U.S. Food and Drug Administration (FDA), the American Medical Association (AMA), the National Institutes of Health (NIH), which contain the National Cancer Institute (NCI). In addition, there are the American Cancer Society (ACS), the Memorial Sloan Kettering Hospital, the Mayo Clinic, the M.D. Anderson in Houston, Roswell Park in Buffalo, N.Y., and others. These organizations constitute Official Medicine, the American medical establishment. It decides, yes, pontificates what medicines and therapies will be available to Americans, and harshly disciplines doctors who venture outside its guidelines.

This book is a collection of stories which should not have happened, stories which will not be heard from Official Medicine, stories about dark undercurrents in American medicine. Political patterns of misuse of both public and private power are seen through what happened to ten little-known healers of the 20th century. Many of them produced breakthroughs of Nobel Prize quality. Most of these therapies are no longer available to help with our numerous health challenges as we begin the new millennium - not because they didn't work, but for political reasons. These stories show how governmental and prestigious private institutions have deliberately misrepresented, held back, discouraged, ignored, and suppressed important inexpensive and non-toxic healing breakthroughs. While government can be expected to be inept, the decisions and actions described in this book were intentional and deliberate, and many people have died as a result.

This book takes as a given that there is a war going on (of which the public is largely unaware) between toxic and non-toxic therapies, and that the non-toxic ones have been getting clobbered. There has been a long attempt to sell a bill of goods that the only real medicine is strong, toxic medicine, almost always patented, produced by pharmaceutical companies, and that only this should be used by doctors or paid for by health insurance programs either public or private. Key to maintaining this status quo is the FDA, which tilts predictably and continuously against non-toxic medicines. Created in 1906 by Congress at the urging of the visionary Dr. Harvey Wiley, the FDA throughout most of the 20th century had little in common with what Dr. Wiley intended. Its original purpose was to make sure that foods are pure and drugs are safe, but it has drifted way off course. The FDA frequently appears less interested in protecting Americans from harmful drugs than from harmless ones, especially those capable of competing with prescription drugs.

Indeed, as we enter the 21st century, the fourth leading cause of death in the U.S. is from reactions to FDA-approved drugs. On April 14, 1998, the JAMA (*Journal of the American Medical Association*) published a shocking report, a painstaking analysis of 39 studies conducted over 30 years. The study showed that an average of 106,000 people die in hospitals each year - that's one every five minutes - from drugs approved by the FDA. The study does not include cases where drugs were misprescribed. When considering deaths from the same cause outside hospitals, *i.e.*, at home, the number rises to around 140,000 a year, according to Centers for Disease Control statistics. These are not deaths from illegal street drugs; those cause only a small fraction of the deaths from FDA-approved drugs, which kill three times the number dying each year from automobile accidents.

And there's more. The fourth leading cause of hospital admissions in the U.S. is from reactions to prescription drugs. About 2.2 million Americans suffer such severe side effects from FDA-approved drugs that some are permanently disabled or require long hospital stays, reported *USA Today* on April 24, 1998. These side effects were estimated to have cost $78 billion in 1997.

When ABC News Director Peter Jennings announced the JAMA study, he presented a doctor whose wife had complained that her pain medication was not taking effect. "My words have come back to haunt me", he told Jennings. "'Take another pill', I told her. 'It won't kill you'". But it did; the next morning she didn't wake up. Only then did the doctor learn that the drug was capable of causing heart problems.

The cost of the American healthcare system has passed one trillion dollars per year - about 1/5 of the U.S. gross domestic product. We spend more per capita on health care than any country on earth. Despite that, some of our statistics are embarrassing: the infant mortality rate in the U.S. is higher than that in Cuba. The number of infants who died before their first birthday is 13.3 per 1000 births in New York City but 10.9 in Shanghai (*Townsend Letter*, May 1998).

A study issued in June, 2000, by the United Nations World Health Organization (WHO) measured a new concept: *healthy* life expectancy. The WHO found Japan leading the world with the U.S. at #20, falling behind every country in Europe as well as Canada, Australia, and Israel. The WHO also ranked national health systems for overall quality. The WHO found that the U.S. system places a heavier financial burden on individuals than do other developed countries, and so rated the U.S. #37. France was ranked #1.

Perhaps its costliness results from the fact that the U.S. has one of the most bureaucratically controlled and over-regulated medical systems in the world. Manufacturers are not free to produce effective non-toxic products or to inform the public on what their products can do. Doctors are only free to prescribe for their patients what has been approved or accepted by Official Medicine.

Because of overuse of antibiotics, many strains of bacteria have developed resistance against any of them. When Jim Henson, creator of the Muppets, lay dying from just such bacteria, Official Medicine had nothing for him. In Texas in early 1998, eight people were suddenly dead from a new strain of Strep A, and doctors were helpless to save them. Old types of bacteria have mutated; new strains of the tuberculosis bacillus do not respond to existing antibiotics. Of those who go into hospitals, 14% to 30% come out with infections they did not have when they were admitted. Some don't come out - 21,000 die each year from such infections (*USA Today*, April 14, 1998). Do effective medicines for such situations exist which could never make it out of the closet in the current over-regulated environment?

The FDA tries to control more than it needs to. It claims regulatory authority over drugs, but defines a drug as anything that is used to diagnose or treat disease. Carried to the logical extreme, prune juice could be considered a drug, since it definitely treats constipation. A 1997 study by Tufts University found that the cost of getting FDA approval for a new drug costs upwards of $200,000,000 and may take ten years or longer. In May, 2000, an article in the *New England Journal of Medicine* stated that getting a new drug approved could cost between $300 and 600 million. The pharmaceutical industry is the richest in the world - yes, richer than the oil industry. However, given such rules, even the richest drug company cannot afford to introduce a new medicine without patent protection. Consequently, more than ever before we live in the era of Patent Medicine, once not a very complimentary term. Securing FDA approval allows a manufacturer to advertise what the approved product will do - *i.e.*, to make health claims, which are forbidden without FDA approval. For instance, it is well established through clinical studies that the saw palmetto herb is more effective - and safer - at shrinking a swollen male prostate gland than the "approved" brands whose advertisements are everywhere (*Health and Healing*, June 1999). If a manufacturer of saw palmetto wished to state this known truth on its label, the FDA would haul that manufacturer into court in short order for having committed the sin of making health claims. The fact that they might be true is beside the point, for the FDA has arrogated unto itself the right to censor them. In a nation which finds it cannot censor pornography under the free speech right of the First Amendment, the FDA finds it can censor a manufacturer and prevent it from telling the public the truth about a product. On January 15, 1999, the U.S. District of Columbia Circuit Court of Appeals held that the FDA had violated the First Amendment of the Constitution by denying four health claims conveying information; the Court also held that the FDA cannot constitutionally deny a health claim conveying information. Paying no attention to the Constitution or the Court, on November 30, 1999, the FDA denied a health claim concerning the herb saw palmetto's ability to reduce a swollen prostate, stating that it considered the claim to be one requiring the filing of a new drug application. Congressman Peter DeFazio wrote the FDA a stern letter protesting its unconstitutional acts. For the FDA, if you want to make health claims, the solution is simple: get in line, spend your $200,000,000 +, and in ten years or so perhaps you can do so. Since the saw palmetto herb cannot be patented, the American male consumer is out of luck at learning about that effective, harmless, and far cheaper product, unless someone can persuade the FDA to obey the Court of Appeals.

In many countries, people think that if they want the best medicine in the world, they need to come to the United States. This is certainly the case for catastrophic injuries. If you're broken to pieces, you've got a much better chance of being put back together properly in the U.S. However, most Americans do not die of accidents but of degenerative diseases. One American dies of cancer every minute, 1,500 a day, 10,000 a week, 500,000 a year. This is the equivalent of three fully-loaded 747's crashing and killing everyone aboard every day, all year long. An American Cancer Society study of cancer mortality rates in 46 countries shows the U.S. as #25, just a little below the middle.

Pretty regularly, someone makes an appeal for more money for medical research. But what about the effective, non-toxic therapies already discovered which have been suppressed, discouraged, outlawed or driven out of the U.S. by Official Medicine? This book deals with those medicines, all non-toxic and mostly not available - not because they didn't work, but for political reasons. But if something is non-toxic, why should the government (FDA) need to "protect" us from it? Or is the protection for companies who do not want competition from inexpensive, effective, non-toxic therapies? The FDA spent eight years of effort and untold millions trying to jail Dr. Burzynski (Chapter 11), discoverer of an effective and NON-toxic cancer therapy.

The FDA's involvement with pharmaceutical companies has been called the most notorious "revolving door" in Washington; upon retirement, about 65% to 75% of FDA employees go to work for drug companies. Upon hearing this, one person commented, "What's wrong with this picture?"

Eight of the stories in this book deal with cancer therapies. These may be of interest to many, since one American dies of cancer every minute. Money for cancer research goes to those trying to perfect "approved" therapies such as chemotherapy and radiation, but both are very harmful. Those researching such therapies might be out of business and have to find another way to pay the mortgage if an effective, non-toxic therapy were to come on the market. As will be seen in these stories, a great deal of effort has been made to make sure that doesn't happen.

The possible loss of Health Freedom in the U.S. was foreseen by one of the signers of the Declaration of Independence, Dr. Benjamin Rush of Philadelphia, one of the most famous doctors in colonial America. Rush wrote:

> *The Constitution of this Republic should make special provision for medical freedom as well as religious freedom. To restrict the art of healing to one class of men and deny equal privilege to others will constitute the Bastille of medical science. All such laws are un-American and despotic.*

While every other kind of freedom is fought for by both liberals and conservatives, there's strange silence when one brings up Health Freedom - freedom for anyone to consult the doctor of one's choice, to obtain any therapy of one's choice, toxic or non-toxic, and to have it paid for by one's health insurance. Our talk and preaching about free markets helped to bring down the Soviet Union. But we don't practice what we preach, for we have no free market in non-toxic therapies in the U.S. - in things which by definition can't hurt us.

For a layman, it is hard to conceive that some of the most basic organizations in our health establishment would lie and cheat, but lie and cheat they have. Political pounding befell some very remarkable medicines and their proponents, with both governmental and non-governmental institutions brazenly lying as they squelched them. The late Senator Paul Douglas of Illinois declared on the Senate floor on December 6, 1963, "It's a terrible thing that we cannot really trust either the FDA or the NCI!" He was talking about Krebiozen (Chapter 5), one of the most shocking stories of all. People picketed the Kennedy White House in 1963 demanding to retain access to Krebiozen, lest they die. Having bemoaned listening to the "experts" after the Cuban missile crisis, the President apparently was still listening to them, for Krebiozen was lost and forgotten, and shouldn't have been. And people died.

Then there is the story of Dr. William F. Koch of Detroit (Chapter 3). From the 1920's to the 1950's, he was curing cancer with *one shot* of Glyoxylide, a substance he discovered. While the cancer epidemic rages on, Dr. Koch is virtually forgotten.

Persecuted relentlessly by the FDA in two trials in the 1940's, he was repeatedly denounced as a quack by the editor of the AMA's JAMA after he refused to sell his discovery to the AMA. Yet there are people still alive at the beginning of the 21st century who were expected to die momentarily until treated with ONE Koch shot. With one American dying of cancer every minute, many might wish that Official Medicine had not thrown away the Koch therapy and the brilliant science that produced it.

The National Cancer Institute (NCI) steadfastly refused to test the Koch therapy, or the Hoxsey therapy, or Krebiozen, but did test hydrazine sulfate (HS), a very cheap non-toxic chemical which cured many terminal patients after conventional therapy had failed to do so. It might have been better if NCI had not tested hydrazine sulfate, for it cheated in the trials. Dr. Joseph Gold, the chief proponent of HS, has warned for years that certain substances - alcohol, tranquilizers, and barbiturates - were incompatible with HS and would cancel its effect - or even make a harmful combination with it. In the Soviet Union and in four trials within the U.S., Dr. Gold's warnings were scrupulously observed, and the average results were 40-50% success in terminal cancer patients - people got better. However, the NCI maintained that the "incompatibles" were a "non-issue" and gave barbiturates to 94% of the 600 patients it treated with HS from 1989 to 1993. Instead of a 40-50% recovery, there were more survivors of the Titanic than there were of the NCI's trials, where no one got better, all died. *Penthouse* magazine blew the whistle on the scandal and suggested that the families of the deceased patients should sue the NCI for genocide. As a cancer treatment, hydrazine sulfate costs about 60 cents a day. Dr. Gold estimates that the cost of one session of chemotherapy would pay for a year's supply of HS (Chapter 10).

Chapter 7 on colostrum (a mother's first milk) tells how former Congressman Berkley Bedell of Iowa was cured of lyme disease, after antibiotics proved ineffective, by a colostrum "targeted" against the spirochete which causes Lyme disease. This was achieved by injecting a killed lyme spirochete into the udder of a cow three weeks before her calf was born. The cow's colostrum then contained antibodies against the lyme spirochete, and this cured the Congressman. There is no known limit to what can be produced by the targeted colostrum method; it presumably could provide a cure for TB, or for various bacteria - even protection against anthrax. It has been used successfully against cancer in animals. The NCI and the NIH have shown no interest in this method, and the FDA discourages the private sector from developing it. When a colostrum drink was shown to be effective against arthritis, the FDA squelched it. The trial of the Minnesota farmer who helped Congressman Bedell to recover is described.

In fact, there is a trial in almost every chapter of the book, as the stories tell what befell the protagonists of various non-toxic, non-pharmaceutical therapies.

The lessons of the ten stories show that there are two principal impediments to non-toxic health breakthroughs: 1) the FDA, and 2) doctors' fear of losing their licenses for using unapproved medicines. There are two simple solutions: 1) remove the FDA's regulatory authority over anything no more toxic than aspirin (everything in this book would pass that test) and 2) pass the Access to Medical Treatment Act, which is already introduced in both houses of Congress. This bill was conceived by Congressman Berkley Bedell so that all Americans might have access to the sorts of unconventional therapies which he believes saved his life twice; lyme disease, as noted, and then from a threatened recurrence of prostate cancer, described in Chapter 8. The "Access" Act provides a procedure for putting on the market medicines not approved by the FDA and protects from prosecution doctors who use them. Doctors would need to obtain the "informed consent" of a patient, who signs a statement that he/she realizes the treatment to be given is not approved by the FDA.

Had these two changes been the law of the land, this book would not have been written, for the stories that follow would not have happened. Legislating these two simple changes would permit the return of most of the therapies described except for those

which have been lost. Since all were inexpensive, with their
return and the appearance of other breakthroughs waiting in the
wings, the costs of American healthcare would plummet.

These changes would permit open competition and a free
market in NON-toxic therapies. The U.S. has had a rigidly controlled market in health products, including non-toxic ones, (to
"protect" us) for most of the past century. The results are a high
death toll from cancer, the absence of effective medicine against
viral diseases such as AIDS and against many bacterial infections, and the most costly health system on the planet. How could
we do worse with Health Freedom? While American emergency
medicine is indeed the best in the world, most Americans do not
die from accidents, but from degenerative disease. Many treatments for the latter are excluded from the market, or their capabilities censored by the FDA, which has usurped for itself the
right to dictate to manufacturers what they can say about their
products. Gradually, before anyone realized it was happening, the
FDA clamped upon the U.S. a harsh regime of censorship and
repression of anything that could compete with the giant drug
companies. Prescription drugs have become so expensive that it
has been proposed that the government pay for them, instead of
forcing the drug companies to reduce prices to the level charged
in other countries such as Mexico and Canada. But there's a better idea; let's give the drug companies some real competition by
removing all governmental controls over anything non-toxic.
Since this would permit truthful advertising of what non-toxic
medicines (nutritional supplements, herbs, etc.) can do, it would
not be surprising to see the cost of prescription drugs come down,
way down, corrected in the way that free markets and open competition regularly do.

We have been warned many times about socialized medicine.
The problem, we're told, is that its overly centralized control sti-
fles innovation. With too much dictation from the top down, with
over-regulation by the FDA, with doctors not free to use effective
non-toxic therapies, a form of socialized medicine is just what we
have, functioning just as badly as we were warned to expect.

While the computer industry is free to make breakthroughs that are the envy of the world, and which happen so rapidly as to leave people breathless, no such freedom exists in the medical field. Instead, such discoveries as the antineoplaston cancer treatment of Dr. Stanislaw Burzynski in Houston are discouraged; the FDA tried very hard to put him in jail. In contrast to so many FDA-approved drugs, antineoplastons never hurt anyone, but instead put many cancers in remission. In addition, here too, the NCI cheated in trials of antineoplastons, diluting them to the point of ineffectiveness. NCI even filed for and obtained a patent on one of Dr. Burzynski's compounds when it discovered he had not patented it (Chapter 11).

Open competition and a free market in non-toxic health products will solve a multitude of problems. In such a market, wondrous things can and will appear, many returning from the oblivion into which they have been cast. How could there be politics in cancer and healing? Surely, one presumes, the best medical discoveries are adopted and the doctors use them. The tragic truth is that it is not that simple.

The Hoxsey Story

Who would have thought that a sick horse grazing in a pasture would give rise to one of the most effective and persecuted cancer therapies of the 20th century? The year was 1840, the place a horse farm in downstate Illinois owned by John Hoxsey. He had put one of his best Percheron stallions out to pasture rather than shoot him after the veterinarian had diagnosed a growing sore on the horse's leg as a hopelessly far-advanced cancer.

But the sore began to heal and John Hoxsey noticed that each morning the horse went directly to one particular spot where he would graze for hours at a time. When the tumor dried up and eventually fell out with a little assist from Hoxsey, he gathered up samples of every plant and herb in the horse's favorite corner of the pasture. Experimenting for months, he finally came up with three formulations; a tonic taken orally, and a red salve and a yellow powder, both applied externally, which he used with success on his and neighbors' horses. So it was horse sense that gave birth to the Hoxsey therapy.

"And that", Harry Hoxsey wrote in *You Don't Have to Die*, published in 1956, "is the story of the origin of the Hoxsey treatment for cancer as it was related to me by my father, who heard it from his father, the son of the man who discovered it". Each of his ancestors kept the formulas secret, passing them on only on his deathbed.

It is still possible to be treated with the Hoxsey formulas - not in the United States, but in Mexico. The fact that the formulas are available at all is a tribute to two very extraordinary people; Harry Hoxsey and his head nurse, Mildred Nelson. While Dr. William Koch (Chapter 3) was a brilliant and highly trained research scientist, Harry Hoxsey inherited rather than discovered a cancer treatment and was a scrappy, resourceful, persistent entrepreneur. Forced to close his large Dallas clinic in 1957, Hoxsey and Mildred Nelson made unsuccessful attempts to keep it going in Utah and Nevada. Then in 1962, after Hoxsey's health broke, Mildred Nelson moved the clinic to Tijuana, Mexico, where it functions to the present.

What happened along the way is an incredible story of dynamic healings, bitter persecutions, many fights, some victories, and some losses. One wonders why it has never been made into a Hollywood movie. (There is, however, a fine video: "Quacks Who Cure Cancer", which tells much of the story.) The usual approach might be to regard *You Don't Have to Die* with a certain skepticism, since it is was written by the chief protagonist for the Hoxsey therapies. However, I take a somewhat different attitude, having interviewed a number of patients at the Hoxsey Clinic in Tijuana. Over and over I heard variations of this story, "I came here 20 years ago with 6 months to live and now I've come back for a check-up and to bring a friend (or a neighbor or a relative) who has cancer". There's no advertising for the Clinic (known as the Centro Bio-Medico); everything is word-of-mouth, patient-to-patient referrals, people who have been helped - yes, cured - telling others in need of help. Talking to patients in Mildred Nelson's waiting room is an impressive experience. It gives a great deal of credibility to the Hoxsey story, so in telling that story, I've quoted liberally from Harry Hoxsey's book. While somebody else may want to pick it apart, I decided to tell it straight from him. Until the Tijuana part begins, most of the Hoxsey story and the quotes are from *You Don't Have to Die*.

Harry Hoxsey was born in 1901 as the youngest of 12 children of Dr. John Hoxsey, a veterinarian surgeon and, like his grandfather John Hoxsey, owner of a horse farm near Girard, Illinois. Dr. Hoxsey occasionally treated humans and gradually turned the veterinary business over to an assistant so as to spend all his time on human cancer. Word-of-mouth brought him an increasing number of patients, most of whom were poor, but Dr. Hoxsey never turned anyone away. Harry remembered his father saying, "Son, cancer don't pick and choose. It hits rich and poor alike, black, and white, Catholic, Protestant, and Jew. All of them have a right to be treated, whether they can pay for it or not. Healing the sick and saving lives shouldn't be a business; it's a duty and a privilege". Alone of the children, Harry liked to help his father. It was assumed that Harry would go to college and medical school and become a doctor.

Sadly, it was not to be. When Harry was 15, his father had an accident, could no longer work, and had to sell his farm and horses to survive. Harry quit school and went to work in the nearby coal mines to help support the family. Three years later, Dr. John Hoxsey, growing weaker, called his son in for a talk.

Taking an envelope from his lockbox, the elder Hoxsey told Harry that he had chosen him of his 12 children to inherit the formulas because of Harry's interest in the treatment. "When you were just a little shaver asking questions and watching me treat patients, I knew you had the call to be a doctor. When I got sick, you didn't say a word; you just went out and got a job in the mines. That took guts and I knew you had what it took to carry on the good work. That's why I picked you, the youngest, to inherit the family formulas." He then required Harry to copy each formula 100 times until he had memorized it, after which his father destroyed the original. Then he told Harry, "I've cured a few hundred people - you can cure thousands. This is a great responsibility. Abe Lincoln once said God must love the common people because he made so many of them. We're common, ordinary people. No matter how high you go, you must never lose touch with the common people. You must never refuse to treat anybody because he can't pay. Promise me that!" Harry promised. A few days later, Dr. John Hoxsey was dead and Harry, not quite 18, was on his own.

In order to put the formulas to use, Harry knew that he had to go to medical school and become a doctor. Since that took money, he worked harder than ever. Two years later, his life changed when S. T. Larkin, a wealthy retired insurance broker, came to Harry with his lower lip and chin disfigured by a running sore.

Larkin told Harry that three doctors had told him he had cancer and would be dead in a year, but that he'd seen Harry's father treat similar sores successfully. Harry told him what he'd told numerous others; that he didn't have a medical license and that it was against the law for him to treat Larkin, and this was why he was saving money for medical school. "People will just have to wait until I finish school". Larkin replied "Son, I can't wait. I'm 84 now but these few years I have left are as precious to me as a whole lifetime is to you. The first thing they teach doctors is that human life is sacred. You have the power to save mine, if you treat me now. If you don't, I'll surely die and you'll be guilty of murder!"

Harry Hoxsey agreed to treat the retired broker on the condition that he keep the treatment secret. But when Larkin came back for his second treatment, he brought a bank director with a cancer diagnosed as terminal. When Harry protested that he couldn't take any more patients until he completed his medical degree, the banker said "Son, you save my life and I'll give you a check big enough to see you through the best college in the country". The banker too was sworn to secrecy but kept the secret as well as Larkin, soon bringing yet another cancer victim. All three had been told by their doctors that they were terminal but they all recovered, wrote Hoxsey in *You Don't Have to Die*.

Harry was soon besieged with patients, one of whom he described in his book as one of the worst cases he ever saw, a Mrs. Stroud, age 45, a farmer's wife. In February, 1924, the local undertaker, whom Harry had treated for cancer of the mouth, took him to see Mrs. Stroud, who had been given up as terminal several months before. Harry was convinced that the case was hopeless but Mr. Stroud begged him to try, so he did. To his amazement Mrs. Stroud recovered. Hoxsey reported her to be alive and well at 75 when he published his book in 1956.

Hoxsey needed to find a college with a good pre-med course that would accept his correspondence course high school diploma. While looking, he was introduced to a Chicago doctor who asked him to treat a few patients under the doctor's supervision at his sanitarium before the fall college semester started. Dr. Bruce Miller, one of the physicians at the private hospital, was so impressed by the results that he went home with Harry to Taylorville to interview some of Harry's patients and some of his late father's in nearby Girard. Dr. Miller returned to Chicago tremendously impressed.

Then Miller laid a bombshell on Harry, telling him that he had no chance ever to be admitted to medical school because "the doctors in Taylorville and Girard are out to get you. They've already complained to the State Medical Board that you're practicing medicine without a license and are seeking a warrant for your arrest. You're blackballed; no medical school will let you in the door". Having a hard time accepting this, Harry asked "How can they keep me from going to school?" He quoted Dr. Miller's answer, **"Few outsiders realize that the medical profession in this country has been organized into a closely-knit association for the protection and benefit of its members...They can't keep you from going to college, but they can keep you out of medical school, and they'll make damned sure that you never get a license to practice medicine in this country".**

Thus Harry Hoxsey's plans to become a doctor collapsed. "What can I do now?" he asked. Miller offered to set up a clinic in Taylorville with himself as medical director and Harry as his assistant, applying the treatment under Miller's supervision. "Then", said Miller, "in a few years if we can produce a few hundred cured cases, the medical profession will have to acknowledge that the Hoxsey treatment is an effective cure for cancer". On March 24, 1924, Hoxsey and Dr. Bruce Miller opened their clinic in Taylorville. So many patients came that within two months they had to find larger quarters.

In the excitement over the new clinic, someone offered to introduce Dr. Miller and Harry to a Dr. Malcolm L. Harris in Chicago, a power in the American Medical Association (AMA), headquartered in that city. Dr. Harris would become its president in 1929. Dr. Miller described to Dr. Harris the results he had seen from the Hoxsey treatment. Harris proposed they treat a clearly hopeless cancer patient, a Sgt. Mannix of the Chicago Police, who had a six-inch open cancerous sore on his left shoulder. Hoxsey tells what happened, "Dr. Harris watched intently as I applied a thick coating of the yellow powder to the gaping lesion, and Dr. Miller put a dressing over it. We left a bottle of our internal medicine with directions that the patient receive a teaspoonful three times a day, and advised the doctor that we would be back in a week to administer another treatment.... Within two weeks the surface of the pustulant sore turned black and started to dry, a sure sign that our medicine was working on the malignancy. Within four weeks, a hard crust had formed, the cancer was shrinking and pulling way at the edges from the normal tissue. Moreover, the rapid improvement in the patient's general physical condition amazed all who saw him. He was able to sit up now, his eyes were bright and alert and the pain had vanished; he no longer needed morphine to sustain him. His appetite had returned...two weeks later, he was walking around.... That same day, we informed Dr. Harris that necrosis (death) of the cancerous mass in the policeman's shoulder was complete, that it had separated from the normal tissue, and could be lifted out within two days."

Dr. Harris invited Hoxsey and Dr. Miller to perform the operation in the hospital amphitheater before the entire staff. So a few days later, Hoxsey writes, "Dr. Miller removed the bandages from Sgt. Mannix' shoulder... I picked up the forceps, scraped and probed the black mass of necrosed tissue. It moved freely at the perimeter but was still anchored at the base. I worked it loose, lifted it out with the forceps and deposited it on the white enamel tray provided for that purpose. And that's all there was to the operation. Dr. Harris inspected the cavity left by the tumor. There was no sign of blood, pus, or abnormal tissue; clean scar tissue had already begun to form. 'In time it will heal level with the surrounding flesh', I told him...Shaking his head incredulously, he declared 'It's amazing; if I hadn't seen it I wouldn't believe it'...The entire demonstration took less than a half hour."

The next morning, Dr. Harris invited Harry Hoxsey to his

office. Hoxsey wrote in *You Don't Have to Die* that Harris stated that he and his colleagues agreed that Mannix' recovery was "convincing evidence that chemical compounds such as you use offer the best hope to eradicate this disease. It's not just the yellow powder you used; it's the amazing improvement in his general condition as the result of the medicine you've been giving him". Dr. Harris then proposed that they set up large-scale trials with absolute medical controls, to which Hoxsey quickly agreed. Harris then told Hoxsey that he had felt sure Hoxsey would agree and accordingly had drawn up a contract for him to sign so that they could get started. When Harry read the contract, "I discovered that I was to turn over all the formulas of the Hoxsey treatment to Dr. Harris and his associates, and relinquish all claims to them. They would become the personal property of the doctors named in the contract.... Further along, I was to agree to close my cancer clinic and henceforth take no active part in the treatment of cancer. My reward for all this was set forth on next to the last page. It appeared that during a ten-year experimental period I would receive no financial remuneration. After that I was to get 10% of the net profits. Dr. Harris and his associates would set the fees - and collect 90% of the proceeds. Stunned and appalled by this incredible document", Hoxsey said he wanted to show it to his lawyer, who might suggest some changes. Dr. Harris' response was "There won't be any changes. We've set forth the only conditions under which your treatment can be ethically established. Unless you accept them in their entirety no reputable doctor will have anything to do with you or your treatment...Hoxsey, until you sign that contract you can't see Sgt. Mannix again." Harris then called the hospital and gave orders that neither Hoxsey nor Dr. Miller was to be admitted to the hospital again, or to communicate with Sgt. Mannix. Harry describes what he did then, "I waited until he hung up the receiver, then seized the telephone and called the Mannix home. Before I could be connected, Dr. Harris reached over the desk and tried to take the telephone away from me. My left elbow flipped up, caught him squarely in the chest, and sent him flying into his chair. It promptly toppled over, depositing him in a most undignified position on the floor. Miss Mannix came on the phone and I explained the situation to her. ' If you want your father to get well, you'd better get him out of the hospital and take him home'…She assured me she'd get him home immediately. Dr. Harris picked himself off the floor, his dignity considerably ruffled, his face red as a broiled lobster. 'You'll never get away with this', he shrilled. 'If you so much as touch that patient, I'll have you arrested for practicing medicine without a license. As long as you live, you'll never treat cancer again. We'll close down your clinic, run you and that quack doctor of yours out of Illinois. Try and set up anywhere in the country and you'll wind up in jail.'" Harry Hoxsey's war with the AMA began that day. In his book, Hoxsey wrote that Dr. William F. Koch's problems with the AMA also started when he refused to assign all rights to his cancer treatment to the AMA (Chapter 3).

When Hoxsey told Dr. Miller what had happened, Miller told him "Harris won't rest now until he's put us out of business. You've made yourself a powerful enemy. It's not just a few local doctors you have to reckon with now, it's the whole American Medical Association. They'll hound you and blacken your name and that of everyone associated with you from one end of the country to another. You're young and brash, but how long do you think you can go on bucking the entire medical profession?" Harry told him "Don't worry about me, Doc; I can take anything they dish out. How about you?" Hoxsey writes that Dr. Miller replied, "I still say a doctor's first duty is to his patients".

After Sgt. Mannix' daughter got her father home, they continued to treat him for three months until he had fully recovered. Sgt. Mannix returned to duty until he retired, dying ten years later. In his book, Hoxsey wrote that he had a copy of Mannix' death certificate, which gives the cause of death as coronary sclerosis, not cancer.

Following the debacle with Dr. Harris, the Taylorville businessman who had introduced him to Harry offered to set up a big clinic in Chicago with Dr. Miller as medical director and Harry as technical adviser. Within a month, Hoxsey discovered that his new partners were charging fees of $500 to $1,000 per patient and were turning away charity cases. Hoxsey protested, telling them that either the poor would get in or he would get out. Dr. Miller attempted to placate him, pointing out that "You can't fight the world single-handed, Harry. We've got to be practical. It takes money to fight the AMA. These people are your friends and will help you put over your treatment". But Hoxsey severed his connections with what he deemed to be a rich man's clinic. Returning to Taylorville, local business friends helped him open a new clinic early in 1925 with a Dr. Washburn as medical director. The maximum fee was $300 and no one was turned away for inability to pay. The Taylorville Chamber of Commerce prepared a booklet with affidavits from 30 former Hoxsey patients which it sent to chambers of commerce around the country, with the result that patients poured in from all over the U.S. and Canada.

On January 2, 1926, the *Journal of the American Medical Association* (JAMA) published a 3 ½ page blast against Hoxsey, his treatment, and everyone associated with him, denouncing them all as quacks. Hoxsey immediately wrote a long letter to Dr. Morris Fishbein, editor of the JAMA, daring him to publish the case of Sgt. Mannix and inviting him to inspect the Hoxsey files. Fishbein never replied, but sent copies of his attack to the Taylorville Chamber of Commerce, which paid no attention. But in July, things got rougher when the Illinois Medical Board obtained a warrant for Harry Hoxsey's arrest on charges of practicing medicine without a license. The sheriff alerted Harry as to how much he'd need for bond money, which Harry obtained. About a week later, the case came before the Grand Jury, two of whose members had been cured of cancer by the Hoxsey treatment, with the others having friends or relatives who'd taken the treatment. Their prompt verdict on hearing the charges, "It's not against the law to save people's lives. Indictment not warranted." His clinic continued to operate.

Then attack came from a totally unexpected quarter. Harry was served with a summons and a complaint signed by all but one of his brothers and sisters suing him for $500,000, the alleged value of their father's estate, *i.e.*, the herbal formulas. When he confronted them, they all had similar stories; tremendous pressure from lawyers from Chicago and Springfield, assuring them that if they didn't sign the lawsuit that it would be directed at them too and they'd then lose their homes, their cars, and their jobs. When the suit was settled and they'd won their shares in the cancer treatment formula, the lawyers told them, a group of prominent Chicago physicians would buy them out for $50,000 apiece. Bond covering the $500,000 demanded in the suit had to be raised immediately or all Harry's assets would be forfeited. The clinic closed when all its equipment was removed, at which point at least some of his brothers and sisters withdrew. No doctor dared to be involved in the clinic for fear of being dragged into the suit. Without a doctor, the clinic stayed closed during the 18 months the lawsuit was pending. But what was Harry to do about the patients? As he puts it in his book, "Sure enough, within 18 months three separate complaints charging me with practicing medicine without a license were sworn out against me. I pleaded guilty to all of them, was fined $100 and costs on each charge, paid up with a clear conscience and no regrets. And I went right on treating my patients". The family case finally came to court in August 1929. Hoxsey's lawyer cited two precedents where plaintiffs sued unsuccessfully for rights to a process they had once abandoned and the judge found in Harry Hoxsey's favor.

It was a costly victory, leaving Harry broke and his clinic closed. His problem was soon resolved when old friends from his nearby hometown, Girard, put up money and opened a new clinic in July 1929. The AMA came out with another blast at the Hoxsey treatment, calling Harry a notorious quack. His reply to the AMA, "I'd rather be notorious and save people's lives than famous and bury them".

In February 1930, Hoxsey got a call from Norman Baker, a flamboyant promoter who had a radio station and a clinic in Muscatine, Iowa. Baker invited him to come show what he could do, and Harry did a broadcast telling of his cancer treatment. Commuting between Girard and Muscatine, Hoxsey treated 50 patients a day, finally closing the Girard clinic upon Baker's promise to offer free treatment to the poor.

One of Hoxsey's most famous cases occurred at Muscatine, a Mandus Johnson of Galesburg, Illinois. The entire top of Johnson's head was covered by a basal cell carcinoma, with biopsy by a Galesburg doctor. It was the worst cancer Harry Hoxsey had ever seen. He told Johnson there wasn't one chance in a million he would survive but agreed to try to help him. Hoxsey applied the yellow powder as he had with Sgt. Mannix, a procedure which would cause the cancer to dry up and then separate from the body, as it had with Mannix and with the horse in 1840. Five weeks later, Hoxsey went on radio and announced that the next night, April 8, 1930, he and the doctors at the Baker hospital would remove the cancer from the top of Mandus Johnson's skull. Hoxsey says, "People came from as far as 800 miles to witness the operation. When Dr. Rasmussen and I lifted the cancer from the sick man's head, exposing the brain, 14 people in the audience fainted. …The AMA Journal immediately published a vicious attack, asserting that Johnson had died as the result of our treatment. We quickly spiked that lie. On May 30, the 'dead man' (Johnson) made a personal appearance, along with 100 other patients, before a giant outdoor rally attended by a crowd of 32,000 (by actual count)….Mandus Johnson lived on until 1950". Hoxsey severed his association with Norman Barker after just five months when he found Baker charging $750 to $1,200 per treatment and refusing treatment to patients unwilling or unable to pay. Leaving Baker, Hoxsey opened his own clinic at Muscatine, treating people whether they could afford it or not.

Shortly after, he received an invitation from some prominent people in Detroit to open a free clinic which they would finance. Jumping at the chance, he and Dr. Rasmussen, who had been with him at the Muscatine Clinic, moved to Detroit. But it was not to be. The long arm of the AMA reached out; Harry Hoxsey was quickly charged with practicing medicine without a license and convicted of the charge before a jury. After 17 months, his appeal was heard and on December 6, 1932, the Michigan Supreme Court reversed the conviction. The Court found that "the physician had charge of the case and the assistance given the physician by the defendant did not constitute practicing the profession of physician". Before his vindication, the Michigan State Medical Board had revoked the license of the Detroit doctor who planned to supervise the clinic, so the free clinic never got off the ground.

After a similar experience in Wheeling, West Virginia, Hoxsey took a vacation at Atlantic City and soon was offered help to set up a clinic there with a local doctor. While in Atlantic City, Judge Thompson, one of his sponsors, arranged a meeting with a cancer doctor in Philadelphia, who expressed great interest. When Hoxsey and his friends went to Philadelphia, the doctor met them at his hospital and Hoxsey writes "He said he'd been in touch with the AMA; before I could treat any patients at his hospital, I'd have to give him my formulas in writing. Recalling my experience with Dr. Harris, I refused, but offered a compromise, 'Let me treat 25 patients. If they get well, and you officially state that my treatment cured them, I'll release my formulas to the entire medical profession.' The doctor repeated that he had to have the formulas first. Judge Thompson urged him to accept my offer; after all, there were 25 lives at stake. The doctor replied, 'Twenty-five more or less makes little difference. We lose them by the hundreds here'". Harry and Judge Thompson returned to Atlantic City.

Soon after, Hoxsey met a Philadelphia osteopath, Dr. Ira Drew, who invited him to come to Philadelphia and work in his clinic. "The AMA can't touch us, scare us, or buy us off", said the osteopath, a member of a branch of medicine different from that controlled by the AMA. This was the spring of 1933, the depth of the Great Depression, and 90% of the patients were charity cases. One day Dr. Drew asked Hoxsey if he would treat an "Ethel Dennis, a colored lady". Hoxsey agreed, noting that "suffering doesn't recognize race, color, or creed". Mrs. Dennis had an "enormously swollen left breast...with glands under the arm and neck involved....Dr. Drew took a biopsy specimen....back came a diagnosis of 'tubular carcinoma'. After several weeks of treatment with internal tonic and the external powder and salve, the entire cancerous mass dried up and fell out, clean scar tissue started to form, and she was well again". Dr. Drew later wrote about Hoxsey, "During the nearly two years that Hoxsey was with me, we cared for many cases of cancer, people coming from all parts of the country. Cancers of the face, arms, legs, breasts, and nearly all parts of the body were presented. The results were astonishing. Many of these patents are alive and well today, more than 20 years later".

In 1936, Hoxsey, nearly 35, had been treating cancer for 15 years yet his goal of recognition and acceptance by the medical profession was as distant as ever. Hearing about the Spann Sanitarium in Dallas, he signed a 6-month contract with Dr. Spann and moved to Dallas.

After six months of intensive work, Hoxsey teamed up with Dr. C. M. Hartzog, one of Dr. Spann's assistants, and opened his own clinic on December 5, 1936. Two days later, Dr. T. J. Crowe, secretary of the Texas Board of Medical Examiners, showed up and threatened Hartzog with the loss of his license and jail, at which point Harry Hoxsey ordered him off the premises. On December 22, an investigator from the Board arrived with warrants for the arrest of Dr. Hartzog, Harry Hoxsey, and Martha Hoxsey, his wife, all charged with practicing medicine without a license. Displaying his license, Dr. Hartzog was informed that it had been cancelled the day before. Both Hoxseys and Dr. Hartzog spent a night in prison before bail could be obtained. When trial was to start on January 4, the State requested indefinite continuance; the next day the three were arrested again on the same charge. After posting bond, Hoxsey obtained an injunction against the Medical Board from further arrests until the cases at issue had been tried.

A few days later, Hoxsey learned that four more warrants for his arrest had been issued by the district attorney of a county where he had never set foot. The same day, Mrs. W. L. Jones, listed as a complaining witness, called Hoxsey and told him that Dr. T. J. Crowe had visited her and urged her to sign a complaint, which she refused to do. Hoxsey writes "She informed them that she was dying of cancer of the intestines at the time she came to our clinic in Dallas for treatment, indeed was so far gone that the doctor advised her husband to call an undertaker. Now, she was entirely well, her weight had increased from 90 to nearly 180 pounds, and our treatment had saved her life". Both Mrs. Jones and another "complaining witness", who'd also refused to sign the complaint, found their names used by Dr. Crowe in yet another county where the witnesses did not even reside. All complaints were quickly vacated.

Hoxsey writes, "And so it went. During the three years 1937 through 1939, more than 100 separate charges of practicing medicine without a license were filed against me. Not a single one resulted in a conviction". In those days, Hoxsey made a practice of carrying $10,000 in cash so that he could quickly bail himself out.

Hoxsey's main foe in the Prosecutor's office was an assistant DA named Al Templeton, who worked up most of the cases against Hoxsey. After Templeton's brother, dying of rectal cancer, was cured by Hoxsey, Al paid Hoxsey a call to thank him. He then resigned from the DA's office and represented Hoxsey from then on, to the consternation of Dr. Crowe. The Templeton case got Hoxsey favorable press for once. A few days later another assistant DA resigned and told the press he was convinced that the Hoxsey treatment really cured cancer. He also later defended Hoxsey in court.

Finally, obtaining a letter Dr. Crowe was circulating to various counties, Hoxsey secured an injunction that put a stop to the swearing out of phony warrants. Hoxsey wrote to Dr. Crowe, "In the name of suffering humanity…let's once and for all allow the facts about our clinic, whether good or bad, to be brought out into the open". There was no reply. Instead, Hoxsey learned that pathologists who had been making biopsies for him had been told by the AMA to stop doing so. He found that "doctors, hospitals, and laboratories all over the country had been warned not to send us any data relating to patients who came to us for treatment".

In July 1941, Dr. Crowe won one for the Texas Board of Medical Examiners. Again charging Hoxsey with practicing medicine without a license, he finally secured a conviction. It was not overturned until 1942, when a new trial was ordered. In point of fact, it was not Hoxsey who was practicing medicine but rather the doctors who worked with him, as had been found in 1932 by the Michigan Supreme Court. A new judge threw out the case and directed the Texas Board of Medical Examiners to cease molesting Hoxsey until and unless it was prepared to present a bona fide case. This victory turned the tide for Hoxsey for several years. With World War II going on, it seemed that the press had better things to report on than Hoxsey's problems with the AMA and the State Medical Board.

In 1946, learning that Dr. Spann was to retire, Hoxsey bought his 60-room building at the corner of Gaston and Peak just east of downtown Dallas and moved there on June 1, 1946.

In 1946, something else happened that would affect the future of the Hoxsey treatment until the present day. Della Mae Nelson of the Nelson Ranch near Jacksboro, Texas, diagnosed with cancer of the uterus and given about 90 days to live, announced that she was going to the Hoxsey Clinic. Her daughter Mildred, a young registered nurse, told her not to waste her money, for everyone knew that Hoxsey was a quack. Her mother replied that she was going anyhow, and Mildred could either come along or stay at home. Mildred said "I'll go along to protect you". At the Clinic, Mrs. Nelson introduced her daughter, an RN, who had come along to protect her. Harry Hoxsey said "I need a nurse. Come work for me", to which Mildred replied "If I were to go to work for you, it would be just to prove that you're a quack". Ninety days later, Della Mae Nelson was not dead but getting well and Mildred went to work for Harry Hoxsey, soon becoming his head nurse. With a lot of Cherokee blood and a family history that traced its ancestry back to Pocahontas, Della Mae Nelson lived on until August 1997, dying at the age of 97. So Mildred

Nelson is descended from Pocahontas.

After the end of the war, Harry Hoxsey went to Washington seeking U.S. government approval but not looking for money. Various members of Congress agreed that an official investigation of the Hoxsey treatment was warranted and referred him to the National Cancer Institute. Hoxsey was told that if he submitted 50 cured cases, he'd get an official NCI investigation. Since the AMA had stopped labs from sending him biopsies (which prove whether or not a patient has cancer) Hoxsey told the NCI where to locate them. NCI rejected his 50 cases on the basis that he had not supplied biopsies, even though he'd told them why he didn't have them, and where they could be obtained.

In 1946, Tom Chapman, a wealthy contractor from Lawton, Oklahoma, brought his 12-year-old son to the Hoxsey Clinic after doctors had told him that the boy was dying and that there was nothing more they could do for his cancer of the lymph glands. Hoxsey agreed to try but, as he put it, "this was one case we did not cure. However, the improvement in the boy's condition prior to death convinced his parents that we could have saved him had he been brought to us earlier". A few months later, nodes began to swell on the Chapman's remaining son. Bringing him to the Hoxsey Clinic, treatment was started; after four days, the nodes stopped growing and in two months they disappeared. When Hoxsey wrote of the case ten years later, there had been no recurrence.

Tom Chapman then got in touch with the Oklahoma Medical Society (in effect a branch of the AMA) and offered to arrange for treatment under the Society's supervision of 25 patients at the Hoxsey Clinic. His offer was rejected. He then addressed the same offer to the American Cancer Society in New York, and again was rejected. Then he got in touch with Senator Elmer Thomas, who had been one of Oklahoma's senators for 20 years. Senator Thomas contacted the Surgeon General and made a valiant attempt to have a government investigation of the Hoxsey treatment. The Surgeon General replied that the AMA had sent him unfavorable articles on the Hoxsey Clinic; therefore he would hesitate to spend federal funds on such an investigation. Hoxsey then wrote to the Surgeon General saying that there would be no need to spend public funds, since Hoxsey himself would pay all the costs. The Surgeon General never replied to Hoxsey's offer. Finally, Senator Thomas wrote Hoxsey on Sept. 2, 1947, "It seems that the medical fraternity is highly organized and that they have decided to crush you and your institution, if at all possible. I have had a few 'rounds' with the heads of all the medical organizations as well as the Public Health Service here in Washington. It seems that the public officials are afraid that if they make any move, or say anything antagonistic to the wishes of the medical organization, that they will be pounced upon and destroyed". Then, wrote Hoxsey, "Senator Thomas discovered that the fears of public officials were not unfounded. When he came up for reelection, the AMA and the Oklahoma Medical Society campaigned vigorously against him and he was defeated".

About the same time, two members of the Oklahoma Legislature, learning that 150 Oklahomans were then taking the Hoxsey treatment, introduced a resolution calling for a joint legislative investigation of the Hoxsey treatment. The Oklahoma State Medical Society and the AMA showered the Legislature with negative telegrams and reprints of JAMA editorials denouncing Hoxsey, but to no avail. The resolution was adopted and a committee was formed of five members from each house who then appointed three medical advisers. When the group arrived at the Clinic on March 11, 1947, the medical advisers did not show up for the meeting to select medical records to be examined. Hoxsey selected them anyhow and the records were turned over to the doctors. When nothing happened for two weeks, Hoxsey contacted one of the state reps. He in turn contacted one of the doctors, who told him that the matter had been submitted to the AMA. Finally, a medical report was submitted to the Legislature which stated that Hoxsey's refusal to divulge the ingredients of his medicines "makes it impossible to evaluate its possible effects".

But the ingredients were known and have all subsequently been shown to have anti-cancer effect. Hoxsey pointed out that one of them:

Potassium iodide, is commonly used in chronic diseases like syphilis to dissolve fibrous tissue in lesions caused by these diseases... The tonic is taken 4 teaspoons a day, 1 after each meal and 1 at bedtime.

We have another type of medication which we apply locally in external cases. Its purpose is to halt the spread of the disease and speed the necrosis (death) of cancer cells. It is employed either as a yellow powder, a red paste, or a clear solution, in accordance with the location and type of the cancer.

All of its ingredients are 'escharotics', and in one form or another were commonly used by the medical profession in the treatment of external cancer long before the development of 'more scientific' (and more lucrative) x-ray and radium treatment. We have adopted techniques which result in effective therapy with much less pain and mutilation than that caused by surgery or irradiation. The yellow powder employed in our clinic is highly selective; it reacts only on malignant tissue, does not affect normal tissue...

In practice, we have found that a small amount of our compounds, when placed on a large cancerous mass, causes a chain reaction which extends an inch or two beyond the point of application. The mass dies, dries, separates from normal, healthy tissue, and falls out.

Hoxsey described as a typical external case:

H. W. Robbins of Rush Springs, Oklahoma. He first came to our clinic in April 1948 with a large sore on the lower

*lip. A biopsy taken at that time revealed epidermoid car-
cinoma Grade 2. Two months after he was put on our
treatment, the cancer dried up and fell out. Five months
later, clean scar tissue had entirely filled the hole in his
lip. When extensive tests showed no evidence of malignancy he was discharged as 'clinically cured'.*

*As a typical internal case, take Mrs. Laura Bullock of
Macon, Georgia. She first came to our clinic in November
1953 with a biopsy report showing cancer of the rectum.
Her doctor said it was inoperable. She was having as
many as 19 hemorrhages a day, during the preceding year
she had received a total of 152 blood transfusions, was
unable to do any of her household chores. A week after
beginning our treatment the hemorrhages ceased; within
two weeks she could get around the house without difficulty; within four months, she gained 26 lbs. In April
1954, physical examination, laboratory tests and x-rays
showed no evidence of cancer anywhere in her system,
and we discharged her as 'clinically cured'. She is directed to come back every year for a check-up. If at the end of
five years there has been no recurrence of bleeding, pain,
or other symptoms of the disease, and she continues to
lead a normal life, and our tests fail to turn up any signs
of cancer, we will consider her absolutely cured.*

Mildred Nelson still recalls a case from her early years at the
Dallas Clinic. A Mr. Burleson was brought in by his wife in an
ambulance, effectively dead. His wife said that he'd been in the
Graford, Texas, hospital for a month and nobody would tell her
what was wrong. Finally, a doctor told her to call the kids, for her
husband was dying of stomach cancer. She said no, she'd prefer
to take him home. She signed him out, called an ambulance, and
took him a hundred miles into Dallas to the Hoxsey Clinic.
Mildred was convinced that nothing would help, but it was Harry
Hoxsey's policy not to refuse treatment to anyone who wanted it.

Mrs. Burleson wanted treatment for her husband, so she got a bottle of the tonic and took Mr. Burleson home to Graford. Four months later, Mildred looked up from her desk and saw both Mrs. and Mr. Burleson walking toward her. Mildred says she had to hold onto her desk when she saw him, so sure she'd been that he had no chance, but there he was! "I was dumbfounded", Mildred recalls. "You could have knocked me over with a feather." Mrs. Burleson told Mildred that she'd used a medicine dropper to feed her husband the tonic with his head in her lap. One day three weeks later, she said, "he woke up".

Mildred Nelson recalls the years from 1946 to 1957 as turbulent and tumultuous (just as had been the previous ten), with Harry Hoxsey being sued, and suing, sometimes losing, and sometimes winning.

In the March 15, 1947, issue of the JAMA, the AMA published another attack on Hoxsey entitled "Hoxsey, Cancer Charlatan". On February 15, 1949, Dr. Morris Fishbein put together an article lifted from his JAMA editorials and got it published in the American Weekly, a Hearst paper Sunday supplement. Since one of the Hearst papers was in Texas, Hoxsey immediately sued the Hearst papers for libel. (Libel being a state, not federal offense, Hoxsey had not been able to file suit against Morris Fishbein for the JAMA editorials, never having been able to catch him in Texas.) As soon as Hoxsey's suit against the Hearst papers was announced on radio, the Texas Board of Medical Examiners slapped 16 separate charges against Hoxsey for practicing medicine without a license, the same charges the Board had failed to make stick on so many previous occasions. The move was apparently intended to take attention away from Hoxsey's suit against the Hearst papers, since all the charges were later dropped.

The Hearst trial started on March 16, 1949. Hoxsey's lawyers put 57 cured patients on the witness stand. Hoxsey writes in his book:

They cited the names of doctors who had treated them

with surgery, x-rays, and radium and finally given them up as hopeless; they told how they'd come to the Hoxsey Clinic and been cured. Some of them had been discharged as long ago as 12 years, and showed no signs of malignancy. To support their testimony, we put into the record biopsy reports, hospital records, case histories, x-ray negatives, and before-and-after photographs.

We'd subpoenaed three prominent pathologists - Dr. May Owen, Dr. Marvin Bell, and Dr. John L. Goforth - all good members of the AMA. They testified reluctantly that they'd analyzed tissue taken from many of those witnesses, and that it was definitely malignant.

The defense in turn put on a great number of doctors to testify that the ingredients of the Hoxsey treatment, individually and collectively, were 'worthless' and had no effect whatsoever on cancer. On cross-examination each was forced to admit that he himself had never tested our treatment on patients, that his testimony was based on theory and not on practical tests.

Mildred Nelson attended every day of the trial. "Sometimes Harry knew things and there was no telling how he knew them", she recalled. "One day in court, Harry suddenly dashed off, saying 'I'll be back in half an hour', and he was." Then Hoxsey got a break. Into the courtroom marched none other than the editor of the JAMA, Dr. Morris Fishbein, himself. When he took the stand to denounce Hoxsey as a quack, he opened himself up for the first time to cross-examination by Hoxsey's lawyers. Under oath, Fishbein was forced to admit that he had never administered the Hoxsey treatment; that was not surprising. However, he was also forced to admit that he had never treated a cancer patient in his life, while insisting he was an authority on the disease. And it got worse; devastatingly, he was forced to admit under oath that he had never practiced medicine one single day in his life, and had even failed his anatomy course in medical school. He did graduate, but he had never completed his internship. This was the so-called "Arbiter of American Medicine". And it got even worse yet for Fishbein. Having a hunch Fishbein might appear, when Hoxsey dashed out, he'd had a subpoena for Fishbein drawn up. When Fishbein left the stand, Hoxsey's subpoena was served on him.

The court found that Hoxsey had indeed been libeled by the Hearst article. It was a great victory, but Hoxsey felt that his real victory was in finally succeeding in suing Fishbein personally. While Fishbein's admissions in the Hearst trial were damaging, there was no question that when Fishbein was the sole defendant, the trial would receive enormous publicity. Realizing that their 25-year Arbiter of American Medicine was going to be exposed as never having treated a single patient in his life, the AMA dumped Fishbein shortly after the Hearst trial. A book called "Medical Mussolini" also helped to dethrone him.

Thus when Fishbein finally appeared in Dallas to defend himself, he no longer was the head of the AMA but just a private citizen accused of libeling and slandering another private citizen. Fishbein got his trial put off until July 14, but it was indeed to prove his Bastille Day.

Hoxsey relates with relish how they put Fishbein to the third degree, "We turned the spotlight on his scholastic pretensions, made him confess that he was unable to get a passing grade in anatomy in his final exams. We forced him to admit that although he never completed his internship, practiced medicine or treated a single patient in all his life, he had amassed a small fortune advising millions of Americans 'What to do until the doctor comes'."

Fishbein made one very momentous concession during the trial which has never received appropriate attention. As the

Hoxsey side was presenting cures of external cancer, Fishbein's lawyer stated "We'll admit you can cure external cancer. We're not arguing about external cases; it's internal cancer we're interested in". It was a tremendous admission by the one-time head of the AMA, that the Hoxsey treatment cures external cancers such as melanoma and basal cell carcinoma. How could the knowledge of that admission be gotten to the many sufferers from those kinds of cancer - people like Sgt. Mannix and Mandus Johnson?

At the conclusion of the three-week trial, the judge handed the jury 34 issues to decide; all 34 were decided in Hoxsey's favor. The jury ruled that Fishbein's statement that "Hoxsey had more than 20 years in which to prove such virtues as might have existed in his method; such proof has never been forthcoming" was false. It ruled that his statement that "diagnosis has never been made by scientific methods" was false. The jury found that Fishbein had "acted with malice in doing the things inquired about". It found that practically every phrase referring to Hoxsey in the *American Weekly* article was false and tended to injure the reputation of the plaintiff and impeach his honesty, integrity, and virtue, and expose him to "public hatred, contempt, ridicule, or financial injury".

Judge Thornton's written opinion in the case should be of interest to anyone interested in evaluating the Hoxsey treatment. Wrote the judge:

This is my second jury of 12 that has found in my court that the Hoxsey treatment cures cancer. I have sat here and listened to over fifty (50) witnesses from all walks of life who say that they have been cured. They have showed their scars; they have given the names of the doctors who operated on them or treated them with x-ray or radium. I have heard the testimony of prominent and eminent pathologists, some of whom I know personally, saying that these patients were suffering from cancer before they went to Hoxsey.

*I am of the firm opinion and belief that Hoxsey has cured
these people of cancer. And the fact that this jury has
answered all questions proves that Hoxsey has been done
a great injustice and that the articles and utterances by
defendant Morris Fishbein were false, slanderous, and
libelous.*

It has been reported, impossible to confirm, that before his
death Morris Fishbein admitted that he had lied about the Hoxsey
treatment.

After these victories, Harry Hoxsey again tried to interest the
federal government. In 1950, he was once more turned down by
the National Cancer Institute, this time on the grounds that the
method of treatment must be fully explained, and that there can
be no secrecy about the composition of the treatment.
Accordingly, Hoxsey submitted to the NCI all of his formulas -
but the NCI turned him down again, returning all of his submis-
sions with no explanation. Instead of an investigation of the
Hoxsey treatment, what happened next was that the U.S. Public
Health Service decided to charge him with distributing misleading information. They stated that his pamphlets falsely represented his medicine as an effective cure for cancer, and sought an
injunction prohibiting Hoxsey from shipping "mislabeled medicine" across state lines. The U.S. Public Health Service was evidently not impressed by Judge Thornton's decision. It succeeded
in obtaining an injunction prohibiting Hoxsey from sending out
pamphlets describing the cures, and from sending medicine to
doctors in other states. That is where matters stood for several
years.

Very little about the success of the Hoxsey treatment ever
made it into the national press. In his book, Hoxsey explains why:

*On Oct. 30, 1937, the AMA Board of Trustees played host
to the National Association of Science Writers at a special
conference to discuss ways and means 'to keep the public
informed of progress in medical science'. The aim, of*

course, was exactly the opposite. Soon thereafter, the writers' association adopted as part of its 'code of ethics' the following principle:

> *'Science writers are incapable of judging the facts of phenomena involved in medical and scientific discovery. Therefore they only report 'discoveries' approved by medical authorities, or those presented before a body of scientific peers.'*

This voluntary censorship of medical news NOT approved by 'medical authorities' (i.e. the AMA) was accepted by the leading news services. For example, in 1940 the United Press sent out a bulletin to its various bureaus which ordered, in part:

> *'Under no circumstances put any story on the leased wire about a remedy. If the bureau manager is convinced that the story has merit, he should overhead it to New York for investigation and consideration there.'*

The conspiracy to censor vital medical news was exposed August 1954 in testimony before the House Committee on Veterans Affairs, when Arthur J. Connell, the National Commander of the American Legion, told Congress that:

> *'a contract exists between the State medical associations and the newspapers which makes it virtually impossible for the veterans' side of medical questions to reach the reading public'*

He read the contract into the record. It stipulated that 'on all matters of health and medical news' no publication or radio broadcast would be made until 'authentic information' is obtained from 'qualified sources' named in the agreement (i.e., AMA officials).

Although most concerned about suppression and distortion of news affecting veterans, Connell pointed out that all other medical news not approved by the AMA is handled in the same manner, and has no way of reaching the public.

No wonder the Hoxsey treatment, and other unorthodox methods, never get a favorable hearing in our 'free' but medically-censored press.

One wonders how many vestiges of this policy are still quietly in place as we enter the 21st century.

But patients still flocked to the Dallas Clinic. Harry Hoxsey was proud to point out that it was the largest independent cancer clinic in the world, with 10,000 cases under review, and not one cent of support from the government. He was also proud that his standard fee in the 1950's was $400 for lifetime treatment, with no charge for the poor who, he stated, made up 25% of his patients.

In 1953, Hoxsey received an important visitor, Benedict Fitzgerald, special counsel to the Senate Interstate Commerce Committee. Fitzgerald had been assigned the mission of investigating various cancer controversies around the country (Hoxsey, Krebiozen) to see if there were any evidence of a conspiracy to restrain trade. His report to the committee discusses the two Hoxsey court trials and confirms that Morris Fishbein admitted that the Hoxsey treatment could cure external cancer. The Appendix of this book (on pages 443-447) contains excerpts from the Fitzgerald Report relevant to Hoxsey and Krebiozen (Chapter 5). Fitzgerald concludes his report stating: "My investigation to date should convince this committee that a conspiracy does exist to stop the free flow and use of drugs in interstate commerce which allegedly have solid therapeutic value".

Even in periods of normalcy, there were tensions. Mildred

Nelson remembers one afternoon when Harry stopped by her office to say he was leaving early to go out to his ranch. He was back in 20 minutes. "I thought you were going to the ranch", she said. "I started", he replied. "Come outside and see something." When she went out with him to his pickup, he pointed to holes where a bullet had gone through the windshield and out the other window.

So in addition to false arrests and trials, Hoxsey had to survive threats as well - but he had the satisfaction of knowing that Judge Thornton had ruled that he was curing cancer. Obviously, Hoxsey, a coal miner as a boy, was tough and a fighter. In his book, he wrote, "I frequently have been accused of being a flamboyant showman and promoter, as well as a healer. If I am all of these things, it is because the AMA forced these roles upon me...I had to find some way to get my cases before the public and promote what my enemies were anxiously avoiding - a public showdown on the true merits of the Hoxsey treatment. The plain truth is I had to become both showman and promoter in order to continue to treat cancer by unorthodox methods and survive."

There were some good moments, too. Hoxsey writes with pride of a group which visited the clinic in 1954, "Ten physicians from all over the nation assembled at our clinic for an independent, impartial investigation of our treatment. They spent two days inspecting the facilities, going over hundreds of case histories and interrogating patients and former patients. On April 12, 1954, they issued a unanimous statement, declaring:

We find as a fact that our investigation has demonstrated to our satisfaction that the Hoxsey Cancer Clinic in Dallas, Texas, is successfully treating pathologically proven cases of cancer, both internal and external, without the use of surgery, radium or x-ray.

Accepting the standard yardstick of cases that have remained symptom-free in excess of five to six years after treatment, established by medical authorities, we have seen sufficient cases to warrant such a conclusion. Some of these presented before us have been free of symptoms as long as twenty-four years, and the physical evidence indicates that they are all enjoying exceptional health at this time.

We as a Committee feel that the Hoxsey treatment is superior to such conventional methods of treatment as x-ray, radium, and surgery. We are willing to assist this Clinic in any way possible in bringing this treatment to the American public. We are willing to use it in our offices, in our practices on our own patients when, at our discretion, it is deemed necessary.

The above statement represents the unanimous findings of this Committee. In testimony thereof we hereby attach our signatures.

S. Edgar Bond, MD	*Richmond, Indiana*
Willard G. Palmer, MD	*Seattle, Washington*
Hans Kalm, MD	*Aiken, South Carolina*
A. C. Timbs, MD	*Knoxville, Tennessee*
Frederick H. Thurston, MD, DO	*Boise, Idaho*
E. E. Loffler, MD	*Spokane, Washington*
H. B. Mueller, MD	*Cleveland, Ohio*
R. C. Bowie, MD	*Fort Morgan, Colorado*
Benjamin F. Bowers, MD	*Ebensburg, Pennsylvania*
Roy O. Yeats, MD	*Hardin, Montana*

Hoxsey summed up the philosophy of his clinic in these words, "We offer the condemned victim what many other doctors deny him; hope, and a fighting chance to conquer the dread disease. They tell him 'You are going to die.' We say, 'You have a chance to live'."

Harry Hoxsey's book provocatively entitled *You Don't Have to Die* came out in 1956 and, after having won so many battles, it appeared that he was ahead of the wave. But the end of the Dallas Clinic, the largest independent cancer clinic in the world, was only one year away.

In 1957, the Texas Legislature was persuaded to pass a law stating that no doctor could work for a non-doctor. As far as is known, the law was only used one time. On its effective date, no doctors were legally allowed to work for Harry Hoxsey. So, after over twenty years in Dallas offering treatments found effective by two juries, the Hoxsey Clinic was finally closed down. With Mildred Nelson, Hoxsey planned to move the clinic to Nevada or Utah, but neither move was successful. Finally, Hoxsey decided that they must move to Mexico and went to Tijuana to make preparations. He would have moved there but after a heart attack, his health broke. He told Mildred "You go and open the clinic but keep my name off of it, for it would just be a lightning rod for trouble".

In 1963, reluctantly obeying Harry's instructions and leaving off the Hoxsey name, Mildred Nelson opened the Centro Bio-Medico in Tijuana, Mexico, in a small building on a hill over-looking the city and the bay of San Diego. With no advertising other than word-of-mouth, patients continued to come in an end-less stream. By opening the clinic, which everybody knew to be the Hoxsey Clinic, Mildred Nelson helped to change the history of Tijuana. The Centro Bio-Medico and Dr. Ernesto Contreras' clinic were the first two "alternative" clinics to locate there. Later came Dr. Max Gerson with his nutrition-based therapy and then others. In the 21st century, with so many clinics in Tijuana, it has largely been forgotten that Mildred Nelson's Centro Bio-Medico - the Hoxsey Clinic - was one of the first two pioneers.

Harry Hoxsey, who had won and lost so many battles, who had even won from the former head of the AMA an admission that the Hoxsey treatment cures external cancer, had another heart attack and then a stroke from which he never really recovered, losing much of his memory. He lived another eleven years after Mildred Nelson opened the Tijuana clinic and died in 1974.

Meanwhile the narco-queen of Tijuana built a large, palatial residence up the hill from the Centro Bio-Medico but was busted and jailed almost immediately upon its completion. From her cell she wrote Mildred Nelson offering her the building for a reasonable price saying, "If I can't enjoy it, I want you to have it". Mildred managed to come up with the purchase price and as a result the Hoxsey Clinic (as most people still call it) is installed in the finest quarters of any of the Tijuana clinics.

To go with the Hoxsey therapy, the following diet is recommended; no pork, tomatoes, vinegar, alcohol, carbonated drinks, white sugar, or white flour, all of which have been observed to nullify the tonic.

Until fairly recently, when one rang the Clinic one was likely to hear "This is Mildred". Almost everyone calls her Mildred and most do so with a lot of love, for she has become something of a Living Legend, this descendant of Pocahontas. On the wall of her office hangs this word for the day, "Lord, help me to remember that nothing is going to happen today that you and I can't handle". Another is equally memorable, "They found something to do the work of five men; a WOMAN".

On my two visits to the Clinic, Mildred said in her no-nonsense manner, "Don't talk to me; go talk to the patients!" And these talks were fascinating. Wondering why one healthy-looking young man was there, I learned that he was from Canberra, Australia. He had first come to the Clinic five years before with a brain tumor and a prognosis of six months to live at the most. Using the tonic, he had become cancer-free. On this visit, he'd come back for a check-up and to bring a friend with the same problem. When I told Mildred about this interesting case, she said "Well, did you think the tonic had stopped working?"

In recent years, Mildred has observed that it's taking longer to cure certain cancers than it used to. Mildred has been dealing hands-on with advanced cancer cases since 1956 - 42 years as of 1998 - a level of in-depth experience equalled by few if any. "Twenty years ago, the tonic would cure a certain type of cancer at a certain stage in six weeks. Now, the tonic will still cure such a cancer, but will take six months. Why does it take longer?" she wonders. "What's different? Is the energy from the herbs weaker, perhaps from minerally-depleted soil? Or is everyone's immune system weaker?"

Maybe it's the latter. In 1958, Nobel Laureate Dr. Linus Pauling predicted that nuclear bomb tests in the atmosphere would ultimately produce about one million seriously defective children and about one million embryonic and neonatal deaths. Pauling then had his passport lifted by the State Department. Also in 1958, Soviet scientist and later Nobel Laureate Andrei Sakharov warned (as reported by Dr. Jay Gould in *Deadly Deceit*) that every 50 megatons of nuclear explosives tested in the atmosphere would cause between a half million and one million deaths worldwide. He then was exiled in Siberia for the next 20 or so years. The Natural Resources Defense Council reported in 1988 that the total of U.S. and Soviet atmospheric nuclear bomb tests amounted to 585 megatons (the fall-out equivalent of 40,000 Hiroshimas). Using Sakharov's rule of thumb, this would translate into between 5,850,000 and 11,700,000 eventual deaths caused by the bomb tests. Such tests were banned by international treaty during the Kennedy Administration in 1963.

This may explain Mildred Nelson's observation that people's immune systems seem to be weaker, and that it takes longer to heal them. Could whatever is causing this phenomenon also be responsible for the relentless rise in cancer cases every year?

Certain grudging recognition for the Hoxsey herbal tonic has developed as herbal medicine has won more respect in recent years. In 1987, Dr. James Duke, Ph.D., former chief botanist at the U.S. Department of Agriculture's Medicinal Plants Laboratory, showed that all the ingredients in the Hoxsey formula have exhibited anti-cancer activity. In his video, "Quacks Who Cure Cancer", Ken Ausabel reported that all the Hoxsey herbs are listed in Jonathan Hartwell's "Plants Against Cancer".

Beyond the effectiveness of the herbs, there is another aspect that may explain some of the tonic's success. Harry Hoxsey wrote that it contained potassium iodide which "is used....to dissolve fibrous tissue" (in other diseases). In *Medical Hypotheses*, 1991,

36, Egyud and Lipinski wrote on the "Significance of Fibrin Formation and Dissolution in the Pathogenesis and Treatment of Cancer". The authors reported that they had microscopically observed the presence of fibrin-like material coating tumor cells. They stated that "the fibrin coat causes neoplastic (cancer) cells not to be recognized by the immunological system and thus makes them immune to attack from the natural killer cells...Consequently, removal of the fibrin coat from tumor cells makes them vulnerable to the attack of killer cells and their subsequent elimination." This is borne out by several studies and anecdotal reports where the use of drugs such as warfarin and streptokinase to dissolve fibrin clots in heart attack victims has been seen to lower cancer rates and to reverse tumors. This fibrin protection of a tumor cell from attack by a body's immune system was not known in Hoxsey's day - or was it? Hoxsey pointed out that the tonic contains a fibrin-dissolving substance. Conceivably, the potassium iodide could dissolve the fibrin coating on tumor cells, thus exposing them to attack by the body's immune system, and to the anti-cancer effects of the herbs.

Mildred Nelson observes that as far as she knows the Hoxsey treatment is still the best available for melanoma and basal cell carcinoma, the external cancers that the AMA's one-time spokesman admitted in a Dallas courtroom that the Hoxsey treatment could cure. The curious ability of the Hoxsey treatment first to kill the (external) tumor and then dry it up until it can easily be separated from the body appears to be without parallel in conventional cancer treatment. Doctors tell of having seen Mildred Nelson do incredible things at the Clinic - "lifting tumors right off" - just like Sgt. Mannix in Chicago and Mandus Johnson in Iowa, and John Hoxsey's horse in 1840, where it all started.

There has never been a report of toxicity from the Hoxsey treatment, which has been used in humans throughout the 20th century (including the work of Harry Hoxsey's father) and in animals since 1840. However, there have been many reports of its effectiveness, above all the evidence presented in the jury trials.

Mildred Nelson states that her success rate with patients

whose immune systems have not been wrecked by chemotherapy runs around 80%. Of course, the treatment doesn't always work, but nothing else always works, either. Mildred does not rest on her laurels. She never stops studying and if she finds something else that works well, she uses that too.

Not knowing what to expect at a Tijuana clinic, a recent patient came back from the Hoxsey Clinic commenting on the high order of professionalism she found and on the cheerfulness of both the staff and the patients. Driving through the gates into the courtyard of the Centro-Biomedico, the first sight other than the handsome mansion itself is a huge screened aviary about 30' in diameter and 15' high, filled with dozens of birds singing at the top of their lungs. That joyful, uplifting sound sets the note for the atmosphere at the Clinic. After being examined, the recent patient first received intravenous administration of cytokines, a new therapy which supplements the immune system. Within two days, the pain from her lymphoma vanished. In addition, she takes the Hoxsey tonic.

During all the years of the U.S. Government's multi-billion dollar War on Cancer, about which little is heard anymore, no move was ever made by the National Cancer Institute to evaluate the Hoxsey treatment. The private American Cancer Society (ACS) states in its Unproven Therapies List that it has no information as to the effectiveness of the Hoxsey herbal therapy, but it's not likely to unless it looks. No ACS representative ever visited the Hoxsey Clinic, either in Dallas or in Tijuana, or made any contact whatsoever.

At long last, a study of the Hoxsey therapy is being undertaken. In 1992, at the suggestion of former Congressman Berkley Bedell and with the sponsorship in Congress of Senators Tom Harkin and Orrin Hatch, legislation was enacted establishing an Office of Alternative Medicine (OAM) in the office of the Director of the National Institutes of Health (NIH). In 1997, the OAM funded a small study of the Hoxsey treatment to be carried out by a group from the University of Texas School of Public Health at the M. D. Anderson Clinic in Houston. The study will focus first on melanoma, an external cancer, which Morris Fishbein granted the Hoxsey treatment could cure. Perhaps finally the results of this excellent non-toxic herbal therapy will become more widely known.

Harry Hoxsey would be pleased, and Mildred Nelson definitely was pleased. Yes, was. Mildred Nelson went to her well-deserved reward on January 28, 1999, so her vast body of knowledge and experience is gone. To have known her strength and gutsiness was to have known what many of the pioneers who opened the West in the 19th century must have been like. The Clinic continues under the direction of Mildred's sister, Liz Jonas, who maintains the policy of a lifetime fee. This was $400 in Harry Hoxsey's time, in the 1950's, and is subject to adjustment as costs rise. In the Year 2000, it is $3,500, and entitles a patient to free checkups as long as needed. In contrast, some other Tijuana Clinics ask from $2,000 to $4,000 a week. The Hoxsey Clinic does not regard cancer as a Money Game.

After Mildred's death, two of her former patients decided to make a video of the clinic and its patients as a tribute to her. Carol and Bernie Main live in Soldotna, Alaska, about 150 miles from Anchorage. In 1985, Carol developed an enlarged pancreas. A local doctor told her it was either pancreatitis or pancreatic cancer. There was no test that could tell the difference, he said. Even if there were, he said, it would make little difference, since there was no treatment for either, and she probably had no more than six months to live. Carol called a laetrile clinic in Tijuana. They wanted $6,000 for two weeks, and were uninterested when they learned Carol had no money. Someone told her to call Mildred, and the story of what happened then is "vintage Mildred Nelson". Upon hearing her condition, Mildred said, "You get down here immediately!" Carol said "But I have no money to pay you." Mildred replied, "Let's worry about how you'll pay after we get you well. Have you got enough money to get here?" Carol said yes and was in the Clinic three days later. She stayed just long enough to pick up the tonic and instructions before heading back to Alaska. For the next two weeks, Mildred had her take nothing but diluted grape juice, half juice and half distilled water, explaining that this would flush out the pancreas. At the end of the two weeks, she felt so much better she painted her living room. Then she started the tonic, continuing the grape juice. Much improved, she returned to Tijuana six months later for a checkup. Her pancreas was no longer swollen, she was essentially well, and she was able to pay Mildred.

Six years later, her husband, Bernie, lost his voice completely. A doctor found several tumors of various sizes. This time it was Bernie Main's turn to go to Tijuana. After he returned with the tonic, Mildred told Carol by phone, "If he does exactly what he's been told, he should get his voice back in six months and the tumor should be gone in five years". The voice came back in six and a half months - Mildred was off by two weeks - and the tumor was gone in four years instead of five.

Carol learned of Mildred's death in the middle of a crowd and could not help breaking down and sobbing. "After all", she says, "she kept my children from being orphans". She and Bernie then decided to make an excellent video about the Hoxsey treatment. Both it and the earlier one by Ken Ausabel can be obtained from the Centro Biomedico, the address of which is in the Appendix.

Harry Hoxsey was hoping to have a study made of the Hoxsey tonic as a possible way to prevent cancer. This is an aspect of the Hoxsey story which should be looked at. Perhaps it might be found that one could do well to use a little horse sense and take 3 teaspoons of tonic one day a week. It would certainly do no harm. As a matter of fact, that was the first rule of Hippocrates, the father of medicine; do no harm.

There are a million new cancer cases every year in the United States and 500,000 annual deaths from cancer. One wonders when the policies of the U.S. Government will change so that the Hoxsey treatment, as American as apple pie, can come home to the U.S. Then the voice of the people will be able to be heard through their free choices as to whether or not they prefer non-toxic cancer therapies such as this one.

BIRTH OF A SCIENCE - OR DEATH OF A SCIENCE?

In Columbus, Ohio, one day in August 1949, Mary Lou Barnes, an attractive 19-year-old blonde student at Ohio State University, developed a headache and a sore throat. A little while later, her right leg felt strange and then gave way under her. Alarmed, her mother called Dr. Harold Wilson, their family doctor, who came that evening. Returning in the morning, he found the right leg completely paralyzed and told Mary Lou's mother the dreaded words, "It's polio". With infantile paralysis (polio) largely vanquished in the 1990's, most people have forgotten the horror of the disease, usually crippling in varying degrees and often fatal.

Dr. Wilson then administered intramuscularly a 2cc shot of a drug called Glyoxylide. The next morning, he found that he could move Mary Lou's leg although she had no control over it. That evening, he phoned and Mrs. Barnes told him that Mary Lou was beginning to be able to move her leg and sensation was returning. Going over as soon as he could, Dr. Wilson found it to be true. She began to improve very rapidly and was able to go down to dinner the next day.

Since Mary Lou was a popular co-ed, newspapers began to hear of the story. Dr. Wilson requested them to hold off for 24 hours while he asked city hospital authorities for permission to try the drug on more polio cases. Permission was denied and it was only then that he learned that the drug was not only not approved by the American Medical Association (AMA), but was actually blacklisted by them.

Wire services carried the story across the country and into Canada, where the *Toronto Daily Star* picked it up for their August 22, 1949 edition, from which article the above details were taken.

In the 1980's and 1990's, we became accustomed to hearing about drugs that can't be sold because they're not approved by the U.S. Food and Drug Administration (FDA). But blacklisted? What's that? And by the AMA, a private organization? Who gave the AMA the right to approve or disapprove of drugs in the U.S.? It seems that at that time they gave themselves the right. They enforced their decisions through their influence with State Medical Boards, which might reprimand or even revoke the license of a doctor using drugs not approved by the AMA. Currently, this might happen to doctors using drugs not approved by the FDA. But in 1949, Dr. Harold Wilson found himself in trouble with the Columbus Academy of Medicine (the local chapter of the AMA). He had saved Mary Lou Barnes from being crippled for life with a legally marketed drug, but one not "approved" by the AMA. It was the first time Dr. Wilson had ever used Glyoxylide in his practice, and the results turned out to be front-page news all across the country. Several years later, in December 1952, the Columbus Academy expelled Dr. Wilson from membership. This sanction denied him hospital privileges - i.e., he could no longer admit patients to Columbus hospitals and treat them there. He did not lose his license, but his reputation was damaged.

Returning to classes after her close call, Mary Lou Barnes was amazed to learn that something that saved her from being crippled was frowned on by top medical authorities. Her comment was "it worked for me!" Her mother said "It was a miracle". Glyoxylide, the *Toronto Star* reported, "is described as an oxidation catalyst, an agent which increases the oxidation process of the body, one of the prime processes of life", and was discovered by Dr. William Frederick Koch of Detroit. By the time Mary Lou Barnes profited from his therapy, Dr. Koch was no longer in Detroit. He had closed his practice, where he had dispensed Glyoxylide to patients for 30 years, and had gone to live in Rio de Janeiro, Brazil.

The long fight that caused his departure is one of the most dramatic in American medical history. The results Dr. Koch achieved with the drugs he developed are extremely well documented. He presented 200 cases of cures of cancer, mostly terminal, complete with hospital diagnoses and biopsies, in two trials. He had been hauled into federal court by the FDA on charges of offering a worthless treatment. FDA failed to prove its case twice and he was not found guilty. The court records and the testimony of the cured patients leave no doubt about the effectiveness of Koch's Glyoxylide, a chemical which the FDA claimed did not exist.

How could it happen that such an accomplishment was not greeted with open arms? How can it be that an effective therapy which was offered legally for 30 years is no longer available?

Dr. William Frederick Koch (1885-1967) received his BA in 1909, MA in 1910, and his Ph.D. in biochemistry in 1916 all from the University of Michigan, where he was instructor of histology and embryology from 1910 to 1914. While at the University, Dr. Koch studied chemistry under Dr. Moses Gomberg, who had already made his discovery of free radicals. Dr. Koch took Gomberg's research one step further by realizing that in the right situation a free radical could prove beneficial in the treatment of disease. In 1914 he became professor of physiology at the Detroit College of Medicine (now Wayne State University) from which he received his MD in 1918. In 1919, he left the college to open a medical practice. Since his parents had emigrated from Germany, they pronounced the name in the old country way, to sound like "coke".

Dr. Koch started a lifelong career of research by investigating the parathyroid glands. These were sometimes removed during operations for goiter, an iodine deficiency disease rarely seen after salt was iodized. After he published in the *Journal of Biological Chemistry* in 1912 and 1913 his findings that parathyroid removal endangered the life of the patient, that surgical practice stopped. This resulted in a laudatory editorial in the *Journal of the American Medical Association* (JAMA) on September 27, 1913 on the discoveries of the brilliant young William F. Koch. He was then just 28, and praised as a researcher by the JAMA before receiving either his PhD or his MD.

Based on what he had learned in his parathyroid research, Koch came up with a startling hypothesis: 1) that cancer and other diseases result from a breakdown in the body's oxidation system (by which cells produce energy from food and oxygen), and 2) that where there is healthy oxidation there is no disease. Observing that heart and brain tissues are extremely resistant to starvation, he deduced that they must be rich in some substances that produce energy. He discovered these substances to be carbonyl compounds and then perceived that these same chemicals were fundamental to the body's oxidation process. He found that when toxins interfered with or removed these carbonyls, oxidation declined and disease resulted. He speculated that if he could substitute the missing or impaired carbonyls, he could restore the oxidation system to normal, thus affecting disease.

Having witnessed the damage caused by conventional cancer treatments, Dr. Koch was determined to develop a drug that would be non-destructive. He wanted something that would work with and complement the body's normal chemistry, such as the naturally occurring carbonyls.

In November 1917, he was given a chance to test his theory on a woman in the last stages of metastatic liver cancer at St. Mary's Hospital in Detroit. The doctor who referred him the case expected the patient to live no more than a week. Dr. Koch was offered the case so that he could do the autopsy. Thus he would be able to see the effects of his treatment, a carbonyl-rich extract of heart and brain tissue. When Koch went to visit her the following week, he found her bed empty, assumed she had died, and that he had not received the body for autopsy through some mixup at the hospital. The following June on a street in Ann Arbor, Koch was astounded when the same woman threw her arms around him, thanking him for saving her life. She had tried to find him earlier, but the hospital had told her that Dr. Koch had left his patients and gone off to work for the U.S. Army. No one at the hospital had told him of her recovery. Until then, his treatment had been an untested theory, and he'd achieved success the first time he'd tried it.

He reported this and other similar results in "A New and Successful Treatment for Cancer" in the *Detroit Medical Journal* of July 1919. A fuller version was printed in the October 1920 issue of the *New York Medical Record*. Then the trouble started.

Shortly after the first article appeared, Dr. Koch received a visit from Dr. Henry Carstens, representing Dr. George Simmons, then editor of the JAMA and the man who laid the foundations of the 20th century AMA. Koch later told friends that Carstens praised him for his successful cancer treatment and then made a startling proposition, "Koch, you're starting a brilliant career, one which we've already noted a few years ago. Here's what we're going to do for you. We'll take this new cancer treatment of yours and run with it. We'll make you famous all over the world!" Dr. Koch answered that this sounded very interesting. However, he pointed out, his compound was difficult to make and deteriorated rapidly. He needed more time to perfect the process and conduct additional research. In addition, he would want to work out arrangements so that people who could not afford to pay would be treated free (a policy he used in his own practice). The AMA representative refused to consider such an arrangement and, Koch wrote later, "he pressured me to turn over to him my whole research including methods of producing the treatment. I refused". (*Psychosomatic Judgment*, Dr. Wm. F. Koch, c. 1960). Koch's long war with the AMA started that day. A couple of months after being denied control of Koch's therapy, Dr. George Simmons denounced in the JAMA as a quack the young doctor he had praised in 1913.

Shortly after this encounter, Koch found a much simpler way to supply carbonyls. This was important, since producing the heart and brain tissue extract (the effectiveness of which he had demonstrated) was laborious and expensive. Very well trained in chemistry, Koch devised a way to create synthetic carbonyl catalysts from inexpensive chemicals. These would have the effect of replacing or restoring carbonyls that had been removed from or blocked in the body's oxidation process. Restoration of the carbonyls enabled the oxidation process to start again and healthy energy production to resume. This meant the difference between disease and health, since with a reinvigorated oxidation system and vigorous energy production, disease could be eliminated. (Research in the 1990's found that oxidation can turn on the immune system, causing killer cells to attack tumors and other infectious agents.)

The two synthetic carbonyl catalysts which Koch used most frequently were called Glyoxylide and Malonide.

Dr. Koch was soon to see the repercussions of his refusal to sell out to the AMA. First, he noted that his scientific theories and results were no longer being accepted for publication in medical journals. Then, in the fall of 1919, he requested the Wayne County (Detroit area) Medical Society (of which he was a member) to appoint a five-member committee to do a test of his catalysts in five undoubted terminal cancer cases to be selected by the committee. As Dr. Koch tells the story (*Psychosomatic Judgment*):

The committee selected terminal cases that had no chance to live. The committee was required to sign their names to the examinations of the patients before I could treat them. These patients were stretcher cases, in danger of dying, and they lay in the ward three weeks waiting for treatment...I was waiting for the patients to be recorded and duly signed by the members of the committee so that I could treat them. Finally, their danger of dying was becoming imminent and I appealed to the president of the Society to force his committee to do their duty so that I could treat the patients...He ordered the committee to be at the hospital the next morning at 10 AM. Two members of the committee showed up and made an examination of one patient. After this one patient was signed up by the two members, they decided it was getting late...They left and that was the end of the committee's signatures on patients. I treated all five patients with a prayer for the

Lord's help and I was not long in waiting. In three weeks, these patients were up and around, no more hemorrhages, no more pain, cheerful, gaining strength, and joyfully encouraging each other.

Startled to see such progress, Koch wrote, the committee ordered the patients back to their distant homes (he noticed that they were all from hundreds of miles away) and forbade them any more care from Koch. One patient up in the 70's, riddled with thousands of metastatic sarcomas of the very virulent neurosarcoma made such a rapid improvement that one of the committee members warned him that he should hurry back home as fast as possible, for if I gave him another dose he would melt away like the tumors had done. He went in a hurry. Of the five cases treated, three were completely cured that I myself found as well as did their own doctors. The fourth, recovering from neurosarcomas, seems also to have recovered as for five years or more other patients came to me on the strength of the good results they observed in his case. Then the committee closed the investigation on the grounds that I had neglected the patients. They gave out a report of no results.

During the 30 years of Dr. Koch's use of his therapies in the United States, that was the only "official" test ever carried out. Every other request Koch made for a test was refused.

Writing in 1955 (*Survival Factor*, Dr. William F. Koch) about the Wayne County trial, Dr. Koch described one of the test patients, "Mrs. Edith Fritts had cancer of the uterus proven by laporotomy as extending throughout the abdomen and perforating the stomach so as to cause severe bleeding. She lived fifteen years in good health after the treatment and died from an accident. The coroner's autopsy showed no cancer was present, and the cause of death had been a brain injury." The treatment was one shot of Glyoxylide.

In 1923, Dr. Koch appealed to the Wayne County Medical Society Cancer Committee to change its false report of 1919. Not only did they refuse to do so but summarily denied the diagnoses made by the 1919 official committee. In all, fifteen affidavits were submitted for the 1923 review. Dr. W. A. Dewey M.D., a professor of homeopathy at the University of Michigan and an independent observer during the Cancer Committee's official review, wrote Dr. Koch on October 25, 1924 (Koch Family Archives):

> *I have received what is termed the latest report on your treatment. This claims to be an account of the séance held on Nov. 5, 1923, at which I was present and took notes of each case. For a studied intent to falsify, a premeditated determination to condemn everything, and an unscientific, un-American assumption to be judge, jury, and prosecuting witnesses, the report of this so-called committee outstrips in bias, unfairness, and mendacity anything that has ever been my lot to observe in a medical practice of forty-two years.*

> *The frankness with which you presented these cases, giving to the committee all the details and referring them to original records and to the family physicians, showed your honest desire to have an honest investigation of your method.*

> *The composition of the committee being for the most part surgeons and radium or X-ray "experts", a class that assumes cancer to be curable only by these methods, was unfortunate in the first place. In the second place, no member of the committee was, in my opinion, qualified to sit in judgment on your treatment by education, experience, or by right. I hope that some day your treatment will have an investigation before a body of seekers after the truth. These you will not find in American official medi-*

cine, which is a trust to keep all progress not coming from its own out of the field.

Dr. C. Everett Field of the Radium Institute of New York became interested in Dr. Koch's work. After reviewing the Radium Institute's October 1923 "Investigation of Thirty-Four Koch Cases", Dr. Field wrote, "The exhibit without doubt formed the most remarkable experience of my medical career". Dr. Field became so supportive of Koch's new scientific philosophy that he ultimately spent years documenting and publishing his findings on numerous Koch case histories. In his book *Is a Cure for Cancer Possible by Antitoxin and Serum Treatment?*, Dr. Field delineated the characteristics of the Koch catalysts:

1) *Used as a means of diagnosis in doubtful cases, it can be of the greatest service in determining the presence of cancer in its incipiency before it manifests itself locally.*
2) *It not only destroys the germ which is the cause of the disease, but it also causes a complete disintegration of its results, the cancer mass and its metastases, while through its powerful antitoxic action, it continues to neutralize the toxemia until all the elements of which the cancer consists are moved from the body and blood stream with the results the sufferer is cured.*
3) *Neither the location of the disease or the existence of secondary metastases affects the success associated with its use.*
4) *It is effective in all types of cancer, carcinoma, sarcoma, and epithelioma.*
5) *There are absolutely no harmful effects following its use.*
6) *It can be used for prophylactic purposes in preventing the development of the disease in those who are now in the early latent stages.*
7) *Its use means the saving of millions of lives and an*

end to one of the greatest scourges of humanity.

Dr. Field met with a stern rebuke from the AMA and his practice was negatively affected by his support of Dr. Koch.

In 1924, Dr. Morris Fishbein replaced Dr. Simmons as editor of the JAMA and defacto head of the AMA. Continuing Simmons' policy of hostility, Fishbein denounced Koch with growing shrillness, repeating the AMA version of the Wayne County Medical Society test of 1919. Koch and the people of Detroit and environs paid little attention. Word of mouth spread the news of Dr. Koch's catalysts, and he never lacked patients.

In *Survival Factor*, Dr. Koch reported that cancer mortality statistics for the decade 1920 through 1929 inclusive showed that while Philadelphia and Los Angeles showed a 30% increase in this decade, Detroit showed a drop of over 20%, and it was the only large city in the US that showed any fall whatever in the death rate from cancer. Wrote Dr. Koch, "Since the only variable that entered the picture was our own therapy, we take credit for the drop in the cancer rate in Detroit".

In his practice during those years, Dr. Koch proved what he had been postulating, that, "cell functions…are provided with energy that is produced and received…in accord with one and the same pattern, and when interrupted so as to produce disease, the fault is the same in pattern and subject to the same type of correction" (*Survival Factor*). So, he stated, the method of correction is the same, whether the problem is asthma, hay fever, tuberculosis, or cancer, all of which he was curing, usually with one shot of his carbonyl catalyst. When a second shot was given, it was at intervals of three months.

Dr. Koch was convinced that the body needed to be nourished and detoxified in order for the catalyst to work properly. Therefore, he preferred to give his treatment after a patient had spent a week on a strict pre-treatment regime. This included a series of colonic irrigations in order to remove toxins lining the intestinal walls. The patient would eat mostly raw fruits, vegetables, and whole grains. Certain foods would be avoided, especially animal protein, coffee, tea, soda, and any processed food. To obtain a successful reaction to Dr. Koch's catalysts, patients were warned to avoid exposure to certain chemicals such as gas fumes, tobacco smoke, solvents, turpenes, drugs, perfumes, and alcohol. Failure to comply with these instructions was found to drastically reduce the success rate. Dr Koch explained that the forbidden substances would interfere with the optimal function of the oxidation mechanism.

Occasionally, a case was so urgent that Dr. Koch would give a shot without the preferred week of preparation. One such patient was Mrs. George Grove, who was diagnosed at the Miami Valley Hospital in Dayton, Ohio, with lymphosarcoma. A mass the size of a cherry was removed from her neck on April 27, 1937, but within three weeks a growth at least five times as large as the original one had recurred in the same spot. It had become as large as half an egg by the time she arrived at the Koch Clinic on May 17, 1937. Dr. Koch gave her one dose of Glyoxylide the same day and upon examination three weeks later, no trace of the growth could be found. Mrs. Grove remained in good health until she was killed in an automobile accident four years later. An autopsy showed no trace of cancer.

Dr. Koch taught that when a toxin interferes with the body's normal oxidation process, cancer and other diseases may manifest. By supplying missing carbonyls, his catalyst could restart the impaired oxidation process, which would then destroy the toxin. He taught that cancer developed in response to a toxin. Therefore, destruction of the toxin would be followed by complete absorption of all cancerous tissues, healing and restoration of the regions involved, and return to health. A restored and invigorated oxidation system would prevent recurrence.

The catalyst worked with only three days of preparation in the case of Mrs. Sparling, She had become afflicted with the lymphocytic cell type of lymphosarcoma, a rapidly fatal illness. After seeing one of Dr. Koch's assistants, she was put on a three-day raw foods diet with enemas twice a day before Dr. Koch came to see her late in the evening of October 27, 1944. Large tumors were bulging from her neck and abdomen and it was clear that the disease was very far along. At Dr. Koch's second trial in 1946, Mrs. Sparling testified, "I received the shot at 11 PM, and the next day at 2 PM I felt a relaxation in my neck, which had been very stiff". In a week, there was a definite reduction in the size of the tumors and in the degree of cachexia, the wasting away which characterizes the final stages of cancer. In six months, Mrs. Sparling's tumors could no longer be felt by physical examination. She had some severe reactions at the 3rd, 6th, 9th, and 12th weeks and at the 24th and 36th weeks. These consisted of chills, fever, and general aches and soreness in the affected areas.

The reactions were what told Dr. Koch that his treatment was working. Sometimes patients would call him and complain that they were feeling badly, fearful of a relapse. Looking at his records, Dr. Koch would say, "The timing is right. You're reacting to the treatment, and this is just what we want. Hang on, since it won't last more than a day or two." Patients would call back a few days later to report that the reaction was over and they were feeling better. Reactions gradually decreased in severity until the toxins were eliminated or the chain reaction was interrupted. Interruption could be caused by breaking Dr. Koch's protocol (*i.e.*, his program).

Here is how Abram Johnson, a patient of Dr. Koch in 1932, described his reaction to the catalyst shot during the FDA's 1942 trial, "About the third day after the shot I felt pretty bad. I became cold. I thought I was going to freeze. The wife put me to bed. We had hot water bottles and about all the blankets we had on me. It lasted possibly an hour. About three weeks later, I had another cold spell, not as bad as the first. I had these cold spells for, I'd say, six months, I believe, every three weeks, but they kept getting lighter". Over that period, he testified, the little growths that had covered the roof of his mouth began to disappear and were all gone in about 6-8 months.

Thus way back in the 1920's, Dr. Koch was observing, predicting, and working with the body's own energy cycles, which we now call circadian. As Dr. Koch observed in *Survival Factor*, these healing reactions were unknown in western medicine.

A fundamental part of the new science which Dr. Koch discovered was the chain reaction which the catalyst would set off, going from cell to cell, inactivating the toxins in each and transforming them into an agent which would go to another cell, causing the same process until all toxins had been inactivated. As Dr. Koch explained it:

> *The toxin...undergoes a chain reaction in which the toxin molecule is dehydrogenated (i.e., it loses an atom of hydrogen) to form a free radical and this combines with oxygen to form a peroxide free radical, and the latter dehydrogenates the next toxin molecule with which it collides to form another peroxide free radical. Thus the oxidation chain is perpetuated until all toxin has been converted. It is evident then that the toxin is converted to antitoxin. The cause is converted into the curative agent. (Carbonyl Therapy by Dr. Wm. F. Koch)*

Dr. Koch's catalyst thus appropriately turned the toxin into the instrument of its own demise, *i.e.*, letting the punishment fit the crime. At his first trial in 1942, a government lawyer asked Koch how one shot could possibly set off a process which would heal so many things; cancer, polio, even leprosy. Dr. Koch replied "It only takes a single match to start a forest fire". A forest fire is a good analogy because what he was doing was to kick-start the body's oxidation system. To set off that internal forest fire required the catalyst and oxygen, which was provided by the raw fruits and vegetables in the diet he recommended. The elimination of particular foods and chemicals in the Koch program is analogous to the removal of water from kindling wood to permit it to ignite more readily.

In 1926 Dr. David Arnott of London, Ontario, visited Koch and returned on a frequent basis. He began to use the catalyst in his own practice and became one of Dr. Koch's most valued collaborators, spreading news of the treatment in Canada. Dr. Arnott documented the versatility of the Koch shot when his brother, Dr.

Henry Arnott, recovered completely from a cardiac thrombosis after one injection of Glyoxylide.

As Dr. Koch's fame grew, the extent of the negative influence of AMA head Dr. Morris Fishbein became increasingly apparent. In 1927, a woman bedridden with cancer of the uterus, a patient of Dr. Carroll Allen of New Orleans, was told by the Mayo Clinic that nothing more could be done. Dr. Allen was amazed when she recovered after a treatment by Dr. Koch. Then a second patient went to Detroit on a stretcher with multiple tubes draining his body and a colostomy opening because of cancer surgery. Three months later, he returned with no tubes, openings healed, natural functions restored, and carrying his own suitcase. Dr. Allen decided he too should go to Detroit, where he spent two weeks with Dr Koch, learning about the treatment. He hoped to spread the news of Koch's discoveries because of his professorship of surgery at Tulane University and through his position as chief of staff at New Baptist Hospital in New Orleans. After securing several cures in hopeless cases, Dr. Allen was pressured to retract a medical paper on the efficacy of the Koch therapy under pain of losing his professorship and his post at the hospital. One of Dr. Allen's friends, Dr. Bryan, professor of surgery at Vanderbilt University, achieved some cures in hopeless cases of cancer and received the same treatment as Allen, being forced to withdraw from use of the Koch catalysts.

In August 1934 the effectiveness of Dr. Koch's medicine was appreciated at home when his son John was suddenly stricken by polio. Koch was away so Dr. Arnott was called. By the time he arrived from Ontario, John was extensively paralyzed throughout his body and close to death, with swallowing paralyzed and no discernible breathing. Dr. Arnott gave him a shot of Glyoxylide.

In ten minutes John began to breathe and within a few hours all the paralysis had gone except for the right arm and leg. The next morning he could swallow and talk, but even then he was still close to death. Eventually, he made a good recovery, walking almost normally.

In 1935, Dr. Koch traveled to Belgium at the invitation of Dr.

W. Maisin, director of the Cancer Institute of the University of Louvain, who was considered a world authority on cancer. Koch had been aware of Maisin's work since the 1920's.

Six weeks after Koch arrived, several wealthy American doctors came to Belgium to attempt to convince the University of Louvain to send Dr. Koch back to Detroit, denouncing him as one of the world's great charlatans. Even the American Ambassador got into the act. Dr. Maisin refused them all, stating that the Rector of the University had told him to stand behind the Koch treatment if it were the truth. "I am convinced it is scientifically sound and clinically efficient", Dr. Maisin told the visitors. He added, "If Belgian charlatans were to go to America, no Belgian doctor would spend one cent trying to get them back". It turned out that one of the Americans had large investments in radium and was concerned about competition from the Koch treatment.

The research in Louvain was published by Maisin and Koch in July 1935 in two articles in the *C. D. de la Societe Francaise de Biologie*, at that time considered one of the world's best scientific journals. These reports were included in Koch's *Chemistry of Natural Immunity*, published in 1939.

Animal experiments were conducted with the various infections of interest to the Belgian government such as leprosy, sleeping sickness, tuberculosis, and venereal disease, proving efficacious in all. As a result, Maisin arranged to have the treatment tested in leprosy, where it achieved an 87% cure rate, in what was then the Belgian Congo, later called Zaire, or the Congo.

Because of the good results achieved on leprosy in the Congo, in 1937, a former U.S. Assistant Surgeon General and several prominent citizens requested then Surgeon General Parran to give Dr. Koch permission to treat lepers at a leper colony in Carville, Louisiana. Dr. Parran wrote the group that he was refusing permission because he had been told by his technical adviser, Dr. Voegtlin, that there was no such treatment. Five years later, in Dr. Koch's first trial, Dr. Voegtlin, in military uniform, testified as an "opinion" witness against Dr. Koch. Confronted by the statement he had made to the Surgeon General, he admitted under oath that he had lied to Dr. Parran. Shortly after, he was promoted.

Also acquainted with Dr. Maisin, Dr. Arnott reported to an Ontario Cancer Commission in 1939 what Maisin had told him (Report of the Ontario Cancer Commission):

> Dr. Koch's formula is a new method for treating disease. It is opening the door to the development of immunity to disease. The Koch formula should not be called merely a cure for cancer. It is a very important step and is likely to change the whole picture of medicine and pathology because of the clinical results. I do not know how Dr. Koch ever came to hit upon this new compound we are using. Not only is it a compound that is new to medicine, but it is also new to chemistry.

For the Ontario Cancer Commission, Maisin wrote a letter dated September 8, 1939 (*ibid*) stating:

> I have spent the last five years in the study and development of the Koch treatment in allergies, infections, and experimental cancer in animals....I am willing to state that over this short period of five years I have seen cancer disappear in animals and man with a return to health as a result of its use, in real cancer proven malignant microscopically...Sometimes the results have been so startling that we feel fully justified to continue the research in this field.

In June 1939, Dr. Koch received an urgent phone call from a member of the British peerage close to the Royal Family asking him to come to London at once. There he treated a person of such prominence that the name has never been released. On the negative side, when he landed, he was intensely questioned by the port authorities. Koch suspected they had been alerted that a "dangerous charlatan" was coming to the U.K. Koch was released when his important patient's chauffeur arrived.

In May, 1941, Dr. Koch sailed for Brazil for research and a little vacation. An hour before departure, it was learned that the ship's doctor would be unable to make the trip. Dr. Koch, the only doctor on board, was drafted for the job. The second day out, an important Brazilian diplomat suffered a hemorrhage of the stomach so severe that when Dr. Koch arrived no pulse could be found. Dr. Koch found a large tumor in the stomach region and the patient later confirmed that he had already been diagnosed with advanced cancer of the stomach. He was returning to Brazil after being told at an American clinic that his condition was hopeless. Dr. Koch gave him a shot of Glyoxylide, made arrangements for his diet, and before they arrived in Rio the man was again eating in the dining room. His recovery amazed his personal physician in Rio, Dr. Renato Souza Lopes. Lopes became very interested in Koch's work and asked him to treat other patients. Soon various cases considered incurable were on the road to recovery, including men high in the government. The Minister of War arranged for Koch to establish the treatment at a large military hospital in Rio where he was to teach the doctors its clinical use and the chemists its manner of preparation. A large number of leprosy and tuberculosis cases were treated, even a few patients in an insane asylum. Suspecting that one case of acute dementia was the result of toxic agents, Dr. Koch administered Glyoxylide with the hope that restored oxidation would destroy the toxins. Five days after treatment the patient returned to normal and was discharged from the hospital.

On Dr. Koch's next visit to the hospital a week later, he was met by a man who shook his fist in the doctor's face and made threatening remarks. Dr. Koch said "I didn't know they taught the patients English in this institution". The man replied "I'm not a patient; I'm a representative of (a pharmaceutical company) and we're going to see to it that you don't interfere in our business in South America any more".

Dr. Koch proceeded about his business of curing illness and thought little of the incident. A few weeks later, he received notice from the U.S. Food and Drug Administration (FDA) that they wanted to discuss his labels with him personally. Koch then left his research in Brazil and returned to the United States in November 1941.

One of the principal responsibilities of the FDA is to make sure that labels on food and drugs are not deceptive. In February, 1942, Dr. Koch met with FDA officials in Washington, presenting proofs of the correctness of his labels, but was told that the FDA planned to take him to court.

Meanwhile, Dr. David Arnott, after considerable opposition from the radium interests in Ontario, was promoting the Koch therapies in other provinces with more success. Results in Alberta were so successful that in mid-March 1942, it was agreed at a caucus of the governing party to invite Dr. Koch and Dr. Arnott to Alberta. They were to put on clinical demonstrations of Glyoxylide with the government providing all needed facilities. This decision became fairly well known in political circles in Edmonton, and Drs. Koch and Arnott were expected at an early date. Had a province of Canada officially accepted and approved the Koch treatments, the cat would have been out of the bag.

FDA had let Koch know that it intended to prosecute him and he probably expected papers to be filed demanding his appearance in court. Nothing prepared him for what happened next. One week after the decision on the Alberta invitation, on the evening of Good Friday, April 4, 1942, too late to get bail money from a bank, Dr. Koch was suddenly arrested in Delray Beach, Florida, and thrown into a Miami jail. Upon his arraignment the next day to set bond, the district attorney demanded a $10,000 bond. This was a very great amount of money in 1942, at the tail end of the depression. The judge asked why such a large sum, since this was not a murder charge but an argument over a label. The district attorney then admitted that the DA in Detroit, who had obtained the indictment at the request of the FDA, had telephoned him requesting that he insist on a $10,000 bond. Dr. Koch had started work in Brazil, his Detroit colleague had told him, and they did not want him to go back and finish it. Then he added "When the United States Government gets through with Koch, he will be all washed up and won't be able to go anywhere". Koch was later told by a high government official that the government was out to get him and used the label strategy as a convenient way to do the job. Koch was the first person ever indicted under the Federal Food, Drug, and Cosmetics Act of 1938, which was the first federal law to bar "unsafe" medicines. The FDA never asserted that the Koch therapies were unsafe, but went after him under its powers to regulate labeling.

Dr. Koch's labels stated that Glyoxylide and Malonide were for cancer and asthma; both were sold only to physicians. The AMA, however, had denied for the previous 22 years that his products had any effect on cancer or anything else. Parroting the AMA line, the FDA charged that his labels were false, fraudulent, and deceptive. The FDA claimed that the remedies were indistinguishable from distilled water and therefore had no effect whatsoever on any disease.

The distilled water charge brought up a very interesting point. In producing his catalysts, Dr. Koch first prepared what is called a "mother liquor", a dark liquid composed of the combination of chemicals he'd discovered in his early research. Then he diluted the mother liquor by one million times, so his catalysts only contained one one-millionth of the original liquid. This is a process well known in homeopathy, a branch of medicine which had been very well accepted in the United States in the 19th century. Perhaps because homeopathy avoids the use of toxic drugs, it has remained popular in Europe, where it is covered by government health insurance programs.

In the 19th century, the AMA took the lead in rejecting homeopathy as a bona fide medical science and threw its lot in with "allopathy", or the use of sometimes toxic pharmaceutical drugs. After an AMA campaign against homeopathic medical schools early in the 20th century, only one survived. Homeopathic medicines are highly diluted, with often no more than one part of the original substance to one million or more parts of distilled water. Conventional or allopathic medicine grants that homeopathic dilutions are harmless, but holds that they are useless, being too weak to contain any real medicine. In other words, they're just distilled water, the charge the FDA threw at Dr. Koch. (Nobody ever said Dr. Koch's catalysts were harmful.)

Dr. Koch, an MD, not a homeopath, had no desire to make a point of calling his preparations homeopathic (although in effect they were) and inviting persecution on those grounds too. He explains in *Survival Factor* that, as a practical researcher, he was looking for what worked. "The question not only is how dilute must the solution...be, but also how concentrated dare it be and still retain physiological activity", *i.e.*, the ability to produce the desired effects. The answer he came up with was a dilution of one part per million. This dilution, he pointed out, "carries thousands of billions of molecules in each cubic centimeter...and only one molecule is required to start a catalytic action which can grow with geometric progression", *i.e.*, the awesome chain reaction.

In the mid-19th century, Michael Faraday, the father of electricity, said that "every schoolboy knows that the important thing about any chemical is the electrical charge which it carries". Dr. Koch was well aware of the electrical properties of his chemicals. Describing the dilutions to produce his catalysts, he wrote in *Natural Immunity* that "the electrons are made more active with dilution". With "only one molecule required" to start Koch's chain reaction, a molecule whose electrons were thus activated was likely to do a more effective job in oxidation. Oxidation involves a transfer of electrons, and increasing oxidation was the objective of the catalyst.

In his February 1942 conversations with FDA scientists in Washington, Dr. Koch told them that "all cancer producing substances are oxidizable. This has been my theory from the start." He explained that he had found the carbonyl group, with its detoxifying action as an oxidizing agent, to be the least common denominator to disease in general; this was why his catalysts were effective in so many different conditions.

Asked by the FDA doctors if he regarded his theory as part of homeopathy, Dr. Koch answered "yes. My rule is this; for a first dose in a rapidly developing malignancy, I send a lower dilution. If it is an old, prolonged affair, I give a very high dilution".

Speaking in good faith as one scientist to others, Dr. Koch might as well have saved his explanations, for the FDA had not acted against him for scientific reasons. In the April 18, 1942 issue of the JAMA, editor Dr. Morris Fishbein claimed credit for having convinced the FDA to attack Dr. Koch. In contemporary language, we'd say the fix was in.

The first trial started in January 1943 and continued until May 23. Even while it was going on, Dr. Koch was having to defend himself on a second front. Soon after the FDA indictment, in a carefully coordinated move, the Federal Trade Commission (FTC) also attacked. The FTC challenged Dr. Koch's theories of toxin destruction by increased tissue oxidation, and presented "experts" who knew nothing of oxidation, the Koch remedies or their track record. The FTC asked a federal court to grant a temporary injunction against Koch's professional advertising until the matter could be settled through an FTC investigation. The injunction was granted. Again, we could say the fix was in.

In retrospect, it is strange to think that all this was happening during World War II, when the U.S. was fighting totalitarian states. Meanwhile, its government was using tax dollars to "protect" Americans from a therapy which had benefited thousands and never harmed anyone, and to foist on the American people a politicized official medicine and official science.

If the trials had not happened, and if Dr. Koch had had success in Alberta and been accepted there, things might have turned out very differently. But the trials did happen and we know a great deal about the effectiveness of the Koch therapies because of them. In his defense Dr. Koch was forced to organize a huge amount of cases histories, diagnoses, biopsies, and a large number of patients who testified to their cures. Two hundred cases were thus presented during the two trials.

One of the government investigators was questioned under oath as to whether or not he had been told anything good about Dr. Koch. He answered in the affirmative. Why, then, he was asked, was there nothing about such good results in his notes? His answer was very simple; he had only been sent out to find adverse comments.

A doctor took the stand and testified that he had used the Koch treatment on one case unsuccessfully. On cross examination, he discovered that he had a faulty memory when confronted with a letter he had written to Dr. Koch reporting the cure of the case in question.

The case of Rita Long was presented by Dr. Koch. In March, 1934, at the age of 14 months, she showed signs of losing the vision in her left eye. A specialist diagnosed her problem as glioma (cancer) of the retina, and removed her eye. Several months later, her right eye began to exhibit similar symptoms. The same specialist gave the same diagnosis again and recommended the same operation again, which would have left Rita blind. Her parents sought out another surgeon for a second opinion. This time, they were given a recommendation that Rita get a Gloxylide treatment from Dr. Koch. Willing to try anything before having their daughter permanently blinded, the parents took Rita to Detroit.

The Glyoxylide injection was given on November 25, 1935, and a second given on August 18, 1936. The results were dramatic. The eye stopped being irritated, the paralyzed, diluted pupil normalized, vision returned, and recovery followed.

Doctors' reports and hospital records were presented as evidence. Corroborating testimony was offered by Rita's aunt, Mrs. Bonnie Mann, her parents, Romaine and Mildred Long, and by Rita herself:

> *I am in the seventh grade and I got all A's. I always tie for about top or second in my grade. I rarely study at home because I can get my lessons at school. I read library books at home. My eye never bothers me at all. I read everything the teachers give me. I have no trouble seeing motion pictures.*

The prosecution's rebuttal witness, Dr. De Long, ignored the bald fact of Rita's recovery. He stated, "There is no treatment, X-ray or anything that we know of in scientific work that can fight this. He then went on to say that the only means of an exact diagnosis of the right eye would have been to insert a hypodermic needle directly into the growth in the center of the eye, macerate the growth, and then extract tissue that would then be viewed microscopically.

Dr. Koch's response was riveting. He pointed out that Dr. De Long's suggested technique would shoot cancer cells into the blood and lymph nodes as well as into the brain, hastening the spread of the disease. He also noted that the procedure would have blinded Rita's remaining eye.

Another patient, Wesley Roebuck, was operated on June 28, 1926, for cancer of the stomach to remove an obstruction that was threatening him with starvation. A few weeks later, the disease returned, causing another obstruction. He then sought out Dr. Koch and received an injection of Glyoxylide. Recovery was rapid and within six to nine months, the large cancer masses were absorbed, and the stomach healed. He testified at the trial about his dramatic cure. In 1950, at age 92, Mr. Roebuck was still in good health and was known for taking seven-mile walks into town from his farm. He testified at the trial about his dramatic cure.

An astounding aspect of the Koch therapy was its ability to cause the regrowth to normalcy of tissues and organs badly damaged by cancer. A remarkable illustration of this was the case of William Schultz, who testified. In the terminal stages of stomach cancer, Schulz underwent an exploratory operation at the Mayo Clinic in the latter part of May 1941. This showed that cancer had destroyed about half the stomach wall and spread to other organs, with x-ray pictures confirming the destruction of the stomach wall. Sent home by the Mayo Clinic as a hopeless and inoperable case, Schultz was taken to a Dr. Mantor in Nebraska, where he received a shot of Glyoxylide on June 16, 1941. The trend of the disease reversed and in six months he was back doing farm work. At the ninth month, he returned to Dr. Mantor and received a second shot.

And so it went. The Koch lawyers presented hard evidence of

cures of cancer of the bone, uterus, stomach, liver, spleen, pancreas, palate, skin, neck, breast, retinoblastoma, lymphosarcoma, hypernephroma, as well as cures of TB, polio, asthma, heart thrombosis, leprosy, hyperthropic arthritis, psoriasis, and rheumatic fever. The government lawyers presented various experts who admitted they had no experience with the Koch therapies. Still, they testified, Glyoxylide and Malonide could not be effective "in their opinion".

There was extensive newspaper coverage of the first trial. The *Detroit Times* from February 6 to March 12, 1943, and the Detroit *Free Press* from February 10 to March 19, 1943, printed a number of articles drawn from sworn testimony at the trial, producing the following headlines:

> *Three Cancer Cures Put in Record at the Koch Trial....Hospital Executive gives Case Histories as Defense Witness... Doctor Testifies Koch Formula Aided 16 cases...Medication Cured His Own Infection, He Informs Court...Koch's Medicine Credited as a Cure for Many Ills...Tampa Doctor Defends Remedies...Koch Medicine Credited with Rebuilding Lung...Cancer Doctor Says Koch Cure Replaced X-Rays...Cancer Claimed Cured by Koch...Koch Remedy Cured Cancer, Nurse Says....Koch Cure Claimed in Heart Case...Koch Drug Praised by Nun...Cancer Cured by Drug, Farmer, 80, Says.*

The Government's charge was very clear; that the Koch remedies were not a cure for cancer, and therefore his labels were fraudulent for so indicating. The Government could not prove its charge and did not win the case.

But neither did Dr. Koch, since the 1942 trial resulted in a hung jury. The U.S. was fighting the Nazis at that point. For many of the jurors, it must have been inconceivable that the government would sponsor an untruthful prosecution, or be involved in a move to eliminate a way to diminish human suffering. So despite the evidence, several of them voted to convict.

When you're not acquitted of an indictment, you're still under indictment. Thus Dr. Koch was not free to leave the country to go to Alberta or to return to Brazil.

Dr. Koch was not idle in the three years before the second trial in 1946. Once upon a time a book banned in Boston was an instant bestseller. Just so, the attacks on Dr. Koch spread the word of his treatment, attracting not just hundreds of patients but many new doctors as well.

In Canada, Dr. Arnott had gotten cattle growers in British Columbia interested in the Koch therapies in 1941. Sufficiently impressed, they convinced the Provincial Ministry of Agriculture to undertake a five-year study over the years 1943 to 1948. As the study progressed, cattlemen found the Koch treatment highly effective in Bang's disease (undulant fever in humans), mastitis, and infertility, thus permitting valuable cows to continue producing longer.

During the three years between the trials, Dr. Koch was contacted by Dr. Willard Dow, president of the Dow Chemical Co. As Dow explained in a letter of June 2, 1946 to Lawrence Thatcher, a friend of Dr. Koch:

> *Some years ago, we decided it was up to us to apply ourselves to the chemistry of such diseases as influenza and find out all we could. During the analysis of the problem entirely from a chemical standpoint, and not from a medical standpoint, we arrived at the conclusion that some medicinal of <u>high oxidizing characteristics</u> should be the method of medical cure (emphasis added). About that same time one of our people here discovered Dr. Koch's activity and found that his chemistry as applied to medical treatment was exactly the thing we were interested in... The government has spent a tremendous amount of money to attempt to prove him (Koch) wrong. It almost seems as if a certain group is attempting to persecute him unjustly... As far as I am personally concerned, I consider him one of the outstanding scientists in the medical profession,*

and he is so far ahead of the thinking of his profession that he is naturally being ridiculed somewhat... I think we all have an opportunity to see something new aborning in Dr. Koch's work.

When the second trial began in February, 1946, government lawyers charged that Dr. Koch's chemistry was bogus, and that there was no such chemistry. (Dr. Koch represented the formula for Glyoxylide as O=C=C=O.) Their witnesses claimed that Glyoxylide and Malonide were really glyoxylic acid and malonic acid. They were surprised when scientists from Dow Chemical testified that there was indeed such a chemistry, which they had verified and put to use in plastics. The Dow scientists pointed out that free radical chemistry (discovered by Dr. Moses Gomberg and used by Dr. Koch) was fundamental to the plastics industry. One of these scientists was Dr. William J. Hale, head of research for Dow Chemical and Dr. Dow's brother-in-law. The other was James Sheridan, Dow's patent attorney.

Sheridan wrote Dr. Arnott on April 21, 1947 about his experiences with the Koch catalysts and his testimony at the trial:

I have been assigned the pleasant task of advising you concerning the nature of the chemical work done by the Dow Chemical Co. on the chemistry of the Koch drugs.

Our activity started in 1944. We had been interested in oxidation and polymerization catalysts. Naturally we were interested when we discovered that Dr. William F. Koch of Detroit was using certain chemicals containing these structures and on the same theoretical basis. Our application was in industrial chemistry and Dr. Koch's was in biochemical systems, but our approaches fell into one category.

We submitted some of the Koch Glyoxylide in concentrated form to analysis. The material submitted was in water solution and therefore, according to FDA expert opinion, should have been a solution of glyoxylic acid. We found, however, that the material was, in fact, a polymer consisting of a chain of carbonyl (i.e.: C=O) groups and that the solution contained no glyoxylic acid. In fact, the solution contained no acid of any kind. We failed to detect acid groups even with spectrum analysis. The Dow chemists who took part in this program testified at the Koch trial in the spring of 1946 in Detroit. It is significant that no rebuttal testimony was offered by the Government.

The FDA had been provided with catalysts from the Koch Laboratories identical to those that the Dow chemists had analyzed. However, the FDA expert, Dr. Wirth, testified under oath that the FDA had not used the material supplied by Koch. Instead, Dr. Wirth stated, the FDA had chosen to produce its own version of Koch's Glyoxylide and Malonide. To do this, it used diluted glyoxylic acid and malonic acid which it claimed were the same as the Koch products. The FDA then proceeded to spend taxpayer money to test its counterfeit products on mice where, not surprisingly, they were ineffective. They then spent more taxpayer dollars conducting tests in hospitals to document the lack of efficacy in human diseases of their version of the Koch catalysts.

Following Wirth's testimony, Dr. Koch explained that there was no glyoxylic acid at all in his catalyst, since Glyoxylide was not glyoxylic acid but the anhydride of glyoxylic acid; hence the name Glyoxylide, a contraction of glyoxylic and anhydride. While that may not mean much to most people, the Dow Co. chemists made it clear that they understood it perfectly and that Glyoxylide performed exactly as Dr. Koch said it did.

In effect, the FDA put Dr. Koch through a second trial over the lack of efficacy not of Dr. Koch's products but of the FDA's fraudulent version of his products. Under cross-examination, FDA witnesses had to admit that they had no working knowledge of or experience with any of Dr. Koch's actual products, or any understanding of homeopathic dilutions.

William Schultz, who had testified in 1942, returned to the witness stand to show X-rays taken since the earlier trial. One from April 1943 showed a 75% improvement in his stomach. One made in June 1944 at the Roche hospital in Sydney, Nebraska, showed a normal stomach. Comparing these to the X-rays taken at the Mayo Clinic in 1941, which showed half the stomach wall destroyed by cancer, Schulz testified that after two Koch shots, his stomach was behaving quite normally.

Would any of the "approved" therapies in the year 2000 accomplish such results?

In addition to many of the cases presented at the first trial was a startling new one, one of the most remarkable of all of Dr. Koch's cures. Walking normally, Violeta Nicola of Bakersfield, California, testified that she was stricken with infantile paralysis at the age of 18 months, had undergone 23 operations and 54 casts, and had worn braces. She stated that she was walking on crutches, dragging the right leg with a brace on it when she visited Dr. Wendell Hendricks, D.O., in Bakersfield in April 1943. Dr. Hendricks testified that on April 7, 1943, he gave her an injection of Glyoxylide. On June 8, she was beginning to move the right leg and could stand by herself, walking around the room with the braces off. On August 13, she had a reaction of chills, fever, and headache. Since then, Dr. Hendricks testified, "she has had complete control over both legs, walking unaided with no crutches or braces." The muscles had developed, the cramps had ceased, and her weight had increased. On June 23, 1944, Dr. Hendricks gave her another shot of Glyoxylide. At the beginning of the treatment, her right leg was 1 ¼" shorter than the left. By September 11, the difference in her legs was reduced to 1/16". While her right calf had measured 4" around in April 1943, it now measured 10 ½", and the left calf had developed from 10" to 11 1/2". He gave her another shot November 11 and testified that "she can now run up and down stairs and walk or run or dance like other normal people". Violeta Nicola's former brother-in-law confirmed in 1998 having heard the story from Violeta, from whom he had not heard in years.

This case appeared to confirm Dr. Koch's teaching that cells invaded by a virus (such as polio) are not dead, but that the virus is interfering with the cell's normal functions. His Glyoxylide stepped up previously blocked oxidation and removed the virus from the cell, which then returned to normal.

Because of the study started in 1943 through Dr. Arnott's efforts in Canada, experts from the British Columbia Government and from the University of British Columbia came to testify on the success of the catalysts in cattle diseases. In addition, British Columbia physicians testified that they had used hundreds and even thousands of the Koch treatments. They depended on the medicines they used for the success of their practices. They could not have afforded to use the Koch shots, they pointed out, unless the shots worked.

While Dr. Arnott had been an extremely effective witness at the first trial, the Government blocked him from testifying at the second trial by the device of calling him as a Government witness. Under the court rules, even had he never actually been called by the Government, he would still have been prevented from testifying for Dr. Koch. Instead, he later calculated, he submitted about 1,000 pages of documentation - in addition to arranging for the witnesses from British Columbia.

During the 1946 trial, Dr. Koch frequently found himself sitting directly behind the Assistant Attorney General sent out from Washington to prosecute him. As the trial progressed, Koch noticed a tumor on the man's neck that was growing larger every week. Finally, Koch spoke to him, "I have observed a dangerous tumor growing on your neck. Even though we're adversaries, I will treat you because I believe your life is in danger." The official replied, "I would never take your quack treatment".

Some of the testimony was quite vociferous. Outspoken Dr. C. E. Phillips, past president of the Orange County, Texas, Medical Society, presented a deposition stating, "I have not many years to live and if I can keep you people from putting this medicine out of the earth, I will prevent one of the most heinous crimes that has ever been perpetrated upon the American public or any other country".

Unlike in 1942, during the second trial the Detroit press carried nothing of Dr. Koch's side of the case, but only the FDA side. The testimony from the British Columbia cattlemen and physicians and from the Dow scientists carried the day. At the first trial, the FDA, *i.e.*, the Government, had asked Judge Ernest O'Brien to direct the jury that if it found the Koch treatment ineffective in even one type of cancer that it must then find it useless in cancer in general. To his credit, Judge O'Brien refused to accept the FDA's request, but the judge at the second trial did so, and made the above charge to the jury.

It must have left the jurors highly confused, and once again they were tending to be a hung jury. Then a juror got sick and a mistrial was declared on July 23. Once again the Government had failed to prove Dr. Koch's therapies were *not* a cure for cancer. But once again, Dr. Koch did not receive an acquittal and was still under indictment.

Not only that, he was very busy attempting to fight the FTC, which was conducting a series of hearings around the country on the temporary injunction they had secured in 1942 against Dr. Koch's advertising (which was only carried in medical trade journals). At that time, FTC rules of evidence were very different from those in a courtroom. Government witnesses were permitted to give "opinions" in rebuttal of hard facts such as x-rays, biopsies, etc. However, Dr. Koch's lawyers were not allowed to cross-examine and challenge these "opinions" or to show that the witnesses were unqualified to testify as expert witnesses. Not too surprisingly, the FTC decided to maintain the temporary injunction and succeeded in making it permanent in 1950. By that time, Dr. Koch had been forced to give up the fight.

During the two years after the end of the second trial, Dr. Koch continued treating patients. His opponents were shaken when one of those who had fought Dr. Koch the most strenuously, the Assistant Attorney General whom Koch had offered to treat, died of cancer a few months after the trial ended.

Lawrence Thatcher, a businessman from Imlay City,

Michigan, not far from Detroit, had read about Dr. Koch in the papers. Then Thatcher's sister was pronounced terminal with cancer of the uterus with 90 days to live. Taking the Koch treatment, in 90 days she was recovering rather than dying. Although Dr. Koch had told her to take precautions if she did not want any more children, she paid no attention, presuming her uterus was out of commission - and six months later, she was pregnant. Thus it happened that Larry Thatcher called Dr. Koch during the second trial. "I'm just a small businessman," he said, "but I'd like to help". Dr. Koch replied that he didn't think his message was getting across to the public and felt that he could use some help in public relations.

In the aftermath of the second trial and the FTC injunction, a great deal of public interest was building up around the Koch treatment. In particular, a number of Christian ministers became involved, aware that Dr. Koch had a long-standing policy of free treatment for any minister. In 1945, a group of Lutheran Ministers led by the Rev. Lawrence Reilly, organized the Lutheran Research Society to support Dr. Koch's work. In 1948, Senator William Langer of North Dakota placed in the Congressional Record an article written by Larry Thatcher about the Koch treatment. The word was spreading.

There were still rumors among government attorneys about even an unheard-of third trial, for the indictment still stood, but the Government was having second thoughts. When a friend of Koch asked the head of the FDA in 1947 what they were planning to do about Koch that year, he replied, "Nothing, absolutely nothing. There's a jinx on him". It had been observed that after the death of the Assistant Attorney General in 1946, the next to go was the director of the FDA office that included Detroit, who had been very energetic in the attacks on Koch. He died of cancer of the stomach soon after the second trial. The next casualty was the judge of the Federal Trade Commission who had conducted the many hearings where hard data presented by the Koch lawyers was allowed to be rebutted by "opinions" of non-expert witnesses. He died of cancer soon after his final reports were written.

Next came the FTC prosecuting attorney who had accompanied
the FTC judge on the nationwide "hearings" or trials. He died of
cancer of the brain shortly after completing his brief.

Perhaps these events were what shaped the next step, which
came as a surprise. On August 17, 1948, the indictments against
Dr. Koch and his brother, Louis, who ran the Koch Laboratories,
were dismissed. When Dr. Koch heard the news, he fell on his
knees in thanksgiving and then prophetically remarked "Even
though this is over, I feel these people will never leave me in
peace. They will keep working until they can find some techni-
cality to bring a new indictment".

The very next day, Dr. Koch's prediction came true. FDA
inspectors came to his Koch Laboratories for a so-called "routine
inspection", and inspected every day for the next three weeks, not
even taking time off for Sundays or Labor Day. Koch insisted on
having witnesses on each visit by the agents and had a stenogra-
pher take down each question and answer. Dr. Koch realized that
the least slip might give the FDA something to turn into a new
indictment.

FDA authority over Koch Laboratories was based on the fact
that the lab was in interstate commerce. By this time, Koch was
no longer young, as he was when the AMA denunciations started
in 1919 after he refused to sell out to Dr. George Simmons.
Remembered by his family as incredibly strong, by 1948, he was
63 and tired of the strain. So Dr. Koch instructed his attorneys to
inform the FDA that as of November 1, 1948, he was out of interstate commerce and that the Koch Laboratories were in the
process of being dissolved.

After Dr. Koch went out of interstate commerce to stop FDA
jurisdiction, both he and the Lutheran Research Society were
inundated with letters, calls, telegrams, and visits from physicians
with patients dying for lack of the treatment. Under the new situation, anyone wanting the Koch treatment would have to come to
Detroit.

A solution was devised. Larry Thatcher organized a group of
ministers, who formed a non-profit corporation called the

Christian Medical Research League. The board of directors was composed of ministers of several denominations and a few businessmen. This new organization took over the manufacture and interstate distribution of the Koch products. It was one thing for the FDA to beat up on Dr. Koch but quite another to go after a group of ministers. The FDA left the League alone.

Ever since 1942, Dr. Koch had been invited to return to Brazil to resume his interrupted research but had been unable to do so because of the indictment. On Thanksgiving Day in 1948, giving his enemies no advance warning, Dr. Koch suddenly left for Brazil. His friends and family wept as he boarded the plane at Detroit's Willow Run Airport. They wondered if he would ever return.

Koch may not have needed to fear another indictment, but who knows? He later told friends "I've spent $400,000 to defend myself (probably like $4,000,000 in 2000). I cannot afford any more legal expenses, so I can no longer afford to live in my own country".

In Brazil, Dr. Koch quickly resumed his research and once again demonstrated remarkable results, this time including aftosa, the still incurable hoof and mouth disease.

Up north, the Christian Medical Research League made an offer to the FDA to set up a public experiment with the Koch treatment. An equal number of League doctors and government-appointed doctors would conduct tests and the results would be made public. The FDA declined.

One of the doctors dedicated to the use of the Koch treaments was Dr. Albert Wahl of Mt. Vision, NY. Dr. Wahl had been a skeptic about Koch for many years, influenced by what he read in the JAMA, as were thousands. Then his sister became terminal with cancer. Their father arranged for her to have the Koch treatment over Wahl's objections. "She promptly recovered in characteristic fashion", Dr. Wahl noted in his *Least Common Denominator*, a carefully documented book published in 1947 on 150 cures he had observed using the Koch therapy. "The most startling element is the utter simplicity of the Koch treatments,"

wrote Dr. Wahl. "After using them, I felt I'd never practiced medicine before". In 1949, Wahl teamed up with Dr. Bessie
Rehwinkel and Dr. Lawrence Reilly to write *Birth of a Science*,
published by the Lutheran Research Society and reprinted in
1957. The book tells the entire Koch saga from the beginning to
where it stood in 1957, and this writer has depended heavily on
this excellent work.

In Brazil, Dr. Koch was working on a book presenting a
definitive exposition of his hypotheses and chemistry, with many
of his case histories. In 1955 he published *Survival Factor in
Neoplastic and Viral Diseases*, with a Portuguese edition in 1960.
This, as well as all his other research, was published privately by
Dr. Koch. The *New York Medical World* article of October 1920
was the last U.S. medical journal to publish his work. No one but
Dr. Koch remembered that the JAMA called him "the brilliant
young Koch" in 1913, but then changed to denouncing him as a
quack in 1919 after he refused to sell his science to the AMA.

By 1950, about 4,000 doctors around the U.S. were using
Koch therapies and holding regular conferences, presenting
papers about their results. At the one in Detroit in 1950, 2-year
old Judy McWhorter was the star. Very ill at six weeks, an
exploratory operation at three months showed a highly malignant
cancer involving 85% of her liver. She was given one to three
weeks to live. A neighbor, Joseph Noah, had been urging the
Koch treatment but the McWhorters' doctor assured them it was
useless. Finally, Judy was near death and Judy's parents took her
to Dr. N. T. Mulloy in Cisco, Texas. He almost did not treat her
for fear she would die at any moment, and that he would then be
held responsible. Mrs. McWhorter absolved him of responsibility and he gave Judy a shot of Glyoxylide on September 18, 1948.
(This was when Dr. Koch was being inspected every day by the
FDA.) In about a week, Judy began to improve, and Mrs.
McWhorter reported this to the doctor who had previously cared
for her. He warned against false hopes, pointing out that it was
impossible for any chemical to destroy such a large growth. Soon
Judy began to gain weight and the tumor began to recede. By

Christmas, a small trace remained but she appeared normal. Another doctor examined her on May 12, 1949, could find nothing wrong, was told of Judy's earlier condition, and still could find nothing wrong. On November 11, Mrs. McWhorter briefed a group of doctors meeting at a cancer convention in Fort Worth on Judy's condition at 12 weeks and then brought in the healthy baby. They all examined her, found nothing at all wrong, and then gave a statement to the press about the amazing case of the little girl who had healed herself with a spontaneous remission. They all were aware that Judy had been given a Koch shot.

In the year 2000, Judy McWhorter is alive and well. All she knows of the case is what she's been told, since she was less than a year old by the time she had fully recovered. However, her mother was only 22 when Judy was born and is also very much alive. She still gets excited and emotional when talking about how she very nearly lost her firstborn but saw her recover miraculously after just one Koch shot. Joseph Noah is no longer alive but his son remembers vividly how his father convinced the McWhorters to try the Koch shot after the doctors had declared that there was absolutely no chance for Judy. He still has pictures of her taken at three months with a tumor half the size of a football growing from her tiny stomach, and then at monthly intervals showing the tumor getting smaller and smaller until by six months nothing more could be seen.

In 1948, the British Columbia Ministry of Agriculture issued a very favorable report on its five-year study of the effectiveness of the Koch catalysts in cattle diseases. Interestingly, the study showed that cattle experienced the same three-week reaction cycles as did humans. The study was the first official recognition of Koch therapy in North America and still the only one to date. Based on the work in British Columbia, in 1948 Larry Thatcher set up Koch Cattle Shots to distribute the medicine in the U.S. Two years later, he issued a report stating that in the previous two years over 3,000 cows had been treated, with results confirming and sometimes surpassing those in British Columbia.

His business flourished and Dr. Harold Wilson of Columbus,

Ohio, who owned three herds of cattle, read of the results. After losing two herds to Bang's disease, he contacted Larry Thatcher, saved the third with Glyoxylide, and learned something of its use in humans. Thus the work in cattle was indirectly responsible for Mary Lou Barnes not succumbing to polio in 1950.

Sometimes there was good publicity. Irving Zweig, editor of the Wellesville, Ohio *Wellesville Press*, headlined his August 11, 1950 edition this way, "Koch Wonder Drug is Not a Fraud, Editor Claims After Trip to Detroit". Zweig titled his article, "Sees Proof of Drug on Cattle Mastitis". Thoroughly briefed by Larry Thatcher, Zweig wrote an imaginary speech by Dr. Koch to medical students saying, "You've been working at medicine from the wrong end. I admit you can mend bones and dope a headache. But how much better to find out why human and animal bodies are subject to disease and then invent some chemical of high oxidizing characteristics to eliminate the cause. That's what I've done". Zweig summarized what he'd learned in this way, "Modern medicine treats the effect and this medicine treats the cause".

In 1955, Dr. Koch was requested by the Secretary of Health of Rio de Janeiro to treat polio cases at the Hospital de Jesus. He was given authority over one ward, to which all polio patients were to be assigned, and impressive results followed. Only later did Dr. Koch learn that the hospital's chief of surgery was on a committee to oversee the distribution of the Salk vaccine in Brazil.

When 6-year-old Florizinha was brought to the Hospital de Jesus in the early stages of polio, she was not placed in Dr. Koch's ward. Left in another section for a month until paralysis was complete, she was only referred to Dr. Koch after the damage was supposedly permanent. She could not move voluntarily and her breathing was faint and shallow. Dr. Koch immediately treated her with Gloxylide. He described what happened:

On my return to the hospital the following week, I entered the hospital ward to find Florizinha sitting up at the foot of her bed dangling her legs over the side. She was engrossed in a conversation with the patient in the next bed. Her arms were moving in gestures to go with her tale and she was kicking her legs. As the doctors gathered around her bed to review the case with me, I noticed an American standing in the rear of the group. He was not dressed in the traditional white robe worn by the doctors in the hospital. The gentleman was a representative of a major U.S. pharmaceutical company with its home office in Detroit.

The atmosphere in the hospital changed, and doctors became difficult to work with. Koch went to the Minister of Health, who found he could not help and resigned in protest. Eventually, hospital administrators were forced to choose between offering Dr. Koch hospital privileges and receiving their routine shipments of pharmaceuticals.

Over the 1950's, Koch Cattle Shots was doing well but doctors using Koch treatments were not. More and more frequently, they were getting into trouble not from their patients but from their state and county medical societies. Criticized by their colleagues, Koch doctors would then find themselves brought up before their state licensing boards. Occasionally their prestige was such that no action was taken, but sometimes they'd lose their licenses. Dr. Morris Fishbein was gone, having been kicked out as head of the AMA after Harry Hoxsey forced damaging admissions from him in a courtroom in Dallas (Chapter 2). But there's an old saying, "the evil men do lives after them". Fishbein or no Fishbein, there's no inertia like that of an adopted policy; the AMA still preached the line that Koch's Glyoxylide was a fraud and that doctors had no business using it. Dr. Julian Baldor, whose studies had shown that oxygen content of tissues increased after contact with the Koch carbonyl catalysts, was forced to give up his practice in Tampa. Dr. Harold Wilson was brought up on charges but survived. Dr. Chester Hardy, who was a prestigious college president as well as a doctor, was taken to court by medical authorities in Tennessee for using Glyoxylide. One of his defenders, Washington lawyer Benedict Fitzgerald, had just authored a report commissioned by the late Senator Tobey dealing with the suppression of several cancer therapies. Dr. Hardy lost his license.

Gradually, doctors began to be afraid to use the Koch therapies and orders began to fall off at the lab in Detroit. Not wanting to tangle with the ministers, the FDA had never given it other than the routine inspection any pharmaceutical facility must expect from time to time. By 1958, there were no more orders, so the Christian Medical Research Society closed the lab. One doctor said "I didn't know how I could continue to practice medicine!"

Something else went wrong in 1958. At a construction site, a girder shifted unexpectedly and hit Larry Thatcher in the head. Although there was no fracture, pains got worse over a period of months and incapacitated him, so he finally agreed to an exploratory operation. The doctors closed him back up and told his wife "Sorry, but Larry's a goner. There's a tumor too big to operate, so just make him comfortable for the few months he has left." When the League's lab closed, Larry Thatcher was very ill and Koch Cattle Shots closed as well.

Some months later, the pains went away and Larry regained his usual robust health. Amazed and wondering how he had survived, his family finally told him what the doctors had said. "Well", said Larry, "I suspected I might have a problem so for awhile there I was putting Glyoxylide under my tongue!"

In 1962, Koch wrote to Larry Thatcher, "I cured diabetes when I was here in 1941 and now we cure it regularly without fail; one or two shots on a full carbohydrate diet with plenty of honey and molasses. And we cure the rapidly fatal juvenile type where insulin's help dwindles from month to month". Extending his research to Argentina in 1964, he became desperately ill while in Buenos Aires and almost succumbed. He survived by managing to give himself a shot of Glyoxylide. In 1965, now 80 years old, Dr. Koch wrote Larry Thatcher that he had been very sick for ten months. Before the illness, he wrote, "I was fairly young, maybe 50 or 60 in health activity. Now my efficiency is only one-third of normal, but I am recovering."

In 1965 Dr. Koch received a visit from Mildred Nelson, who had set up the Hoxsey Clinic in Tijuana in 1962, five years after it had been closed down in Dallas (Chapter 2). Impressed by her, Dr. Koch asked her to stay for another month, during which he would teach her everything. Then she could go back to Tijuana and offer the Koch treatment as well as the Hoxsey. Having planned to be away only two weeks, she felt she couldn't spend an additional month and regretfully turned down his offer. Had she been able to accept, the world might still have the Koch therapy.

Dr. Koch improved enough to travel to Germany in 1966 and observe results obtained by a group of doctors working with his catalysts. In early 1967, he asked Larry Thatcher to recruit a group of 30 to 50 American doctors. He would accompany them to Germany and train them there for three weeks on how to carry on his work. Thatcher soon had 15 lined up, but it was not to be. In June, Dr. Koch suffered a stroke and lost his speech. On December 9, 1967, he died. He had never returned to the United States.

In the U.S., few noticed. The Christian Medical Research League had closed its lab eight years before. There were no more Koch doctors using Glyoxylide or Malonide, but only doctors - and patients - with memories of them.

Larry Thatcher continued his public relations work for the Koch therapy, telling all who would listen about what he had observed and experienced. One night in New York in the offices of Dr. Robert Atkins, Larry, age 84 and in excellent health, held a group from the Foundation for Advancement in Innovative Medicine (FAIM) spellbound for two hours while he related the saga of the Koch therapies. Someone asked him what was the most memorable case he had ever seen. Larry thought a moment and then told of a worker he'd known who had a cancer that had eaten through the bone in his arm. Larry kept urging him to go to Dr. Koch. Finally, with his arm in a sling and the lower arm con-

nected to the upper only by some skin and muscle,, the man
agreed. Dr. Koch gave him a shot of Glyoxylide. When Larry
next saw the man some months later, there was no more sling and
his arm appeared normal. He told Larry that the bone had completely grown back and that he had gone back to his normal work.
Later, Dr. Koch showed Larry the man's X-rays, with the bone
regrown. "I've seen some incredible cases", said Larry, "but that
was probably the best".

Dr. Atkins asked Larry what percentage of success Dr. Koch
had in cancer when he was still in the United States. "About
60%", Larry estimated, "and the other 40% were probably due to
people not following his instructions. Dr. Koch could rev up the
oxidation system with his catalyst, but if people went to eating the
wrong diet, they could quench the chain reaction."

With virtually total recall of Dr. Koch's work until he was 90,
Larry Thatcher, an almost saintly man in his dedication to helping others, passed on at age 94 in April 1997.

It has been estimated that during the Koch era there were
500,000 recoveries from cancer and other diseases. This counted
those treated in Brazil and in the Congo, where there were reports
of 400 cures of leprosy. If the Koch science had been flawed, then
thousands of patients would not have recovered from a whole
host of diseases, with some still alive in 2000.

The effect of his catalysts on cancer has never been paralleled
in modern medicine and takes on huge significance in light of the
worldwide cancer epidemic. The importance of the Koch treatment in cancer almost overshadows its success in asthma, which
has doubled in the U.S. in the last twenty years of the century.
The number of sufferers from asthma rose from 10.4 million in
1990 to 14.6 million in 1994, almost one in twenty, according to
the National Center for Health Statistics. The costs of asthma
were $6.2 billion in 1997, projected to rise to $14.5 billion by the
year 2000. The death rate from asthma jumped 78% from 1980 to
1993. According to Dr. Koch, Glyoxylide burned up the toxins
that cause asthma. Patients who recovered from asthma testified
at both trials.

Dr. William J. Hale, research director of the Dow Chemical Company and one of the few who grasped the chemical reality of Koch's oxidation-enhancing carbonyl catalysts, called Dr. Koch "The Modern Pasteur".

Ironically, in the world after Pasteur, scientists have been taught to look for one microbe as the cause of each disease. But Dr. Koch taught that a healthy person inherits a healthy oxidation system. Finding a carbonyl group of chemicals to be a fundamental part of the oxidation system, he taught that disease occurs when a toxin weakens the carbonyls, diminishing oxidation efficiency. He created potent synthetic carbonyls which he used as catalysts to jump-start inefficient oxidation. He explained in *Survival Factor* how the catalyst works. In the presence of adequate oxygen (oxidation needs oxygen), the catalyst precipitates a chain reaction which, like a continuous fuse, goes from cell to cell destroying toxins until they are all removed, permitting all cell functions to be restored, and only then does the fuse go out - presuming nothing extinguishes it such as fumes or poor diet. He made it very clear that the catalytic reaction was indifferent to what it was oxidizing and therefore was capable of burning up whatever should not be in the body. This, he explained, is why the catalyst affected so many different diseases and conditions. To explain how the chain reaction continued after only one shot, Dr. Koch said "Nobody is surprised that a car keeps running after it starts". Dr. Koch's catalysts had the "utter simplicity", as Dr. Albert Wahl put it, of really elegant solutions.

Recalling the old Chinese saying that one picture is worth a thousand words, computer graphics could simulate Koch's chemistry showing: 1) normal oxidation, with sufficient oxygen and unimpaired carbonyls; 2) disease; the introduction of a toxin and its integration into and disruption of the carbonyl group, thus causing the oxidation process to slow down; 3) the introduction of the catalyst: a) with sufficient oxygen it catches fire, and b) without sufficient oxygen it won't catch fire; 4) the chain reaction, as the peroxide free radical thus produced goes to the first toxin it encounters, changing it in turn to another peroxide free radical, which then goes on to another toxin, etc., in an explosion in every direction; 5) what happens when a toxin capable of stopping the chain reaction, such as automobile exhaust, enters the picture.

In the 1930's, Otto Warburg won the Nobel Prize for showing that impaired utilization of oxygen was associated with cancer. Dr. Koch had been saying and publishing that since 1920.

Nobel Laureate Albert Szent Gyorgi, the discoverer of Vitamin C, was on the track of carbonyls. In an article published in 1974 entitled "The Search for a Natural Cure for Cancer" he wrote "There are atomic groups called carbonyls which contain oxygen....Carbonyls arrest cell division and my laboratory was led to the conclusion that it is still the carbonyls which arrest cell proliferation and it is the carbonyls who make the cell return to the resting state after it completes division. *If the carbonyls are missing, proliferation has to go on and cancer results* (emphasis added). We were not the first to be led to such a conclusion. A decade ago a very intuitive researcher, Dr. William F. Koch, came to the same conclusion."

Once in awhile, something happens to cause people to rethink basic principles, such as the atom bomb in 1945. Something new had happened, whether or not people thought it possible. Similarly, Dr. Koch set off an explosion inside human bodies, which burned up the toxins which cause many diseases. A new science, it was every bit as important as the atomic bomb, a new method of getting the body to heal itself, demonstrated in thousands of cases.

The authors of *Birth of a Science* wrote, "the history of the Koch Treatment is more dramatic than anything which the mind of a Hollywood fiction writer could imagine". When they wrote that, the treatment was still available.

But the Medical Camelot came to an end. It is incredible that it ended, since it lasted thirty years. How could something this important come to an end? But it did. Old Dr. Phillips was right when he said at the 1946 trial that suppression of the Koch science would be "one of the most heinous crimes ever perpetrated upon the American people". Dr. Koch's work indeed represented the Birth of a Science. His discovery of the significance of the carbonyl group was confirmed by Szent Gyorgy. This was a new principle in biochemistry and threw light on a basic body mechanism. Dr. Koch devised a simple and inexpensive way to restore that mechanism when impaired, with vast consequences for the healing of disease. By demonstrating fundamental new principles of biochemistry, Dr. Koch deserved a Nobel Prize and still does. Will anyone ever follow up on his work? Will we ever again hear the name of Dr. William Frederick Koch? Or should this chapter be entitled "Birth and Death of a Science"?

WHAT BECAME OF THE RIFE TECHNOLOGIES?

In 1976, the late Christopher Bird published an article in *East West* Magazine entitled "What Became of the Rife Microscope?" What indeed? And what became of the Rife Ray Tube as well?

In San Diego in the 1920's and 30's, Royal Raymond Rife built several light microscopes capable of seeing viruses and bacteria in their live state with magnification said to be 60,000 times. The best light microscopes of that time - or today - could magnify around 2,500 times, not enough to see virus-size bacteria. The electron microscope with its great magnification came along in 1939 but cannot see live viruses, virus-size microbes, or bacteria because the nature of its process kills the specimen.

Thomas Jefferson defined genius as the infinite capacity for taking pains. In this respect and others, Rife was certainly a genius, first as an intuitive researcher and also as a creator of superb technological instruments, some of which have not seen their equal since his time.

Rife set a goal of finding out if there was a virus capable of causing cancer. After completing his microscope, he spent most of the 1920's in this pursuit. Working with cancerous tissue confirmed by lab analysis to be malignant, Rife found what he deemed to be the guilty microbe and injected it into mice. When they then developed cancer; he removed their cancerous tumors and found the same microbe in them once again. In the late 19th century, German researcher Dr. Robert Koch (apparently no relation to Dr. William Koch) established a procedure for determining the cause of a disease; recovering a suspect microbe from a sick animal, injecting it into a test animal, and then, if that animal develops the same disease, recovering the same microbe from the second animal. Rife had fulfilled the Koch postulates.

Rife named the cancer microbe the Bacillus X, or BX virus, since under his microscope (observing it alive), he could see it change from a bacteria, or bacillus, to a virus-size microbe. Rife asked himself if this live organism producing a purplish red color, and therefore a frequency, could be killed by another frequency which would resonate with the vibratory rate of the microbe. Rife thus created a ray tube which broadcast various frequencies. When it was finally ready, he would sit in front of his microscope tuned to the BX microbe for hours on end, tuning the dial of his frequency device, going through one frequency after another. Finally one day when he reached a certain frequency, he saw the light of the BX microbe glow brighter and then go out, after which it disintegrated. He painstakingly repeated the process and always saw the same result. Then he placed the BX microbe in test mice and, after they had developed cancer, exposed them to the frequency he had discovered. There was no contact between the animals and the ray tube; they were simply in its presence a few feet away. He repeated the process numerous times to double-check his research. In this way, Rife determined what he called the Mortal Oscillatory Rate (MOR) for the cancer microbe. During the summer of 1934, 16 terminal cancer patients sat a few feet away from Rife's Ray Tube for three minutes every third day. After 90 days, 15 were declared fully recovered by attending physicians and in another month, the other one as well.

In a nutshell, that is the essence of the Rife story - a microscope that could see virus-size microbes, which the best electron microscopes cannot see in their live state, and a frequency-emitting ray tube capable of killing the microbe which caused human cancer, thus enabling cancer patients to recover.

This story fired up Christopher Bird to write his 1976 article five years after Rife died at age 83, a forgotten man. The article revived some interest in Rife's work but was largely ignored. Then Bird showed the article to independent scholar/journalist Barry Lynes, who urged Bird to write a book on Rife. Bird, researching for his *Secrets of the Soil*, told Barry "I don't have time - why don't you write it?" The result was Lynes' comprehensive *The Cancer Cure That Worked*, which triggered a Rife revival. Then came *The Royal Rife Report* by Borderland Sciences and later *The Rife Way* by the late Dallas researcher Mark Simpson. An article by Dr. R. E. Seidel and Elizabeth Winter entitled "The New Microscopes", published in the February 1944 *Journal of the Franklin Institute* and later reprinted in the Smithsonian annual report, contains a great deal of information on how the Rife microscope worked and about research done with it.

After reviewing available materials on Rife, one has the same feeling as when reading about Dr. Koch; something is lost, something wonderful.

The tragic story of Royal Raymond Rife started with his birth in 1888 in Elkhorn, Nebraska, but little is known about his very early life. At some point, perhaps 1906, he settled in San Diego, where he lived the rest of his life. *The Rife Way* contains a picture of Royal Rife (called Roy by his friends), as a dapper young man in his early 20's "on the concert stage playing the mellophone, French horn, and cello". Rife met a Chinese American girl, Mamie Quin, and married her in 1912, settling down in a house near the mansion of the Bridges family, who had made carriages until they went out of style. Mrs. Bridges had money of her own as a sister of Henry Timken, an Ohio magnate in ball bearings. During a period when Rife served as the Timkens' chauffeur, Mrs. Bridges became fascinated by Rife's dreams of high technology and set him up a lab above their garage. When Rife was not researching, he shared the Timkens hobby of racing fast cars and fast boats. Rife's skills as a chef were much appreciated, and he was a good musician. It was said of Rife that he was a quiet man, but when he talked, he was fun. Encouraging Rife's idea of building a super microscope, Mrs. Bridges funded a two year sabbatical for him in Germany. Taking Mamie, Rife spent a couple of years in Germany, may have studied at Heidelberg University, and spent some time at the Zeiss Corp. Learning what he needed, he returned to San Diego and completed his first microscope in the early 1920's.

In time, word of his endeavors began to get out. Over the course of the next 20 or so years, Rife's tracks begin to get a lot clearer from the 10-15 newspaper articles that appeared in San Diego newspapers about the young genius Royal Rife and his amazing microscope. An article in the May 6, 1938 San Diego *Evening Tribune* gave a retrospect of Rife's early years:

> *The San Diego man, who is hailed by many as a veritable genius, has experimented with important studies, inventions and discoveries in an unbelievably wide and varied array of subjects. These fields of pursuit range from ballistics and racing car construction to optics and many equally profound sciences. And in 1920 he was investigating the possibilities of electrical treatment of diseases.*
>
> *It was then that he noticed these individualistic differences in the chemical constituents of disease organisms and saw the indication of electrical characteristics, observed electrical polarities in the organisms.*
>
> *Random speculation on the observation suddenly stirred in his mind a startling, astonishing thought: 'What would happen if I subjected these organisms to different electrical frequencies?', he wondered.*

It may have been an article in the July 1931 issue of *Popular Science* which brought Rife to the attention of one of the most prominent medical researchers of the time, Dr. Arthur Isaac Kendall. Kendall was head of the Department of Bacteriology and Director of Medical Research at Northwestern University Medical School in Chicago. In 1904, Kendall had been director of the Panama Canal Commission's Hygienic Laboratory, which evolved into the National Institutes of Health in 1930. Sometime in 1931, Dr. Kendall asked his friend Dr. Milbank Johnson in Los Angeles to investigate what he had heard about Royal Rife and his microscope. Dr. Johnson was medical director of the Pacific Mutual Life Insurance Co., former president of the Los Angeles

Medical Association, a member of the board of directors of the Los Angeles County Pasadena Hospital, and one of the founders of the American Automobile Association, well connected and politically influential.

In November 1931, Dr. Johnson arranged a meeting with Royal Rife and took three other doctors with him. One of them was Dr. Alvin Foord, head of pathology at Pasadena Hospital and later president of the American Association of Pathologists. On November 9, Johnson wrote Rife, "I want to say that we all spent one of the most instructive and interesting afternoons of our lives in your laboratory...I wired Dr. Kendall on what we had seen and our opinion of it and this morning I received the following telegram, 'Expect to start for California Saturday'". Dr. Johnson added "He should arrive in Pasadena November 17, so be sure and have your microscope in perfect condition for the Big Chief when he arrives. I will bring him down to San Diego in my car".

When Kendall arrived, he brought along his "K medium", in which, he reported, he was able to detach dwarf bacteria from normal size bacteria. At the time, these disease-causing microbes were called "filtrable viruses". This claim was considered impossible at the time by many prominent researchers. Working with Rife, Dr. Kendall placed a typhoid germ in his "K medium", triple-filtered it through the finest ceramic filter available and then, under Rife's microscope, they could clearly see tiny microbes glowing with a turquoise blue light as they escaped from the larger bacteria. Rife and Kendall thus proved that bacteria contained smaller pathogens that could be seen under Royal Rife's microscope.

Wasting no time, on November 20 Dr. Milbank Johnson invited 30 of the most prestigious medical figures in southern California to a banquet in honor of Rife and Kendall at "Belbank", his mansion in Pasadena. In an opulent setting, Rife's and Kendall's discoveries were announced and discussed. On November 22, the *Los Angeles Times* reported:

Scientific discoveries of the greatest magnitude, including a discussion of the world's most powerful microscope recently perfected after 14 years of effort by Dr. Royal R. Rife of San Diego, were described Friday evening to members of the medical profession, bacteriologists and pathologists at a dinner given by Dr. Milbank Johnson in honor of Dr. Rife and Dr. A. I. Kendall.

The strongest microscope now in use can magnify between 2,000 and 2,500 times. Dr. Rife, by an ingenious arrangement of lenses applying an entirely new optical principle and by introducing double quartz prisms and powerful illuminating lights, has devised a microscope with a lowest magnification of 5,000 times and a maximum working magnification of 17,000 times.

The new microscope, scientists predict, will prove a development of the first magnitude. Frankly dubious about the perfection of a microscope which appears to transcend the limits set by optic science, Dr. Johnson's guests expressed themselves as delighted with the visual demonstration and heartily accorded both Dr. Rife and Dr. Kendall a foremost place in the world's rank of scientists.

Rife and Kendall wrote up a report on their research, "Observations on Bacillus Typhosus in its Filtrable State". This was published in the December 1931 issue of *California and Western Medicine*, the official publication of the California, Nevada, and Utah medical societies. The discovery was also reported in *Science* magazine on December 1, 1931, and in the *Science News Letter* on December 12, 1931 in an article entitled "Filtrable Germ Forms Seen with New Super Microscope". On December 27, 1931, the *Los Angeles Times* reported that Rife had demonstrated his microscope at a meeting of scientists and that "Dr. Rife has developed an instrument that may revolutionize laboratory methods and enable bacteriologists, like Dr. Kendall, to identify the germs that produce about 50 diseases whose causes are unknown."

In the next step in Rife's growing recognition, Henry Timken, the Ohio industrialist, brought him to the attention of Dr. Edward Rosenow, a senior researcher at the Mayo Clinic. In July 1932, at Dr. Kendall's invitation, a three-day series of experiments were carried out in his Chicago lab by him, Dr. Rosenow, and Royal Rife, who brought his microscope. Working with two other microscopes as well as Rife's, the three reconfirmed what Rife and Kendall had already published and studied some viruses of special interest to Dr. Rosenow. Rosenow published the results in the July 23, 1932 *Proceedings of the Staff Meetings of the Mayo Clinic* and also in an August 26, 1932 article in *Science* magazine entitled "Observations with the Rife Microscope of Filter-Passing Forms of Micro-Organisms".

A bacteria in its normal state is too large to pass through the tiny pores of a ceramic filter, but a virus-size "dwarf bacteria" can. So the orthodox view holds that if something can pass a filter, *i.e.*, is "filtrable", it cannot be a bacteria but must be some smaller form. The title of Rife and Kendall's report was a contradiction in terms for those who accepted as fact that a bacillus cannot be "filtered". Thus some of the outstanding authorities of the time didn't believe Kendall and Rosenow. Strangely, when Dr. Kendall announced his findings at a major scientific meeting in July 1932, he neglected to mention that his observations had been seen and could only be seen through a new and very special microscope to which he had access. This omission left him open to attack, and his critics did not hesitate to do so. As Barry Lynes observes, had Kendall made clear how he arrived at his findings, the JAMA article the following month might have focused on the marvelous new microscope rather than on the dispute between Kendall and his critics. These happened to be the most distinguished bacteriologists of the time, Dr. Rivers of the Rockefeller Foundation and Dr. Zinsser of Harvard. The critics having set the tone, Dr. Rosenbow received the same treatment as Kendall - disbelief, even derision - even though he referred to the Rife microscope in his report in the Mayo Clinic *Proceeding*. This put a damper on the forward momentum of Rife's acceptance.

For lack of a shoe a horse was lost, for lack of a horse a battle was lost...In retrospect, Dr. Kendall's failure to announce the Rife microscope simultaneously with his findings at that conference may have had just that significance; had he done so, probably Drs. Rivers and Zinsser would have left no stone unturned until they too could do research with a Rife microscope (Kendall had one), and things might have turned out very differently.

In the 19th century, Louis Pasteur had pronounced the germ theory - that an external germ was responsible for each disease. His rival, Antoine Bechamp, taught instead that the environment inside the body causes certain normally harmless microorganisms to change forms, after which they become harmful and cause disease. The concept that germs and microbes could change forms is called pleomorphism. In the insect world we see this in the change from caterpillar to cocoon to butterfly. Insects aren't microorganisms, to be sure, but the illustration demonstrates the concept. Pasteur's concept that germs do not change form is called monomorphism and is still the accepted view in bacteriology.

In reality, it would appear that they were both right to some extent. Certainly children at school "catch bugs" that are going around; according to Pasteur, that would be the only way one could catch something, *i.e.*, from an outside source. Almost everyone knows that can't be true, having come down with a cold after becoming overtired or overstressed without having been around anyone who had a cold. There's no question that certain specific microbes cause certain specific diseases but that doesn't prevent them from changing forms - like the butterfly - or evolving if the inner environment of a person's body turns toxic.

Can microbes change within one's body because of stress? One summer during college, I worked in Yosemite Park and climbed Half Dome. Although in good health, I was not in shape for mountain climbing and was exhausted by the time I got to the top, although not so much that I will ever forget the spectacular view. I cannot remember ever having been so tired as when I finally got to bed that night. The next morning I was off to the infirmary with a 104 degree fever. No illness had been going around Yosemite; nobody had flus or colds. It seemed that exhaustion had so weakened my immune system that something which normally had been held in check was able to take over and put me in bed for a couple of days. Considering pleomorphism, it might be that exhaustion produced specific chemicals which changed the environment within my body and caused something that had not harmed me before to change into something that did. Or in Dr. Koch's terms, a toxin (produced as a result of the change in the body's environment) had momentarily broken down my oxidation system.

Under his microscope, Rife was clearly seeing bacteria changing forms. Growing microorganisms with Dr. Kendall's K-medium, Rife, Kendall, and Rosenow all saw a "filtrable" form (hence the titles of their reports) produced from various bacteria, indicating pleomorphism. Even now, this view is not accepted by orthodox scientists; Dr. Robert Gallo, co-discoverer of the HIV virus, said that "pleomorphism is insanity". Gallo doesn't have access to a Rife microscope, so he cannot see for himself any-more than could Kendall's and Rosenow's critics in the 1930's. Solid evidence of pleomorphism has been published since Rife's time by the New York Academy of Sciences on October 30, 1970, in reporting the work of Dr. Virginia Livingston-Wheeler, Dr. Eleanor Alexander-Jackson, Dr. Irene Diller, and Dr. Florence Seibert. Pleomorphism is also confirmed in the work of Gaston Naessens (Chapter 8), inventor of a contemporary supermicro-scope.

In 1932, Royal Rife was not focusing on the pleomorphism argument that had engaged Kendall and Rosenow, but on cancer, and after Kendall's visit, he was now armed with the K medium. After 20,000 tries, he told a friend, he at last succeeded in isolat-ing what he called the "BX virus" (which today might be called a dwarf bacteria or microbe) and establishing it as capable of caus-ing cancer, as noted earlier. He also found a bacterial form of the microbe and wrote in 1953 "this BX 'virus' can be readily changed into different forms of its life cycle by the media upon which it is grown", observing that a variation of as little as two parts per million in the media was sufficient to trigger the change.

Rife's next step was to seek the frequency to kill the BX microbe. Barry Lynes quotes a long-time friend of Rife, who wrote in 1958:

> *I've seen Roy in that doggone seat without moving, watching the changes in the frequency, watching when the time would come when the virus in the slide would be destroyed. Twenty-four hours was nothing for him. Forty-eight hours. He had done it many times. Sit there without moving. He wouldn't touch anything except a little water. His nerves were just like cold steel. He never moved. His hands never quivered.*

> *I've seen the cancer virus. I've seen the polio virus. I've seen the TB virus. Here was a man showing people, showing doctors, these viruses of many different kinds of diseases, especially those three deadly ones - TB, polio, and cancer.*

> *Time and time again since that time some of these medical men had made the proud discovery that they had isolated one of the viruses of polio. Why that was one of the most ridiculous things in the world. Thirty-five years ago (1933) Roy Rife showed them these things.*

Closely following Rife's progress during 1932 and 1933, the years of the breakthroughs in cancer, Dr. Milbank Johnson kept in touch with Dr. Kendall and promoted Rife's work with other researchers. Although his first letter in 1931 was addressed to Mr. Royal Rife, from 1933 on Johnson's letters were addressed to Dr. Royal Rife, later calling him Roy. There is a report that Rife received an honorary degree from the University of Heidelberg for work in photomicroscopy. It is known that in the early 1930's the University of Southern California (USC) scheduled the award of an honorary degree to Rife, writing him a letter asking certain questions. Dr. Johnson wrote Rife urging him to respond to USC; Dr. Kendall wrote that he would attend the ceremony. Not much of a writer, Rife apparently never answered the letter and the offer was withdrawn.

In the spring of 1934, Dr. Johnson asked Rife to meet him in La Jolla (just north of San Diego) to discuss setting up a cancer clinic for humans. Rife agreed since, as he wrote in 1953, he had conducted successful tests "over 400 times with experimental animals before any attempt was made to use this frequency on human cases of carcinoma and sarcoma".

For the clinic, Johnson rented the large home of the recently deceased Ellen Scripps. (She and her brother founded the Scripps newspaper chain). Dr. Johnson persuaded Dr. Kendall to come for part of the summer.

At the end of three months in the summer of 1934, the results, as mentioned, were 15 cures out of 16 terminal cases of cancers of various types, as reported by Rife in 1953. Barry Lynes found evidence that the other one was cured by the fourth month.

We have descriptions of two of the cases. Dr. Kendall described Tom Knight, whose "tumor was on the cheek where it could be seen, watched, and measured from the start to the finish, and this I have done". A year later, Dr. Johnson wrote a letter to two San Diego doctors "to introduce Mr. Thomas Knight. He was the one who had the carcinoma over the malar bone of his left cheek that we treated at the La Jolla clinic last year". Dr. James Couche, a San Diego doctor who became a colleague of Rife as a result of the 1934 clinic, wrote 22 years later about a case he saw there:

The one that impressed me the most was a man who stag-gered onto a table just on the last end of cancer; he was a bag of bones. As he lay on the table, Dr. Rife and Dr. Johnson said 'Just feel that man's stomach'. So I put my hand on the cavity where his stomach was underneath and it was just a cavity, almost, because he was so thin; his backbone and his belly were just about touching each other.

I put my hand on his stomach which was just one solid mass, just about what I could cover with my hand...It was absolutely solid! And I thought to myself well, nothing can be done for that. However, they gave him a treatment with the Rife frequencies and in the course of time over a period of six weeks to two months, to my astonishment, he completely recovered. He got so well that he asked permission to go to El Centro as he had a farm there and he wanted to see about his stock. Dr. Rife said 'Now you haven't got the strength to drive to El Centro'. 'Oh yes', said he. 'I have, but I'll have a man to drive me there.' As a matter of fact, the patient drove his own car there and when he got down to El Centro he had a sick cow and he stayed up all night with it. The next day he drove back without any rest whatsoever - so you can imagine how he had recovered. I finally bought one of those frequency instruments and established it in my office.

A year later, Dr. Johnson wrote in a letter that "the clinic was opened and run by me to satisfy me personally that the Rife Ray would destroy pathogenic organisms in vivo as well as in vitro. The latter we had repeatedly demonstrated in the laboratory. I had to have this information conclusively positive before I could recommend to my friends to get behind the work...I intended to finance it through to the end." Upon the conclusion of the Clinic, Dr. Johnson formed a Special Medical Research Committee at the University of Southern California (USC) to supervise the Rife research and eventually to announce it. Composed of cautious medical professionals, the Committee balked at early release of the Clinic's amazing results, preferring instead to gather more data.

To this end, in 1935, Milbank Johnson arranged for Dr. O.

Cameron Gruner of McGill University, Montreal, to spend May and June with Royal Rife. Dr. Gruner was a renowned researcher in blood and had obtained a fungus organism from the blood of 92% of cancer patients he had examined. Rife took Gruner's fungus, placed it in Dr. Kendall's K medium, and then filtered from that culture Rife's BX virus. Barry Lynes reports, "In 1937, Dr. Milbank Johnson wrote a letter describing what Gruner and Royal Rife had discovered in May-June 1935: 'Dr. Gruner was present at all the experiments and we agreed - I think beyond a doubt - that our BX and the organism which he obtained from the blood, although in a different form from our BX, are one and the same organism. It looks, therefore, as if we know how to produce at will, by means of the appropriate culture, any one of the three forms desired'". (Rife had found a third and later a fourth form of the organism.)

Dr. Gruner's findings, then, would suggest that a simple blood test would indicate the presence of an organism capable of causing cancer if the blood's environment changes. The contemporary Gaston Naessens of Quebec has discovered another version of such a test (Chapter 8).

In November 1935, Dr. Johnson decided to set up a second Clinic using an advanced version of the Frequency Instrument with modifications suggested by Rife's new assistant, Philip Hoyland, an engineer introduced by Johnson. Johnson closed the Clinic in the spring of 1936 to wait for another improved version of the frequency device.

Earlier in the year, Rife had trained Dr. Walker, assistant to Dr. Meyer of the Hooper Foundation in San Francisco. Walker wrote in October: "The copy of the results of the test on typhoid organisms would appear to establish conclusively its efficacy to kill these organisms in the tissues. If the Ray should prove equally efficient in killing other pathogenic micro-organisms, it would be the greatest discovery in the history of therapeutic medicine." Meanwhile, Royal Rife built a newer, smaller microscope. With his "Universal" microscope, completed in 1933, having cost over $30,000, the new one was intended to be able to sell for around

$1,000, so that many more people could be involved in the research. With a magnification of 10,000 to 15,000 times, the new 'scope was still far better than any other light microscope.

In July 1936, Rife moved into a new lab, the lab of his dreams, built with funds supplied by Henry Timken.

In September 1936, Dr. James Couche opened a clinic, having acquired his own Ray Tube Frequency Instrument. Writing in 1956, Dr. Couche stated:

I saw some very remarkable things resulting from (the Frequency Instrument) in the course of over twenty years.

I had a Mexican boy, nine years of age, who had osteomyelitis of the leg. He was treated at the Mercy Hospital by his attending doctors. They scraped the bone every week. It was agonizing to the child because they never gave him anything; they just poked in there and cleaned him out and the terror of that boy was awful. He wore a splint and was on crutches. His family brought him to the office. He was terrified that I would poke him as the other doctors had done. I reassured him and demonstrated the instrument on my own hand to show him that it would not hurt. With the bandage and the splint still on he was given a treatment. In less than two weeks of treatment the wound was completely healed and he took off his splints and threw them away. He is a great big powerful man now and has never had any comeback of his osteomyelitis. He was completely cured. There were many cases such as this.

Among Dr. Couche's 1936 clinical cases was a Mrs. Tobish who was suffering from senile cataract. After six exposures to the frequencies for carcinoma and streptothrix, her vision returned to normal.

In September 1936, Dr. Johnson opened his third clinic, which he continued until May 1937. Johnson had sent Royal Rife, whose eyes were suffering from too many hours at the microscope, to Dr. Joseph Heitger, an eye specialist in Louisville, Kentucky. On June 1, 1937 Milbank Johnson wrote Dr. Heitger: "Our special effort this past winter has been working on cataracts...The application of the Rife Ray as we have used it does, in the great majority of cases, restore the visual function of the eye, that is the portion of visual disturbance due to opacities in the lens. How it does it and why it does it I do not know, but the above statement is an absolute fact supported now by many cases. How I wish we could get together and go over this work. I believe it will result in epochal changes in the profession's handling of cataract cases."

In 1937, Rife agreed to the formation of Beam Ray, a company set up to manufacture the frequency instruments. Ben Cullen, Rife's old friend since 1913, became president; Philip Hoyland, the engineer, and Dr. Couche were also involved. Barry Lynes reports that "Fourteen Frequency Instruments were built by Beam Ray. Two went to England, a third to Dr. Richard Hamer, and a fourth to Dr. Arthur Yale. Two more went to Arizona doctors and the remaining eight went to southern California doctors."

Ben Cullen later reminisced about Dr. Hamer's results in *Cancer Cure that Worked*:

> *Hamer ran an average of 40 cases a day through his place...Hamer was very well known on the Pacific coast... His case histories were absolutely wonderful. We would go in there and see rectal cancers... He cleaned them up completely... people... that had developed cancers, he'd find they had syphilis or gonorrhea. By golly he'd clean those up completely. Not a doggone taint of it in the blood stream at all. Clinically cured.*

In 1937 the Special Medical Research Committee came to a decision that in retrospect could not have been more unwise. Queried by Montreal doctors as to why the results of the 1934 Clinic had not been released, Dr. Johnson replied, "Our Committee has decided that the etiology of cancer must first be established before we publish anything concerning the possible treatment. We are therefore going to let the Rife Ray rest until this most important work is done."

To help establish the etiology (origin, how it develops), Dr. Johnson put a lot of effort into attempting to arrange for Dr. Gruner of McGill to return and spend a year working with Rife. Because he was internationally known for his research with blood, it was thought that his prestige, added to that of Kendall and Rosenow, would help win acceptance once an announcement was made. Johnson sought a grant to fund Gruner's year with Rife from the International Cancer Research Foundation in Philadelphia. However, the Foundation's staff was full of skepticism and pre-conditions, and no grant was ever made.

Recalling Dr. Johnson's statement in 1935 that he "intended to finance (the Rife work) through to the end", one might wonder why he did not finance Dr. Gruner's visit himself when it was clear there would be no grant. Barry Lynes' research discovered that between the famous 1931 dinner for Rife and Kendall and 1944, Dr. Johnson sold Belbank, moved to a smaller house, sold that, moved to a yet smaller house, and sold that, moving to an even smaller house. All of them, Lynes noted, were fine houses, but not as grand as Belbank. It is largely forgotten, Lynes points out, that there was a second stock market crash in 1937, not as severe as that of 1929, but enough to stall recovery from the Great Depression until the Second World War. It may be that Dr. Johnson suffered financial reverses, causing him to reduce his scale of living and making it difficult to carry through on his original plan to finance Rife's work "through to the end".

As Barry Lynes puts it, "funny how men often think they have forever". A power in the CMA (California Medical Association) by virtue of having been head of the Los Angeles Medical Association, it seemed unlikely that there might be anything in the CMA/AMA situation that Dr. Milbank Johnson could not handle.

But clouds were gathering that would upset Dr. Johnson's and Royal Rife's plans. Ben Cullen describes what happened, as quoted by Barry Lynes in *The Cancer Cure That Worked*:

Among Dr. Hamer's cases was this old man from Chicago. He had a malignancy all around his face and neck. It was a gory mass. Just terrible… It had taken over all around his face. It had taken off one eyelid at the bottom of the eye. It had taken off the bottom of the lower lobe of the ear and had also gone into the cheek area, nose, and chin. He was a sight to behold.

But in six months, all that was left was a little black spot on the side of his face and the condition of that was such that it was about to fall off. Now that man was 82 years of age. I never saw anything like it. The delight of having a lovely clean skin again, just like a baby's skin.

Well he went back to Chicago. Naturally, he couldn't keep still and Dr. Morris Fishbein heard about it. Fishbein called him in and the old man was kind of reticent about telling him. So Fishbein wined and dined him and finally learned about his cancer treatment by Dr. Hamer in the San Diego clinic.

Well soon a man from Los Angeles came down. He had several meetings with us. Finally he took us out to dinner and broached the subject about buying Beam Ray. Well we wouldn't do it. The renown was spreading and we weren't even advertising. But of course what did it was the case histories of Dr. Hamer. He said this was the most wonderful development of the age.

Unable to buy Beam Ray, another tactic was devised. Ben Cullen said that a partner in the company was bribed. Philip Hoyland had helped Rife with certain electronic improvements and apparently was the only one beside Rife who knew the frequencies, which were kept as a closely guarded secret. Deeming himself to be more valuable to the company than the others, he demanded more shares, which had been distributed equally among the partners. When he was refused, he cooked up a suit against Beam Ray claiming that he'd discovered the frequencies, apparently hoping to seize control of the company and then cut a deal with the Los Angeles man. Because the Los Angeles law firm he employed was more high-priced than his partners believed Hoyland could afford, they presumed it had been paid for by the Los Angeles man they assumed to be Fishbein's representative.

Hoyland's lawsuit went to trial on June 12, 1939 and Beam Ray won. In giving judgment in favor of the company, Judge Edward Kelly stated of Hoyland "I am not convinced of his blameless character...I am denying the plaintiff has clean hands". It is unlikely that in 1939 Beam Ray was rolling in money. They had built 14 instruments and their hope for fame and fortune was linked to eventual widespread approval and acceptance by the medical profession, the long range campaign Dr. Milbank Johnson was managing. How lucrative Beam Ray could have been can be judged by the rapidity with which hospitals everywhere installed expensive radiation equipment from the 1930's to the present day. By 1939, however, big money had not yet happened for Beam Ray. Ben Cullen had used his own money to set up the company, and by the end of the trial, he was broke.

The biggest problem was that the market had disappeared. During and after the trial, the San Diego Medical Society warned all the doctors who had been involved with the Rife Ray that if they continued using it, they could lose their licenses. Dr. Hamer returned his instrument, which was rented. Dr. Couche stuck it out, did not lose his license, and continued using his machine until the 1950's. With no market, Beam Ray disintegrated. Ben Cullen lost his house and had to take a job.

Before the trial, Rife was planning to leave for England in mid-May to take a microscope to Dr. B. Winter Gonin, who had ordered it and two Frequency Instruments. Gonin and his associates planned to distribute the microscope worldwide. One week before Rife's departure, he was subpoenaed for the Hoyland trial. Of the material available to us about Royal Rife, one gets the impression of a gentle genius, both a gentleman and a gentle man. Ben Cullen, who had known him from the inception of his ideas on cancer through their implementation, described him in 1958 in this way, "In my estimation, Roy was one of the most gentle, genteel, self-effacing, moral men I ever met. Not once in all those years I was going over there to the lab, and that was approximately 30 years, did I ever hear him say one word out of place". A religious man, an accomplished musician, obviously a superb researcher, Roy Rife's pictures show the face of a gentle and brilliant man but not that of a fighter. Not like one-time coal miner Harry Hoxsey, whose pictures show someone who could take it and dish it out, who almost relished a fight.

The main casualty of the trial was not Beam Ray but Royal Rife. Barry Lynes describes what happened at the trial, "Hoyland's lawyer tore into Rife in a way he had never before experienced. His nerves gave". Lynes quotes Ben Cullen, "Rife was called in to testify two or three times…Rife had never been in court and he just became a nervous idiot…in that he couldn't stand it and he did his best to keep calm, his hands shaking like a leaf. He had started smoking pretty heavily and inhaling which he didn't use to do before. Anyway, he took to drinking pretty heavily because the doctor couldn't find anything to stop his nervousness without forcing him into a drug addict."

The pressure had pushed Royal Rife into alcoholism. Ben Cullen recalled, "afterwards, during his clear moments when he wasn't under the influence of liquor, he would endeavor to progress but every doggone day at a certain time he would go and get a little nip out of his car and that was the end of it".

Ben Cullen's statement is the only known evidence linking Dr. Morris Fishbein and the disaster that befell Beam Ray and the Rife technology. Some sources say that Fishbein knew about Royal Rife all the time from Dr Kendall, a thoroughly establishment man there in Chicago. While Fishbein may have heard vaguely about Rife's microscope from Dr. Kendall, it would appear that it was the case of the cured 82-year-old which caused him to focus on Rife's technology. Did Fishbein precipitate the attempt to buy out Beam Ray and then, when that failed, Hoyland's lawsuit? The most important question, however, is who caused the San Diego Medical Society suddenly to come down hard on the Rife doctors, whose work could hardly have been unknown to them. Dr. Fishbein had already been warning in the JAMA against electronic medicine in the 1930's. Did the San Diego Medical Society finally, in 1939, get around to following Fishbein's advice - or were they pushed? With Dr. Milbank Johnson's clear delight in the Rife technology and all he had done to encourage it, he must have been horrified at what happened. Given his changes of residences and the indication that his financial situation may have changed, it may be that he was no longer in a position to exert as much influence as before, and to stave off the disaster. We will probably never know the answers to these questions.

Dr. Johnson conducted no further clinics and in 1942 sent his Frequency Instrument to Dr. Gruner in Montreal, hoping the latter would make use of it to provide corroboration of Rife's great work. However, Gruner at McGill, in an atmosphere of academic orthodoxy, feared to use the device and gave it to a friend who dismantled it for spare parts. It may well have been Johnson's hope to seize a later opportunity to restore the momentum behind Rife's research, and to announce the results of the 1934 and subsequent Clinics. If he had survived until after Harry Hoxsey so thoroughly embarrassed Morris Fishbein that the AMA removed him in 1948, Johnson might have found a way to reverse suppression of the Rife technology.

But he did not survive until then. In 1944, Dr. Milbank Johnson entered the hospital for a routine tonsillectomy and did not come out. He was 73 by then and it may have been that his death was from natural causes, precipitated by the stress of the operation.

That ended the first chapter in Rife's work, during which he achieved his greatest breakthroughs, worked with some of the top medical figures of his day, and nearly saw his technology accepted as standard for the medical profession, Milbank Johnson's goal. This was the period during which, Rife told the San Diego *Evening Tribune* in an article printed May 6, 1938, "the mortal oscillatory rates for many organisms have been found and record- ed. The Ray can be tuned to a germ's recorded frequency and turned upon that organism with the assurance that the organism will be killed".

Little is known of Royal Rife during the World War II years. There was a period from 1946 until 1950 when he virtually dis- appeared, apparently part of it being an attempt to "dry out" from the alcoholism.

In 1949, Dr. James Couche made a trip to Montreal to visit Dr. Gruner. Upon his return, he gave an interview to the *San Diego Union* which appeared in its edition of July 31, 1949:

> *Gruner told Dr. Couche that he was satisfied that Dr. Rife's large microscope had revealed a virus. He said fur- ther that the work he did with Rife at his Point Loma lab- oratory and follow-up researches at McGill University, had confirmed that tumor growths positively could be pro- duced by the virus discovered in San Diego.*

> *In San Diego yesterday...Dr. Rife said... 'I discovered that the virus organism gets in the blood of the victim at one stage of the growth.'*

> *Dr. Couche said...that if cancer is a blood disease it is carried to all parts of the body in the blood stream and surgery would be of little use...It will surely be a great honor for that patient San Diego investigator, Dr. Rife, if his virus turns out to be the entity chiefly responsible for causing this dread disease.*

Rife's comment combined with Dr. Couche's statement would be of significance to those who have undergone surgery to remove tumors only to have cancer materialize somewhere else.

In 1950 Rife advertised for a tool and die maker and John Crane answered the ad. Crane had the needed skills, some knowledge of electronics, and was a good machinist, so Rife hired him. Fascinated by Rife's story, Crane urged him to build more Frequency Instruments. In addition to helping him with these, Crane urged him to write, and several of Rife's few writings are from this period.

In 1954, Crane contacted the National Cancer Institute (NCI) concerning the Rife therapeutic instruments. Barry Lynes writes, "The Committee on Cancer Diagnosis and Therapy of the National Research Council 'evaluated' the Rife discovery. They concluded it couldn't work. No effort was made to contact Rife, Gruner, Couche, or others who had witnessed actual cures (Couche was still curing cancer patients at that time). No physical inspection of the instruments was attempted. Electronic healing was thus bureaucratically determined to be impossible. (In 1972, NCI Director Dr. Carl G. Baker used the superficial 1954 evaluation to dismiss Rife's work when asked for information by Congressman Bob Wilson of San Diego."

In November 1956, Rife was the featured speaker at a meeting of the San Diego section of the Instrument Society of America. The flyer states that "on display for their first public showing will be one of the new 'Frequency Instruments' and a 17,000 power optical microscope developed by Dr. Rife". Rife's speech was on "Optics in Industry and Medicine", and he was identified as Director of Research of Life Labs, which John Crane had organized.

Crane engaged a John Marsh as a sort of traveling salesman for the instruments he and Rife were building. One day in 1957 while visiting his parents in Dayton, Ohio, Marsh came down with a bad sore throat and sought out Dr. Robert Stafford, the family doctor. Having known John since infancy, Dr. Stafford asked him what he was doing. "I'm doing something that will put you out of business", John replied. "Well, then I want to hear all about it", the genial Stafford replied. Marsh told him about the Rife Frequency Instrument, adding "If you ever have a terminal cancer patient, let me know and I'll bring you a machine".

A few years ago, a friend in Ohio told me that there was a

doctor in Dayton who had worked with a Rife device for five years. With the encouragement of former Congressman Berkley Bedell for whom I was doing some research at the time, I was soon on my way to Dayton. There's nothing like talking with someone who's been there to drive home the reality of what we lost with the disappearance of the Rife technology, I realized after talking to Dr. Stafford.

Over lunch at the Country Club where he had invited my friend and me, Stafford told us the above story and about his experiences with the Rife device. Perhaps six months after his conversation with John Marsh, one of his patients, Mrs. Byess, age 82, was nearing death from cancer, so he called Marsh. In 1957, Rife and Crane had finished a new generation device but there were few takers and they were anxious to find reputable doctors who would work with them. Marsh told Stafford "I'll drive across the country and bring you a machine". He arrived at night, Dr. Stafford recalled, too late to go to the hospital. They talked and Marsh told him about the background and accomplishments of the wonderful Rife Ray Tube Frequency Instrument. "From what you tell me, John", said Dr. Stafford, "this machine of yours will do virtually anything. Well, here's a test case for you. Here's our old dog Skip. We have to lift him up onto the couch and lift him into the car. But we can't put him to sleep; he's one of the family. Do you think your machine will do anything for Skip?" They gave Skip three treatments in all, one every three days, Dr. Stafford reminisced. After that, Skip could jump onto the couch and jump into the car, and lived another five years. "If anybody had told me that story", Stafford laughed, "I'd never have believed it. I'd have said 'hogwash!' But I saw it happen to my dog." Later, he said, his nurse's dog had a cancerous tumor which disappeared after Ray Tube treatments.

The day after Skip's first treatment, Stafford and Marsh took the Ray Tube to the hospital to treat Mrs. Byess. Delivery of the frequencies from the early 1930's had always been done through a large bulb, or tube, filled with helium or argon gas. Following instructions sent by Crane, they rigged up an apparatus to pass the bulb slowly up and down the length of Mrs. Byess' body, sus-pended about two feet above. Treatment was every other day for 3-5 minutes. At that point, her life expectancy would have been about 2-3 weeks; she was bleeding extensively and was clearly nearing the end.

Over the course of the next two weeks, to Dr. Stafford's amazement, Mrs. Byess began to recover. The bleeding stopped, she began to feel better enough to complain about the food, got out of bed, walked around, and began to make plans to go home. Despite her remarkable recovery, that didn't happen. Hearing that a friend was on the next floor, she climbed a flight of stairs, missed a step, fell and broke her hip, and was dead in a week. Dr. Stafford secured her husband's permission for an autopsy, which was done by Dr. Zipp, the Dayton coroner. The results; no cancer. The lady in the next bed was also dying of cancer; seeing Mrs. Byess' recovery, she asked if she too might be treated. Dr. Stafford pointed out that she was not his patient but if it was okay with her doctor, it was okay with him.

Dr. Robert Stafford was, and still is, one of the most respect-ed doctors in Dayton. At that time (1958) Chief of Staff of Good Samaritan Hospital and former head of the county medical soci-ety, Stafford was solidly mainstream and anything but far-out. The other doctor quickly gave his permission and treatment began of the second patient. To everyone's amazement, she too quickly recovered in about two weeks and actually went home, but died about a month later. Dr. Stafford again secured permis-sion for an autopsy, also performed by Dr. Zipp. He again report-ed no sign of cancer and that the woman had died of complica-tions caused by radiation treatments.

These results made him a believer, Dr. Stafford told us during our luncheon. Leaving the machine with him, John Marsh drove back to San Diego, and Stafford saw several more dramatic results. One involved his 4-year-old son, who "threw one of those fevers that kids will do, right in the middle of the night before Mrs. Stafford and I were to leave for a convention. I was prepar-ing to cancel our trip but my sister, who had come to take care of the boy, said 'why don't you try the blue light?' That was how we referred to the device, since the Ray Tube glowed blue. She sat beside the glowing bulb with the boy in her lap for an hour. After a half hour, he quieted down and in an hour the fever was gone and he was fine." Another time, Dr. Stafford told us, he had been out shoveling ice and snow on a cold drizzly day. "I should have known better", he said, "since that whole week I'd been tending patients with the flu. Suddenly I began to start feeling sick and getting sicker by the minute. I can't go to the office, I thought, but I must; I'm on duty and my partners have the day off. Well, I con sidered, why not try the blue light, which we usually kept at the house at that time. So I sat in front of it, began to feel better, and after about 45 minutes I was no longer coming down with the flu and went to the office as planned."

Engaging Dr. Zipp's cooperation, the two carried out a series of tests with mice, implanting tumors, treating the mice with the Ray Tube, and seeing tumors disappear.

Dr. Stafford told us another story that is remarkable and puzzling. "You know how Dayton winters are cold and clammy. I was always cold in winter and regularly wore long underwear to keep warm. But after I'd used the blue light for a few months, I was never cold again!" We all agreed that if that device were still available it would sell well up north, even as we wondered what could be the mechanism which would produce such a fortuitous result.

He had use of the machine for five years, Dr. Stafford told us. During that time, the California health authorities cracked down on John Crane and John Marsh for practicing medicine without a license, and both spent three years in jail. Upon his release, Marsh called Stafford and asked for his machine back. "It's yours", Dr. Stafford told him, "so John came and got it and that was the end of my experience with the Rife Frequency Instrument". During the time it was with him, a few of his colleagues gently questioned his use of it but nobody ever made any trouble.

Crane's and Marsh's problems started when authorities sent an undercover agent to buy a machine one day in 1960 after

Crane unknowingly had been taped making medical claims for the instrument. As Crane took a check in payment, he was arrested, the check was snatched back from him, and his machines were seized.

Crane and Marsh brought witnesses to the trial who attested to having been cured by the machines. One case was especially interesting, indicating that the 1950's instruments had the same ability to dissolve cataracts as their 1930's predecessors. As Barry Lynes reports it, "During the trial, James Hannibal, age 76, testified. Blind in one eye, he'd been treated by the Frequency Instrument. After several applications, his cataract disappeared, just as cataracts had disappeared in many of Dr. Milbank Johnson's patients during his 1935-37 clinics."

Royal Rife prepared a deposition in behalf of John Crane, which was not accepted at the trial. Other witnesses at Crane's trial, Barry Lynes reports: "testified to the curing of chronic bladder irritation and the elimination of a throat lump one-half the size of an egg. Also cured were fungus growths on hands, fissures in the anus, pyorrhea, arthritis, ulcerated colon, varicose veins, prostate troubles, tumorous growths over eyes, colitis, pains in the back, and heart attacks. One man testified that for 17 years he had a growth the size of an egg on his spine. After treatment, it had disappeared." It was all to no avail. Crane and Marsh were convicted and sent to jail.

Concerned about being subpoenaed again, Royal Rife spent the time of the trial and a few months more in Tijuana, Mexico, returning in poor health. Around the time of these troubles, someone broke into Rife's lab, set a fire, and destroyed much of his equipment. The concrete building did not burn but gone were the irreplaceable movies Rife had made of various viruses and of their destruction by his Ray.

Until his imprisonment, John Crane was a bold and enterprising man, but upon his release from prison, he was no longer the same. The lab was destroyed, Rife was failing, and Crane was understandably bitter. The second, but lesser, Rife chapter was over.

As a footnote to the story, Dr. Arthur Kendall, who'd played such an important part in the 1930's, retired in 1942; he too was cut out to be a researcher, not a fighter. After buying a ranch in Mexico, he lost it and was living with his son-in-law in La Jolla in 1958, according to Ben Cullen. Barry Lynes reports that he died in 1959 - close to the Scripps Ranch where he had observed the 1934 Clinic, and close to Royal Rife. One wonders if they got together to talk about better times, but there is no record that they ever met again.

Rife's wife Mamie was still alive in 1955 but died before he did. In 1971, Rife quietly passed away, an ill old man, at the age of 82.

John Crane deserves credit for having salvaged many of Rife's files from total oblivion, and for getting Rife to put on paper a record of his achievements. Chris Bird did his usual superb job when he reopened the story. But Barry Lynes deserves even more credit for having tracked down the fading pieces of an almost forgotten story before nearly everyone connected with it had passed away. I have relied heavily on his *The Cancer Cure That Worked* and his helpful advice in the preparation of this chapter.

Where did the Rife microscopes and Frequency Instruments go? Probably some are in the hands of the FDA. A few original ones are in private hands, but are not in commercial use, *i.e.*, in treatment for pay. As for the microscopes, shortly after the 1944 Franklin Institute article by Seidel and Winter appeared, a lab technician stole a vital part from the Universal microscope, rending it inoperable. It still exists and has been partially restored. One microscope, apparently the one bought by Dr. Gonin in England, was in the Wellcome Museum in London, but it is said that parts have been removed from that as well. In other words, there is no place where serious researchers can go and view living organisms (which, as noted, cannot be seen under an electron microscope) and test the effects on them of a Rife frequency Instrument. This capability has not existed since the destruction of the Rife lab.

Could we recreate the Rife technology if there were a focused effort to do so? Steve Ross, Director of the World Research Foundation and very knowledgeable about Rife, states that to his certain knowledge the Ergonom microscope in Germany, invented by Kurt Olbrich, can see viruses in their live state. As for the frequency devices, BK frequency generators are readily available and it is likely that the beam tube through which Rife broadcast his Ray could be reproduced. So it is possible that with an Ergonom microscope, a frequency generator, and a beam tube, the bacteriological research opened by Rife with Kendall, Rosenow, and Gruner could be restarted and move forward again. Since Rife's time numerous researchers, such as those mentioned earlier whose work was published by the New York Academy of Sciences and more recently Dr. Alan Cantwell, have found microorganisms which they have observed to be capable of causing cancer. Thus obtaining a BX microbe or its equivalent should not be difficult. There remains the matter of the frequencies. Lists of them are around, but are they really the ones Rife found? Conceivably, with contemporary computerization and automatic focusing capabilities, it might be possible to test various frequencies without the need to spend 24 or 48 hours at the microscope, as Rife did.

It would be a lot of work, but the conceivable results would justify the investment. In addition to its potential for impacting the cancer epidemic, the Rife Beam Ray would probably put an end to the growing epidemic of tuberculosis. It would have been a lot simpler if our society had taken advantage of the discoveries of the genius Royal Raymond Rife when we still had him around.

At the moment, the Rife technology is as lost as Atlantis, but could it be found again?

Barry Lynes' book contains a letter written in 1953 by a naval officer who had commanded a unit of doctors and bacteriologists, who had known Rife for many years. It is, as Lynes suggests, "a fitting epitaph to the Rife tragedy":

I have been privileged in having known you and having heard from your own lips the story of your work. You gave me a glimpse of science of the year 2000. But often I'm a little sad when I realize that men must struggle so hard to get what you tried to give them, and I am even more sad when I see so many problems for which you alone have the answers. When I see pictures taken with the electron microscope, I have to laugh, because I remember better pictures showing more detail which were hung in the hallway of your laboratory. When I read 'research' reports on genetics, evolution, or any of the fields of microbiology I have to laugh, because years ago the scientists were offered the answer and they refused the gift! The combination of your mind, your will, and your energy is so rare as to skip entire generations. The world has great need for your work.

Perhaps the world will someday rediscover one of the greatest gifts on which it has ever turned its back. Someday we may develop equipment similar to the Rife Ray machine. By then the AMA will be forced to accept its use for the elimination of disease organisms. Man will live a healthier, happier and longer life.

If we reach that millenium in my life, I will have one unhappy memory - that the man most deserving to have his name linked for all time with human happiness will have been all but forgotten because his life's work was lost in a struggle with the AMA and the 'accepted' scientists of his day rather than made available through a new approach; and because when it is rediscovered, it will be given a new name.

The millennium has come, but science of the Year 2000 has still not caught up with Royal Rife. Something lost. Something wonderful.

L'Affaire Krebiozen

Only something of major importance - like civil rights or Vietnam -will bring people out to demonstrate in Washington. On June 5 and 6, 1963, in President John F. Kennedy's last year of life, hundreds of cancer patients and their relatives picketed the White House. Because of new FDA regulations about to go into effect on June 7, they were fearful that they would lose access to Krebiozen, an experimental, non-toxic cancer drug which, they were convinced, was keeping them alive. President Kennedy complained after the disaster at the Bay of Pigs in Cuba, "Why did I listen to the experts?" Apparently he was still listening to them, for he did not intervene, and eventually patients did lose Krebiozen, and they died. In 1964, the FDA indicted its discoverer, Yugoslav Dr. Stefan Durovic, and Dr. Andrew Ivy, one of the most respected scientists in America, who had organized research on the drug.

In 2000, Koch, Hoxsey, and Rife have all been forgotten and Krebiozen too; like the others, it does not deserve to be. After all, how many things will induce people to picket the White House? L'Affaire Krebiozen, we could call it, like l'Affaire Dreyfus which convulsed late 19th century France. In that case, the famous writer Emile Zola set the record straight in his book, *J'Accuse* (I Accuse). Before it was over, l'Affaire Krebiozen resulted in nine months of hearings by a special committee of the Illinois Legislature, and nine months of trial by the FDA ten years later.

What was Krebiozen? And who was Dr. Andrew Ivy? One won't find much in medical libraries, and what is there is written in a condescending tone, "Dr. Ivy, such a fine man, but he was 'taken in' by Krebiozen". Not one word about clinical results;

after all, the drug had been pronounced "worthless" by the American Medical Association. But who would picket the White House for something worthless? Then, in one tiny footnote, there is a passing reference to Dr. Ivy's Zola, Chicago medical journalist Herbert Bailey. Bailey wrote *K-Krebiozen - Key to Cancer?* (1953) and *A Matter of Life and Death - The Incredible Story of Krebiozen* (1958). All quotations are from the latter book unless otherwise noted.

In 1949, Dr. Andrew Ivy, MD and PhD, was 56, Vice President of the University of Illinois in charge of its medical colleges, well known, highly respected, and at the peak of his career. He had taught more than 5,000 students. He discovered several of the body's hormones. He co-authored a text on peptic ulcers. A bold innovator, he started some of the first experiments in space medicine and held the world's first symposium on medical problems that might be encountered when humans started reaching for the stars. It was under his sponsorship that BCG, the tuberculosis vaccine, was made available in the U.S. on a mass scale. During World War II, he was chosen to organize the Naval Medical Research Center in Bethesda, Maryland, serving as its first director. After the war, Dr. Morris Fishbein of the AMA nominated Dr. Ivy to be consultant on medical ethics at the Nuremberg Trials, and served on a committee to advise Ivy.

The Code of Medical Ethics, prepared by Ivy and adopted at Nuremberg, stated that a patient "should be so situated as to be able to exercise free power of choice, without the intervention of any element of force, fraud, deceit, duress, over-reaching or other ulterior form of constraint or coercion". The United States is a signatory to the Nuremberg Code.

Having done extensive research and writing on cancer, Ivy served from 1947 to 1951 as Executive Director of the National Advisory Cancer Council, which advised the U.S. Public Health Service on where to spend money for cancer research. He was also a director of the American Cancer Society. He repeatedly urged the creation of a series of treatment centers where non-toxic therapies could be tried on terminal cancer patients.

As Vice President of the University of Illinois, Dr. Ivy was a legendary fund-raiser. During his seven years in that post, he increased funds for medical research from $85,000 to almost $1,000,000 annually, increased the scientific budget from $2,000,000 to almost $11,000,000 per year, raised $25,000,000 for a huge expansion in the colleges of medicine, dentistry, pharmacy, and nursing, and helped obtain $15,000,000 for clinical facilities. It was Ivy who went to the Legislature to obtain around $90,000,000 every two years. The legislators liked him and usually gave him what he requested.

To give a sense of Dr. Andrew Ivy's renown, *Science Citation Digest* shows that during the period 1964-1971 Dr. Ivy's articles, (1500 over 35 years, or an average of 40 per year or nearly one a week) were cited more than those of any other scientist in the world in his fields of physiology and gastroenterology.

In 1947, Dr. Ivy published a paper in *Science* magazine proposing that there must be some substance in the human body which normally protects it against cancer and which routinely destroys cancer cells. He was right, of course, and Dr. William F. Koch had already discovered one such factor, the carbonyls. The tragedy was that Dr. Koch was never again published in medical journals after his *New York Medical World* article in 1920. Dr. Ivy would probably not have heard about Dr. Koch except in JAMA editorials blasting Koch as a quack, and Hoxsey as well. An article in the *Bulletin of the History of Medicine*, 1984, by the late Patricia Ward Spain, states that in the early 1950's Dr. Ivy "helped to expose the cancer quackery of Harry Hoxsey".

Could there be anyone more qualified than this highly respected member of the scientific establishment to shepherd a cancer breakthrough into acceptance by mainstream American medicine? Could someone so much at the heart of the medical world have a falling out with the AMA? The story of how that happened is so full of intrigue, politics, and drama that it is meat for another movie; Anthony Hopkins would make a wonderful Dr. Ivy.

In Buenos Aires, Dr. Stefan Durovic read Dr. Ivy's article on cancer with interest since he was pursuing the same hypothesis. Born of a Serbian family in Yugoslavia, Durovic was already respected as a dedicated scientist in the 1930's. Early in World War II, Dr. Durovic and his brother Marko, a wealthy industrialist, escaped to Rome and from there to Argentina. Resuming his research and focusing on cancer, Dr. Stefan remembered how horses on their family estate outside of Belgrade would sometimes develop tumors on the neck called "lumpy jaw disease"; either they would become very sick and die, or they would recover and the growth would be gone in two weeks. The cause of the disease was a fungus called actinomyces bovis, and Durovic had worked with fungi at the Pasteur Institute in Paris in the 1930's. Durovic reasoned that the horses which recovered must contain some resistance factor in larger quantities than the ones which didn't. He then inoculated horses with the fungus and developed a process for extracting a substance - only about one milligram per horse - which he hoped was what he was looking for.

Durovic arranged for a colleague to test the material in stray dogs. Then, in 1949, interested in testing another medicine in the U.S., he left for Chicago with an introduction from Buenos Aires businessman Humberto Loretani to businessmen Edward Moore and Kenneth Brainard. They in turn introduced him to a doctor whose tests with his product were not successful.

While in Chicago, Durovic received news from Buenos Aires of favorable results with his compound extracted from horses in 10 cancerous dogs, most so old they had cataracts. Not only had tumors been reversed in 6 of the 10, but their cataracts had disappeared as well. Durovic mentioned his second product to Moore and Brainard and showed them the article by Dr. Ivy which he'd read in Argentina. They quickly arranged to take him to the famous doctor.

In those days, testing experimental drugs was relatively simple. All that was needed was to demonstrate that the drug was non-toxic and then to keep the FDA informed of the results. After satisfying himself that Durovic's substance was non-toxic, Dr. Ivy arranged to give it to several hopelessly terminal cancer patients.

Drs. Ivy and Durovic soon had reason to take the drug seriously. A patient with advanced carcinoma of the vagina was treated September 28, 1950. Pain was gone within hours. Three days later, the cancerous mass was half gone and a second injection was given. By October 9, the mass had completely vanished. In writing of this case, Herbert Bailey reported that on January 15, 1952, a biopsy was taken from the place where the tumor had been and no cancer cells were found. In June 1957, the patient was still well with no sign of cancer.

After several similar results, Ivy and Durovic gave the substance the name Krebiozen, from the Greek meaning that which regulates growth.

Another of their earliest cases was the wife of Dr. John Pick, a famous plastic surgeon and a faculty member at the University of Illinois. Mrs. Pick was expected to die within a week at the most and lay in a coma in the final stages of metastasized breast cancer. She had not eaten in two weeks. She was given an injection of one microgram of Krebiozen at 11 PM. To her husband's amazement, she awoke at 2 AM, very hungry. She ate the lobster he brought her, fell into a deep sleep, and awoke again at 8 AM wanting breakfast. After bacon and eggs, she announced that she was feeling fine and intended to go to the office - and did a week later! She then received Krebiozen every three weeks but evidently it was not enough, for a few weeks later, she suffered a relapse. After a double dose of the drug, she rallied, became her normal self for another two weeks, but then collapsed and died.

Dr. Pick had begged Dr. Durovic to give his wife more injections, but at that time, nobody had a clear idea about proper doses or frequency of injections. Dr. Durovic recalled how, in the cancerous dogs in Buenos Aires, too high a dose would kill off cancer cells too fast, overpower the liver's capacity to process them, and kill the dog as surely as the unchecked cancer. So they lost Mrs. Pick, but she was never in pain again after the first dose. Dr. Ivy wrote, "In retrospect, patient should have received larger doses".

After seeing the last minute results with his wife, Dr. Pick decided to try Krebiozen on other hopeless cases. The first one was a Catholic nun with an extensive brain tumor who had been in terrible pain, had lapsed into a coma, and whose death was expected momentarily. Within 24 hours of the first injection, she regained consciousness and started eating; when Dr. Pick saw her two days later, she was consuming half a chicken. Since her internal organs were too seriously damaged for her to be able to survive, she died a few days later - but with no pain.

With these early cases, Drs. Ivy and Durovic could see that Krebiozen clearly had a biological effect on cancer - but was it a cure? Dr. Ivy knew that in scientific circles one did not talk about a cure until a patient had survived at least five years.

When Dr. Durovic arrived in the U.S. speaking English poorly, Messrs. Moore and Brainard had been a great help, taking him to meet Dr. Ivy and assisting in many ways. In February 1950, Dr. Durovic's brother, Marko, came to Chicago. By then, surprising results had been observed with Krebiozen. Marko spoke English fluently and as soon as he arrived, Moore and Brainard presented their bill for the help they'd given his brother; they wanted distribution rights for Krebiozen. Marko refused since any deal the Durovics might make would need to be with a pharmaceutical company, and Moore and Brainard had no experience in that field. Both Durovics recognized the help Moore and Brainard had provided and offered them a royalty or a partnership in Marko's company, Druga, if they would share in costs of the development of the drug. They refused both, insisting on full distribution rights. A few days later, they asked for a power of attorney, which Marko refused to give. Soon, Dr. Ivy later testified, Moore and Brainard asked him to put pressure on the Durovics to give them distribution rights. Dr. Ivy protested that his role was science, not business, but agreed to try to settle the differences. Feeling that they had an obligation to Moore and Brainard but not that much, the Durovics agreed to Ivy's suggestion to accept the findings of an impartial arbitration board to determine how much they should pay. At first Moore and Brainard accepted, but then refused.

By late 1950, the Durovics' visitors' visas were expiring and they were being pressured to leave the country by May 10, 1951. Senator Paul Douglas, a friend of Ivy, agreed to introduce a bill to give them permanent residence, but felt there would need to be some sort of announcement, if only to doctors.

From 1949 to early 1951, Dr. Ivy had tried Krebiozen in 22 patients. He'd seen beneficial results in 70% of the cases and believed it was time to ask other clinics to join in the research. He had planned to have a small meeting for cancer specialists in June 1951, but because of the problem of the Durovics, he decided to call a group together at the Drake Hotel in Chicago on March 26. Ivy had been getting pressure from various newspapers to give them a story. Word was getting around about several near miraculous recoveries, including someone who worked for one of the major papers. As a researcher, the last thing he wanted was headlines. Among his guests, he invited four medical journalists he trusted not to sensationalize the cautious announcement he would make; one of them was Herbert Bailey.

Explaining that he had been engaged in research with a new experimental drug, Dr. Ivy sent the following invitation to 80 cancer specialists, doctors, and laymen who had been following the research:

> *Up to January 1, 1951, 22 patients have been observed long enough for us to believe that a preliminary report of our observations to a limited group of physicians and lay people who have been connected in some way with our study or who are particularly interested in cancer, is appropriate and warranted. It is my opinion that the substance deserves a thorough clinical study and evaluation, since I believe it shows much promise in the management of the cancer patient. You are cordially invited to attend. (signed) A. C. Ivy*

That was all, not the slightest mention of "cure". Unbeknownst to Ivy, someone who had just lost a relative to cancer without the benefit of Krebiozen, but who was aware of its benefits, sent out a separate press release which stated:

> *The battle of medical science to find a cure for cancer
> achieved its realization today according to the documen-
> tary report... of the discovery of Dr. Stefan Durovic... of a
> substance which has produced successful results follow-
> ing experiments on patients conducted in Chicago for the
> past 18 months. A number of patients who have been
> cured of this disease were present...at a meeting...in the
> Drake Hotel... Krebiozen is no longer a dream. Cancer
> need no longer signify certain and inevitable death,
> according to the clinical report... This dread disease has
> been genetically explained today and its successful cure
> has been realized.*

Dr. Ivy had always conducted his affairs with the restrained
decorum of a scientist and when he entered the crowded meeting
room at the Drake to popping flashbulbs, he wondered if he was
at the right place. Then Dr. Pick showed him the other, unautho-
rized press release and Dr. Ivy almost cancelled the meeting.
After consultation with close advisors, he decided that the cat was
out of the bag and that the press would likely sensationalize
things more if he did cancel, so he decided to go ahead.

Explaining that it was far too early to talk of cures, and that
the purpose of the meeting was to attract more researchers, he
managed to defang most of the sensationalism. But to an extent
far worse than anyone realized at the time, the damage was done,
for Dr. Ivy had enemies, and enemies with an agenda he could not
have imagined. Publicity-seeking is anathema in scientific circles. While Ivy had not sent out the second press release, it stirred
up a lot of noise. This gave his enemies an opening to attack, suggesting that "Ivy is cracking up", and "Ivy's a good man, but he's
been taken in by this Krebiozen".

While the newspapers did not use the word "cure" at Dr. Ivy's
request, they did indicate that a serious new cancer treatment was
at hand. The result was that 1500 calls a week poured into the
bewildered University of Illlinois. The people whom Dr. Ivy had

not invited began to take on significance, because they were miffed at not having been previously informed. These included Dr. George Stoddard, the president of the University of Illinois, Dr. Stanley Olson, Dean of the College of Medicine, Dr. Warren Cole, head of Surgery, and Dr. Danely Slaughter, head of the Illinois Tumor Clinic, who was under Dr. Cole.

The excess of publicity scared off most of the big cancer clinics, whose participation Dr. Ivy had hoped to secure until the paparazzi of his time descended on his meeting. Two hundred physicians, however, did agree to do research with Krebiozen as well as two small but respected cancer clinics. Senator Paul Douglas introduced a bill to provide permanent resident status for the Durovics, so the Immigration people quieted down.

On March 31, 1951, Dr. Ivy received a call to come to Grand Rapids, Michigan, on a mission of mercy. Senator Arthur Vandenberg of Michigan, widely regarded as a great statesman, was dying of cancer. A Republican during a period of Republican control of the Senate and at the time of Senator Joseph McCarthy, Vandenberg, as Chair of the Senate Foreign Relations Committee, had pronounced that politics stopped at the water's edge. He had cooperated with the Truman Administration in establishing a bipartisan foreign policy which endured throughout most of the Cold War. Mostly forgotten now, much of the credit for taking petty politics out of that policy was due to Senator Vandenberg. When Drs. Ivy and Durovic arrived, the Senator's doctor doubted he would last the night, since cancer had invaded almost every part of his body. Mentioning that they had seen some favorable results with patients "in extremis", Dr. Ivy said "If Dr. Durovic is willing, I think we should try. If I were in the Senator's condition, I would want someone to give me some Krebiozen". The shot was given, and not only did the Senator survive the night, he lived another 18 days. His doctors' reports follow:

The day following the injection, the Senator became noticeably more alert and definitely manifested an appearance of well-being. There was also a noticeable reduction in his narcotics requirements that day... We were privileged during these eighteen days to witness a most amazing cyclic response which we can only attribute to the administration of Krebiozen. There were days of profound toxicity and prostration... Alternating with these periods, when he at times seemed in extremis, there were days of uncanny revival during which he would read the papers, listen to the radio, watch television, smoke his beloved cigars, and converse freely and intelligently, and manifest good humor and a feeling of well-being. We were compelled to regard with awe what was transpiring before our eyes... Whether or not the Senator's life could have been saved had Krebiozen been administered at an earlier stage is, of course, a matter of conjecture. The fact is that from the third day following the first injection until his death he was miraculously relieved of practically all pain... and that narcotics... were... abolished is a matter of record. To see a man suffering unbounded pain only partially dulled by maximum doses of morphine abruptly become completely and permanently relieved in the presence of widespread devastating malignancy has been one of the most dramatic therapeutic achievements it has been my privilege to observe.

In 1951, Dr. Josiah J. Moore had been Treasurer of the AMA for ten years. He became a major player in the organization in the power vacuum left after the departure in 1948 of Dr. Morris Fishbein. Shortly after Dr. Ivy's March 26 meeting, Dr. Moore convinced the AMA to appoint a committee to investigate Krebiozen with himself in charge. As the first piece of business, he took Dr. Paul Wermer, secretary of the AMA Committee on Research, and Oliver Field, chief of the AMA Bureau of Investigation, to visit the brothers Durovic. After discussing Krebiozen, Dr. Moore brought up Ed Moore and Ken Brainard and asked, "Don't you think you have an obligation to Moore and Brainard for the distribution rights to Krebiozen?" The Durovics were surprised to learn that Dr. Moore knew Moore and Brainard, but replied in the negative. Then Dr. Moore stated, "You must give the distribution rights to Moore and Brainard!" (This came out in sworn testimony a year later.) Marko Durovic, a lawyer, then said, "Stop. We will discuss the scientific aspects of Krebiozen but the business aspects are no concern of the American Medical Association". After a moment, Dr. Moore commented that Marko was a sharp businessman and then he and his committee left.

In April 1951, the Durovics received offers from two large pharmaceutical companies, Abbott and Lilly, for the right to market Krebiozen. One of the offers was for $100,000 cash plus $1,000,000 in cash upon government approval, plus 5% royalties. In addition, the company offered to purchase the entire stock of Krebiozen at cost ($7.26 per ampule, and there were 200,000 ampules). Further, the Durovics would retain basic rights to Krebiozen and any improvements. However, Dr. Durovic wanted scientific tests done first to determine whether Krebiozen was a permanent or only a temporary help for cancer. In addition, he wanted a maximum price set on the drug. Neither company was willing to do that, so he refused both offers.

Later in the spring of 1951 Dr. Ivy was called before the Cancer Committee of the Chicago Medical Society to explain the March 26 meeting, satisfying them that he had not been responsible for the publicity. He noted that Dr. Josiah Moore, a member of the committee, took a leading role and asked a lot of questions.

Stories like that of Gary Cathcart convinced Drs. Ivy and Durovic that they were on the right track. On June 25, 1951, 12-year-old Gary took his first shot of Krebiozen. He had been brought home to die in a few days or weeks of what his pathologist called the worst type of fast-growing cancer. Herbert Bailey tells the story:

Dr. Pick administered the regular adult dose - one-thousandth of a milligram. Three days later, the head of the tumor had shrunk to one-half its original size.

Unbelievable, implausible... but there the proof was. It was decided to... (give) another shot... double strength. Gary went into almost immediate shock and Dr. Pick spent a worried, sleepless night treating for shock symptoms. Gary rallied, however, and two weeks later no examining doctor - and there were five - could feel the slightest remnant of the once terrible tumor. It had completely dissolved. For the next six weeks, the boy had a huge appetite and then the tumor came back; by August 14, it was back to half its original size. Krebiozen was resumed and the growth halted, but now it took larger doses to cause the same tumor disappearance as before. A year later, however, the tumor could no longer be felt.

In June 1951, Sr. Humberto Loretani, who had introduced Dr. Durovic to Moore and Brainard, appeared in Chicago and visited the Durovics. He told them he came representing Moore and Brainard, who felt they were entitled to the distribution rights for Krebiozen. Marko and Dr. Stefan told him they were willing to pay whatever an arbitration board would recommend, but would not concede the distribution rights. In a second meeting, Loretani told the Durovics that "Moore and Brainard had a very powerful friend at the American Medical Association who would see to it that if they did not get the distribution rights, the Durovics and Krebiozen would be completely and utterly destroyed. Also Dr. Ivy would be eliminated as a potent medical force because he would not help Moore and Brainard obtain the rights. Loretani added that since the AMA governed practically all medical matters in the U.S., naturally anyone who controlled the AMA itself would be able to command anything he wanted. He even went so far as to name this omnipotent official, one Dr. J. J. Moore, Treasurer and member of the Board of Trustees of the AMA. He said Dr. Moore was working in collaboration with his good friends Moore and Brainard and they would ruin Krebiozen and Dr. Ivy. The Durovics would then have no other choice but to sell out cheaply...Loretani asserted that there was a friend of Ed

Moore on the medical faculty of the University of Illinois. This friend even then was preparing an unfavorable report on Krebiozen and it would be published in the AMA Journal. All this could be avoided, he explained, by surrendering the distribution rights to the Moore group now…Loretani stated that in case the Durovics could not give up the distribution rights to Moore and Brainard, the latter would settle for the sum of two and a half million dollars. In return for that sum, all projected and forthcoming attacks on Krebiozen by the AMA would be cancelled. The Durovics would be free to research and develop the anti-cancer drug just as they pleased.

The above paragraph is derived from sworn testimony to an Illinois legislative committee in 1953, as reported by Herbert Bailey in *A Matter of Life and Death*.

A few days later, before Dr. Ivy learned of what Humberto Loretani told the Durovics, Dr. Moore invited Ivy to meet Loretani. The point of the meeting seemed to be when Dr. Moore told Ivy that Moore and Brainard were upset with him for not forcing the Durovics to accept them as distributors. Ivy replied that he had tried to settle the matter but his role as a scientist was to see if the drug had merit, not about how it might be distributed. Dr. Ivy was puzzled as to why Dr. Moore was concerned with Moore and Brainard.

Shortly after, a friend told Ivy that Dr. Moore was "out to get him", and wondered why. About the same time, June 1951, two other friends with contacts at the top of the AMA told Ivy that "unless he disassociated himself from Krebiozen and denied it had value, he would be expelled from the Chicago Medical Society. He would lose all of his national medical positions. Further, he would be 'blasted' by the AMA and be forced to resign from the vice-presidency of the University of Illinois".

"At that time", Herbert Bailey points out, "Dr. Ivy was accorded the respect of the entire medical world and believed that results scientifically obtained would convince anyone. What did he have to worry about?"

On July 11, Ivy was startled to read a press release from the

secretary of the AMA to the effect that a critical report on
Krebiozen would be issued in about six weeks. Knowing that it
would take at least two years to come up with any sort of an evaluation of Krebiozen, Ivy could not see how such a report could be
done so hurriedly, or why. Trying to be helpful, he asked Dr. Pick
to invite Dr. Wermer to look at some of his cases, which Wermer
did. Dr. Pick later testified that Wermer told him one day that
summer, "It's too bad a man of your calibre has to go down with
the ship...I'm sorry, but that's the way it has to be". Puzzled,
Pick asked Wermer what he really thought of Krebiozen. Wermer
replied "If my mother had cancer, I would want you to give her
some Krebiozen".

As a show of the high regard in which Dr. Ivy was held, in
August 1951 Governor Adlai Stevenson appointed him to a three-
year term on the Medical Center Commission, an important post
that expanded Ivy's already considerable political base.

Dr. Ivy then received a letter warning him that the *Journal of
the American Medical Association* (JAMA) did intend to print a
negative report on Krebiozen:

> *When that AMA report - and it will be devastating -
> appears, it is my belief that the following events will
> occur: 1) the newspapers will publicize the AMA report
> not once but repeatedly, and reporters will pester various
> medical bodies for statements about what they are going
> to do about it and about you; 2) the Chicago Medical
> Society will act quickly to declare you a member not in
> good standing; 3) you will quickly be deposed from all
> official connection with national cancer committees, etc.
> 4) your post at the University of Illinois will be taken from
> you. These events will follow in greater or lesser rapidity,
> but they will surely occur, for the AMA report will serve
> as the initiator of a whole chain of reactions...You have
> been in a precarious position ever since the Drake Hotel
> meeting... There is only one constructive thing you can
> do... At the very earliest moment you must have in the*

*hands of the AMA - before their report is set in type - a let-
ter which you will ask them to publish at once... You must
say that critical examination of the records forces you to
the conclusion that your original hopes have not been
realized and that Krebiozen has no value in the treatment
of cancer.*

Dr. Ivy wrote his informant that "I could not write the letter
(you suggest) and keep faith with myself".

After receiving the grim letter of warning, Ivy called a meeting of the Krebiozen Research Foundation, which consisted of
the Durovics, Dr. Pick, and a few others. They realized there was
a battle ahead but felt the only way was to continue on course. Dr.
Durovic decided to send a letter to Dr. Lull at the AMA attempting to dissuade the AMA from making any early statement on
Krebiozen. "It does not improve a situation or a problem", he
wrote, "to add another premature public release to a previous premature announcement accidentally released", *i.e.*, the March 26
meeting. Durovic pointed out that "the public had not been
harmed in any way since Krebiozen, a non-toxic material, was
being distributed free of charge under the regulations of the FDA
only to qualified physicians". Durovic asked the AMA to cooper-
ate in a mutual attempt to establish the truth about Krebiozen. He
added "We have been unable to conceive of an acceptable reason
why the AMA would decide or desire to make a critical report,
favorable or unfavorable, at this time".

The Krebiozen researchers went even another step and told an
AMA sub-committee on October 18 the name of the fungus
which was injected into horses to produce Krebiozen. This had
been held as a trade secret until then and was revealed to lift the
stigma of "secret remedy" which had been applied to Krebiozen.

The Durovics might as well have kept their secrets. By
October 18, the AMA's "Status Report on Krebiozen" was
already in print and was published in the JAMA on October 27,
1951. The report covered 100 patients and stated that "ninety-
eight failed to show objective evidence of improvement...These

findings fail to confirm the beneficial effects reported by Ivy and associates." The *Chicago Tribune* stated in an editorial, "Medically speaking, Krebiozen is dead".

When Dr. Ivy analyzed the "Status Report", he found that one of his own staff members, Dr. Danely Slaughter, head of the University of Illinois Tumor Clinic (whom Ivy had not invited on March 26) had given the AMA a negative report on Krebiozen after observing it only three weeks. Now, Ivy could see that Slaughter turned out to be the person at the University of Illinois who, Loretani had warned the Durovics, was preparing an unfavorable report on Krebiozen. Asked why he didn't fire Slaughter, the kindly and trusting Ivy said "I've never fired anybody in my life except an acknowledged thief; I rehired him and he proved to be honest the rest of his life". It did not bother Ivy that Slaughter was a good friend of Ed Moore and the nephew of Moore's boss.

Drs. Ivy and Durovic knew where every single ampule of Krebiozen went and, following FDA regulations, doctors were obliged to report back to them on the use of each ampule. After some study, Dr. Ivy realized that some of the AMA's 100 cases were from clinics which had not reported back to the Krebiozen Research Foundation but only to the AMA, thus breaking FDA rules. After securing these missing reports, a picture began to emerge. Krebiozen had demonstrated itself to be a medicine of mercy, as in the early cases of Mrs. Pick and the nun and, later, Senator Vandenberg. However, Ivy and Durovic were not trying to be earlier versions of Dr. Kevorkian but to learn what Krebiozen could do to save lives. Thus they preferred not to treat patients whose vital organs had been so damaged that there was no chance of recovery. But it seemed to Dr. Ivy that the AMA must have looked for such patients, for 73 of the 100 cases were so close to death that there was only time for 2 injections 3 days apart in 40 cases and 4 injections in another 33. This seemed to them to be a deliberate attempt to discredit Krebiozen. By comparison, Dr. Ivy's first test run of patients received an average of 80 injections.

Analysis of the AMA "Status Report" took time, and before

Dr. Ivy completed it, he was living through some of the previous summer's predictions. On November 12, less than 3 weeks after publication of the JAMA Status Report, Ivy was put on trial by the Executive Committee of the Chicago Medical Society on the charges of 1) publicity, 2) the JAMA Status Report's denunciation of his work, and 3) the understanding that Krebiozen was a secret remedy. Dr. Warren Cole was a member of the Executive Committee. Dr. Ivy was told to wait outside the chamber and finally brought in to speak for ten minutes, later hearing that the vote had already been taken. He was not told of the verdict, only learning it when a reporter called him that evening to ask his reaction to his suspension for three months from the Chicago Medical Society. The reporter read him a release from the Executive Council which stated that "members were free to associate and fraternize with Dr. Ivy during his suspension". The Chicago *Sun Times* reported that "the vote was 31 to 17, the minority protesting vigorously that the vote should be taken after, not before Dr. Ivy had a chance to speak". There were 6,000 members of the Chicago Medical Society; 31 had voted to smear a world figure in medicine. Many felt that the proposal for suspension would never have passed a vote of the full membership.

One of the letters Ivy soon received stated "My feelings are those of all of us who have had the privilege of associating with you through the years, and who know that your greatness is invulnerable".

Any doubts that the whole series of events had been carefully orchestrated in advance were laid to rest when the November 24 issue of the JAMA printed a letter from the National Research Council dittoing the AMA Status Report, *i.e.*, beginning to fulfill the prediction that national organizations would begin to disavow Andrew Ivy. Within just eight weeks, the AMA had trashed Krebiozen, Dr. Ivy was suspended from the Chicago Medical Society, and the National Research Council echoed the AMA line on Krebiozen. It smacked of being "wired".

At the University of Illinois, President George Stoddard at first backed Ivy, stating that "if Ivy's final report on Krebiozen is favorable, then the Society's action will seem unimportant". Then he changed his position and proposed to set up a "Krebiozen Evaluating Committee", to which Ivy agreed. Ivy accepted the appointment of Dr. Warren Cole as chairman, and it became known as the Cole Committee.

Over the winter of 1952, Dr. Ivy and his wife, a noted scientist in her own right, were busy compiling data. By April, they had completed a two-volume, 700 page report on 500 patients, all except 10 in their last stages where all usual treatments had failed. The results; symptoms were ameliorated in 70%; swelling decreased in 70%; size of tumors decreased in 50%; body weight increased in 66%; pain decreased quickly; there was no evidence of toxicity. Ivy's cautious conclusion was that "Krebiozen is biologically active in the management of a significant number of patients with cancer and deserves a further more detailed and controlled study".

Then someone dropped in on Dr. Ivy and advised him "Do not announce your favorable findings to the Cole Committee or you'll be fired!" - the last part of the previous year's predictions. Ivy replied that "he could not... alter his report to make Krebiozen look good - or bad; his report was a work of science and as a scientist he would be compelled to submit it even if it cost him his job. He told his friend that he must be the victim of a hoax. Surely no one in the American Medical Association could be that immoral - or that crude." He had been told by the Durovics of Loretani's warning about Dr. J. J. Moore, but he had not taken it seriously.

Then a second messenger came with substantially the same message. By this time Dr. Ivy, who had published 1500 papers, was beginning to get rejections saying "we are sorry to hear of your little embarrassment with the Chicago Medical Society recently and for this reason feel it wise to withhold your article from publication until this unfavorable publicity has subsided". Meanwhile, doctors began to back off using Krebiozen. The Status Report and the suspension were taking their toll.

Even Major General Wallace Graham, President Truman's

personal physician, felt the pressure. The sort of public figure to whom Ivy had access, Graham had treated a dozen veterans and their wives with Krebiozen and wrote to a friend of Ivy's, "I have had unusually good results with Krebiozen. Due to the controversy which was stimulated by adverse quarters, it was the Army policy not to allow me to continue with this…research." Bailey reported that as of 1958, Dr. Graham, back in private practice, was again using Krebiozen with excellent results.

The AMA never issued any official directive against Krebiozen; nevertheless, it was effectively blacklisted, just as Dr. Harold Wilson found Dr. William Koch's glyoxylide to be in 1948 in the case of Mary Lou Barnes. The AMA had pronounced that Krebiozen didn't work, so even though some doctors knew it did, they feared to use it.

With positive results coming in from clinics working with him, Dr. Ivy hoped that science would win out in the end and delivered his report to Dr. Cole in June 1952.

On June 14, 1952, Senator Brien McMahon of Connecticut, Chair of the Congressional Committee on Atomic Energy, received a shot of Krebiozen. By the time his cancer was discovered, he was riddled with tumors and was already terminal, inoperable, and untreatable. His doctor had attended Senator Vandenberg and had seen nine other cancer patients respond to Krebiozen. The doctor told Herbert Bailey, "The effect was amazing and unheard of, I believe, in previous methods of cancer therapy. Within six days, Senator McMahon's hip tumor had completely liquefied - that is, it had changed from a solid, fast-growing cancer into a mushy fluid filled with dead cancer cells. We drained off about eight ounces of this material." Improving rapidly, with no pain, it almost seemed as though he might recover, if something could have given him a new set of lungs. Realizing how much Krebiozen had helped him, the Senator learned that Senator Douglas was trying to pass his bill to grant permanent residence to the Durovics so that they could continue their Krebiozen research. He called his friends, including House Speaker Sam Rayburn. The bill passed and Senator McMahon was aware that he was largely responsible for permitting the Durovics to stay in the U.S. before he died a few days later.

On September 20, 1952, the Cole Committee delivered its findings on Krebiozen, and they were strange indeed. The Committee stated "It is our belief that Krebiozen has no curative value in the treatment of cancer"; of course, Dr. Ivy had never claimed that Krebiozen would cure cancer, for it was too early to say that. The Committee added "On the basis of evidence submitted, we cannot state it is entirely devoid of biological activity" and lamely concluded, despite the foregoing, that there should be more research *if* the manufacturing process was made available. The Committee's report contained a "Conclusions" part and a main section labeled "Confidential". This part was ordered withheld by Dr. Stoddard, who claimed it was too technical for the public, but it was no more technical than the Conclusions. The two made weird reading side by side. Conclusions stated that "we have been presented no microscopic examination of tissue evidence" (before and after treatment slides), but the Confidential report states "Microscopic slides were examined on nine patients..." Herbert Bailey pointed out that the Confidential report "is admitting that of nine patients, five were cancer free, according to microscopic tests. But does a hint of this creep into the Conclusions? Indeed not!" It seemed almost as though the Conclusions were based on an entirely different report, since in so many ways they contradicted solid data contained in the Confidential part. In effect, it seemed as though the Conclusions were written by a master of sophistry. It later turned out that Dr. Cole himself wrote the Conclusions and delivered them to Dr. Stoddard without bothering to obtain the signatures of any of the other committee members, as a sort of fait accompli. Again, one could say "the fix was in".

While most Chicago newspapers accepted the Cole report uncritically ("the gods have spoken", as Bailey put it), there was one reporter, Miss Effie Alley of the Chicago *American*, who did not. She called hospitals, she called patients, she was persistent. She even got hold of Dr. Ivy's 500-case report, which he had not released. Her hardest job was convincing her editors, but she did that too. The result, in the fall of 1952, was an 11-day series of solid evidence that belied both the Cole Committee's Conclusions and the earlier AMA Status Report. Near the conclusion of the series, the *American* stated that "in the eleven days of the series, no member of the medical profession and no member of the Cole Committee challenged the truth of this paper's articles". The *American* even pried a quote from Dr. Ivy, "I cannot deny the truth or validity of the articles now appearing in the *American*. It is apparent that they are based on actual hospital records and case histories".

On September 24, President Stoddard accepted the Cole Committee's request for more research and decreed that it would start once the University itself had manufactured Krebiozen and had it chemically analyzed. There would be, he said, no "technical, legal, infringement on the technical, legal, or financial rights of the innovators", *i.e.*, the Durovics. A series of negotiations followed but neither Dr. Stoddard nor his deputies would put such assurances in black and white. Finally, claiming the Durovics were stalling, he announced that there would be no further research with Krebiozen by any University staff member at any time and "I am informing Dr. Ivy of these prohibitions". Stoddard's order boomeranged, being seen as suppression of research.

At a meeting of the Board of Trustees of the University of Illinois on November 28, 1952, Dr. Stoddard asked the Trustees to abolish Dr. Ivy's job as Vice President - *i.e.*, the final piece of the predictions. Since the fuss at the University had begun to sound like a buzzsaw in the newspapers, 18 legislators attended the meeting. State Senator Roland Libonati, the Democratic whip, made a speech and then turned to Dr. Ivy saying "Now let's hear from Dr. Ivy. Now is the time to speak in your defense, Dr. Ivy." Ivy replied that all he had to say was contained in the request he had already made for a six-month leave of absence to study Krebiozen. As a scientist, Ivy was convinced that in the end, science would win out over politics; he thus preferred not to get involved in a political fight. Trustees accepted Dr. Ivy's request for a leave of absence and did not accept Stoddard's request to abolish Ivy's job.

Meanwhile, the Legislature passed a bill to investigate the Krebiozen controversy. While it was being drafted, Herbert Bailey reported, the AMA lobby succeeded in restricting the investigation to the controversy only as it existed at the University of Illinois. The bill passed both houses overwhelmingly and a committee of 7 Senators and 7 Representatives was set up to hold hearings, with powers to subpoena witnesses and documents.

Perhaps the reason Dr. Ivy said no more than he did at the Trustees meeting was because he was sitting on a bombshell which he could not decide how to handle, and which he had withheld while hoping for a favorable recommendation from the Cole Committee. In the previous summer he had been brought sworn affidavits which attested to the strangest story outside of a James Bond movie.

L'Affaire Krebiozen, which started in Argentina, received another injection from Argentina in the spring and summer of 1952 when Commodore Alberto Carlos Barreira, wealthy businessman and former Under-Secretary of the Argentine Air Force, came to Chicago. A very close friend of the Durovics, he was looking after their lab while they were in the U.S. He had observed the initial trials of dogs in Buenos Aires and had attended the ill-fated Drake Hotel meeting. He had followed the progress of Krebiozen and was aware of the remarkable results Ivy and Durovic were seeing. Then came the AMA Status Report, and Commodore Barreira was confused. "Que pasa?" he thought. Smelling a rat, he flew to Chicago without informing the Durovics or Dr. Ivy. He went straight to the AMA and secured an appointment with Dr. J. J. Moore, who, he was told, was handling Krebiozen.

After several meetings with Dr. Moore, on May 22 the Commodore gave the Durovics a sworn affidavit which "completely verified the complaints of Messrs Stefan and Marko

Durovic that they had been victims of commercial conspiracies by people such as Messrs Ed Moore, Kenneth Brainard, and Humberto Loretani in association with Dr. J. J. Moore, who had used the American Medical Association for their own interests." On advice of counsel, Barreira then had his secretary, Anna Schmidt, come up from Buenos Aires to assist him in his meetings with Dr. Moore, so that it would not just be his word against Moore's.

The following is excerpted from sworn affidavits prepared by Commodore Barreira and his secretary, Anna Schmidt, concerning a series of meetings between one or both of them and Dr. J. J. Moore during May, June, and July, 1952. These affidavits are part of the record of the Illinois Legislature's Hearings on Krebiozen. Posing as someone who had had a falling out with the Durovics, the Commodore found Dr. Moore intensely interested. Early on, Moore told him that Krebiozen was a good product. Barreira told Moore that he had documents in Argentina which were quite incriminating against the Durovics; Moore was determined to get hold of them. Then, just like an FBI sting operation, Barreira got Moore to explain his scheme to obtain the distribution rights for Krebiozen. Moore invited Barreira to participate because of his damaging documents, which Moore could use against the Durovics. A plan was laid out. Barreira would join Dr. Moore and Ed Moore and Ken Brainard, highly recommended by Dr. Moore, against the Durovics. The AMA executive would continue to harass Krebiozen scientifically by causing the AMA journal to publish additional unfavorable articles about Krebiozen. Eventually, they would force the Durovics to their knees and make them beg for terms. Then Dr. Moore and the Commodore as the rightful owners of Krebiozen would share the proceeds, which they agreed would be millions. They would work out the exact division with their business partners, Moore and Brainard, and, of course, Humberto Loretani, whom Moore referred to as "our man in Buenos Aires".

According to Barreira's testimony, Moore told the Commodore, "When the Durovics are financially exhausted, they

will have no other choice but to sell their rights and we have a
buyer ready for that time". The game plan was that if they had to
ruin the name of Krebiozen in order to get hold of it, they would
change the name. In one conversation the Commodore prompted
Dr. Moore by saying that he was only interested in the money. Dr.
Moore replied "We are all interested just in the money. We have
to meet together to find the way to obtain it, lots of it, and soon".

Before Miss Schmidt came up from Buenos Aires, Dr. Moore
flew to Buenos Aires, met there with her and Loretani, and then
helped her get a visa to come to the U.S.

In order to prevent Dr. Moore from denying that he'd ever
met the Commodore and Anna Schmidt, after the latter arrived in
Chicago, she regularly taped her telephone conversations when
she called Moore to set up appointments.

The Commodore had resisted Dr. Moore's suggestion that he
meet with Ed Moore. The following comes from the sworn affidavits of Commodore Barreira and Anna Schmidt about their
meeting with Dr. Moore on July 16 in Chicago:

> *Dr. Moore stated that he could not understand why the
> Commodore always refused to meet with Ed Moore.
> Commodore Barreira answered that it was because he
> wanted to come to an arrangement with Dr. Moore and
> sign a pact because he considered him (Dr. Moore) as the
> most important person... Dr. Moore replied that he would
> make all the arrangements but that the Commodore
> should bring his papers first in order to see how useful
> they were and what percentage in this business could be
> assigned to the Commodore, but that he personally could
> not sign any paper because of his position in the AMA and
> that the fight he was carrying on under the name of the
> organization did not permit him to show his face. So it is
> the same if any one of the group signs, and for this reason
> the formal representative of this business was Ed Moore
> with whom Commodore Barreira had to sign any agree-
> ment...*

Further in the affidavit, Dr. Moore was quoted as saying that "in spite of all the warnings to Dr. Ivy of the consequences he would suffer, which had been made to him in various ways, Ivy had remained stubborn in the defense of Krebiozen. He said Dr. Ivy was their principal obstacle. He said they had expelled him from the Chicago Medical Society for three months last year and caused him great damage as a medical authority. He said they were then working to have him removed from his office at the University of Illinois, using their men they have at the same university.

The Commodore and his secretary had concocted a story that the Durovics were considering selling out to an English group, in order to see Dr. Moore's reaction. The following is from another part of the same sworn affidavit of the 5th meeting between Moore, Barreira, and Miss Schmidt:

Commodore Barreira began by telling Dr. Moore that he received the information concerning the England affair of the Durovics through a business friend of his... Dr. Moore answered 'I hope it will be impossible' and went on saying how bad it would be for all of us if the Durovics would make such an arrangement because we would lose all possibility of obtaining their surrender. He said that Krebiozen would escape from our hands and the whole fight would have been useless.

Having obtained the information he was looking for, the Commodore informed Dr. Moore that the supposedly damaging documents had been examined by competent authorities in Buenos Aires, who had come to the conclusion that they would not hold up in court as proof of anything. That was his excuse to break off contact with Moore, and there were no further meetings. The Commodore had obtained proof that everything Loretani had told the Durovics a year before was true.

All these affidavits were in Dr. Ivy's hands in August 1952. He gave copies to Dr. Stoddard, suggesting that the latter give them to Dr. Cole, but Stoddard refused. Finally, Ivy could under-

stand what was going on, and that the events that had befallen
him had all been manipulated, and had nothing to do with science. For the first time, Ivy sought out a journalist and called
Herbert Bailey, giving him the affidavits and a copy of his 500-
case report. That was when Bailey decided to do a book on
Krebiozen.

Dr. Ivy then called John F. Sempower, a Chicago attorney
with whom he had worked in the past, and showed him the affidavits. The latter drew up a legal brief and a complaint to file in
federal court for a cause of action against Dr. Moore, Messrs
Moore and Brainard, and the American Medical Association.
Sempower felt that the AMA should be held responsible for the
action of its executive officers, if they were acting under the cloak
of its authority. Sempower believed that the affidavits proved vio-
lations of federal interstate commerce law. Later, Department of
Justice attorney Benedict Fitzgerald, on loan to Senator Tobey to
investigate the Krebiozen and Hoxsey matters, also came to the
conclusion that interstate commerce laws had been broken.

Attorney Sempower expected at any moment that Dr. Ivy
would give him the go-ahead to file suit. But Ivy held back, hoping for a favorable conclusion from the Cole Committee. It was
not Dr. Ivy's style to sue people, and until that time he had never
sued anyone in his life. He never authorized Sempower to file the
suit.

In the summer and fall of 1952, the AMA was winning the
battle to discredit Krebiozen, but Dr. Ivy said very little, confi-
dent that science would win out. It should have - but who would
publish Dr. Ivy's science on Krebiozen? The AMA would not and
seemed able to persuade other medical journals to follow suit,
just as had happened to Dr. Koch.

The Legislative Hearings opened on April 9, 1953.
Commodore Barreira and his secretary presented their affidavits
and testimony the very first day. Dr. Josiah J. Moore's name was
suddenly all over radio and television surrounded by their sensa-
tional charges. He rushed to a microphone shouting, "A lot of
things have been said against me here today and I want to be

heard". The chair explained that first the witnesses had to be cross-examined and then he would have his turn. Once Dr. Moore understood that he would have to be sworn and then exposed to cross-examination, he never again volunteered to testify.

Throughout the hearings, Dr. Moore's lawyers constantly repeated that their client wanted to take the stand to defend himself - but he never did. Because the Committee's authority was restricted to the controversy only as it affected the University of Illinois, it could not subpoena Dr. Moore and require him to testify under oath.

The main points about Dr. Moore were made the very first day. AMA lawyers insisted that Dr. Moore had acted on his own and never attempted to deny the actions of their Treasurer. Dr. Moore's lawyers and the AMA lawyers then took turns cross-examining Dr. Ivy, the Durovics, the Commodore, and Miss Schmidt, without ever shaking their story.

None of the statements in the affidavits of Commodore Barreira and Anna Schmidt was ever denied by Dr. Moore in written but unsworn testimony he offered the Krebiozen Committee, and he never offered any sworn testimony. He never denied that he had schemed with Moore and Brainard to obtain distribution rights to Krebiozen. He never denied that he had used the JAMA to discredit Krebiozen. He never denied that he was behind all the slaps at Dr. Ivy. Moore frequently repeated that his involvement with Krebiozen was only to protect the American public (even while he sought the distribution rights).

If Dr. Ivy had authorized Sempower to file the lawsuit, Dr. Moore would have had to testify under oath.

In May 1953, Effie Alley of the Chicago *American* ran into Dr. Moore in the press room at a medical convention. Herbert Bailey reports, "She asked Dr. Moore about the Commodore and Miss Schmidt. 'I saw them all the times they said I did, all right', Alley quotes Moore as replying. 'What was your purpose?' she asked. 'I was supposed to get them out of the country', he answered. 'Why would you want to do that?' she asked. Miss Alley says Dr. Moore hesitated at this and finally replied 'Oh I don't know'. Then he shook his finger warningly at her and said 'If you keep on with this, you'll get in trouble, Miss Alley!' With that, he left the press room."

Dr. Ivy took the opportunity of the Hearings to demolish the AMA Status Report. He testified about the 73 patients who seemed to have been selected in proportion to their nearness to death, as mentioned earlier. There remained the core of the report, 24 cases reported by a Dr. Szujewski, a friend of Dr. Moore. Szujewski's role was that of a lab technician, to perform certain enzyme tests on patients to reflect if Krebiozen was bringing their cancers under control; five or six such tests were enough to give a picture but two or three were not. In 11 cases sent to Szujewski, the six enzyme tests performed on each of the 11 patients showed that Krebiozen was working and keeping the cancers under control. Dr. Ivy testified that Scujewski had omitted those 11 completely. Five patients which Scujewski did report as having improved he attributed not to Krebiozen, but to "natural control". This is another way to say spontaneous remission, which is generally agreed to happen only once in 100,000 cases. So Szujewski reported five spontaneous remissions in 24 cases. But the worst thing, Dr. Ivy testified, was that these were Dr. Phillips' patients, not Dr. Szujewski's, which Phillips had sent him simply for enzyme tests.

At that point, Senator Libonati interrupted and said, "Just a minute. I want to ask something. Do you mean to say that Dr. Szujewski faked this report?" Dr. Ivy responded "Yes, it is a dishonest, false, and misleading report. Szujewski has the temerity to take patients Dr. Phillips sent him for blood and enzyme tests and then write this article stating that Krebiozen had no effect on Dr. Phillips' patients, and then furthermore he was so unethical that he told Dr. Phillips' patients they should quit taking Krebiozen and they should come to him for treatment...These were Dr. Phillips' patients. Dr. Szujewski did not give them Krebiozen, he did not supervise them, he did not examine them, he did not study their X-rays. It is outrageous and rank falsification for him to make statements about the course of pain, body weight, and complete or partial inhibition of the cancerous growth, or to say that Krebiozen is or is not effective... It is difficult to understand why the editorial staff of the JAMA published an article which contains so many errors."

Dr. Ivy prepared a chart comparing data submitted by Szujewski about Dr. Phillips' patients and data in Dr. Phillips' files, showing that some patients which Dr. Szujewski claimed received Krebiozen did not get it and some patients received it who he said did not. Dr. Ivy showed that Szujewski had included three patients where only 2 enzyme tests had been done, not enough to form a conclusion.

Ten patients who were categorized by Szujewski as "dead and dying" were anything but, it turned out. They wrote to Senator Pollack who chaired the Hearings, complaining that "such a false report could be a source of serious embarrassment to us in our social or business activities!" All 10 appeared at the hearings and testified. Of the 10, 7 had no sign of cancer and were leading normal lives, this being 2 years after their erroneous inclusion in the Status Report. Herbert Bailey noted in his 1958 book that 6 years after the Report, 7 were still alive; 3 had died, but not of cancer. In other words, by the standard 5-year test, they were cured.

The 24 cases of Dr. Phillips' patients which Szujewski wrote about in the Status Report were written up by him as a separate article and submitted to the JAMA. No fool, Dr. Moore had Dr. Wermer write Szujewski stating, "As Dr. Moore expressed to you, it is of utmost importance that Dr. Phillips' name be attached to this paper" (since these were Phillips' patients). "Nevertheless", Bailey reports, "this paper of Szujewski was accepted and published by the JAMA without Dr. Phillips' name, who alone had authority to write about his own patients".

Dr. Ivy also brought out that the Status Report omitted cases from 140 physicians who had sent their reports to the AMA research committee, as well as to Dr. Ivy. Findings by these doctors closely paralleled what Dr. Ivy was seeing in the 100 cases he was supervising; Krebiozen was subjectively beneficial (less pain) in 70% of the cases, and objectively beneficial (proof by X-rays, tumors measured to shrink) in 50% of the cases. All these cases, Dr. Ivy testified, were in the hands of the AMA and were omitted from their Status Report.

Fakery, falsification, unethical. These were harsh words, but no one ever attempted to deny or correct Dr. Ivy's analysis of the AMA Status Report on Krebiozen, or to sue him.

The Hearings ground on and on, the Committee unable to force Dr. Moore to testify, with his lawyers continuing to insist he was anxious to do so - but he never did. Lawyers for Moore and the AMA effectively filibustered the Hearings away, constantly going over and over points that had already been covered, ignoring complaints of the legislators.

In the spring of 1953, in the midst of the grueling Hearings, Bishop Bernard Sheil, founder of the Catholic Youth Organization, awarded to Dr. Andrew Ivy the Pope Leo XIII award in recognition of those who contribute greatly to humanity. The Bishop later told Herbert Bailey "Dr. Ivy is one of our greatest living scientists. He's been outrageously mistreated (regarding Krebiozen). This problem is not just freedom of research in science or medicine. It's a question of whether our fundamental liberties will remain intact."

On July 25, 1953, at a meeting of the Board of Trustees of the University of Illinois, Trustee "Red" Grange, the famous football star, made a motion of no confidence in Dr. Stoddard. It passed 6 to 3 and Dr. Stoddard immediately resigned. Then the trustees voted not to renew Dr. Ivy's contract as Vice President, in effect firing him. However, they asked him to remain as head of the Department of Clinical Sciences and Distinguished Professor of Physiology. The final prediction had come true.

In Washington, Senator Charles Tobey of New Hampshire, Chair of the Interstate Commerce Committee, learned of the Krebiozen and Hoxsey controversies. Borrowing trial lawyer Benedict Fitzgerald from the Justice Department, Tobey sent him to Chicago for some quiet investigating. Fitzgerald met Drs. Ivy and Durovic, examined Dr. Ivy's 500 cases, saw the affidavits, and returned to Washington to brief Senator Tobey. Tobey knew there were cancer cures that worked which were scorned by Official Medicine. His son, Charles Jr., had recovered from a supposedly hopeless cancer with a "bacteriophage" treatment developed by Dr. Robert Lincoln of Medford, Massachusetts. Goading establishment medicine to test the Lincoln treatment, the Senator had heard many promises but none had materialized.

Tobey was not surprised by Fitzgerald's briefing and directed him to write a report as the basis of a full-scale investigation. Tragically, Senator Tobey then had a heart attack and died soon after. In his last days, he sent Benedict Fitzgerald to Sloan Kettering in New York City where his friend Senator Robert Taft of Ohio lay dying of cancer, to tell Taft and his doctors about Krebiozen. But columnist Drew Pearson reported, "the doctors refused to use it, citing opposition of the AMA". Since Tobey's successor as committee chair was to be Senator John Bricker of Ohio, Tobey sent Bricker a letter requesting him to carry on the Krebiozen investigation because of its importance to the American people. Bricker had other ideas. After Tobey died, when Fitzgerald tried to submit his report to Bricker, the Senator refused to see him. Senator Bricker was guest speaker at the next annual convention of the AMA.

Fitzgerald then asked Senator William Langer of North Dakota to insert his report in the Congressional Record, which Langer did on August 3, 1953. Excerpts from *The Fitzgerald Report* relevant to Hoxsey and Krebiozen are in the Appendix of this book (pages 443-447).

Summing up what he learned about Krebiozen, Fitzgerald stated that "there is reason to believe that the AMA has been hasty, capricious, arbitrary, and outright dishonest, and the alleged machinations of Dr. J. J. Moore (for the past ten years treasurer of the AMA) could involve the AMA and others in an interstate conspiracy of alarming proportions... It is my profound conviction that this substance Krebiozen is one of the most promising materials yet isolated for the management of cancer..."

After Drew Pearson published the entire Fitzgerald Report,

Senator Bricker insisted the investigation did not lie within the scope of his committee and passed the buck to the House Interstate and Foreign Commerce Committee, which held hearings on health in the fall of 1953. Dr. Ivy was not invited but attended. Dr. Paul Wermer was invited and spoke about cancer quack remedies and how the American Medical Association "had always protected the public against such fakes". When he saw Dr. Ivy in the audience, he did not mention Ivy or Krebiozen by name but his press release did - and it was printed all over the U.S. After Dr. Wermer's testimony, the committee chair asked Dr. Ivy if he wished to testify, but Ivy declined.

In early 1953, Dr. Durovic had talked to the New York representative of the giant German pharmaceutical company, Bayer. The Bayer man asked for and received a copy of the Ivy Report (500 cases) which, in addition to case histories, contained a section on the fungus actinomyces bovis, the scientific rationale for Krebiozen, and basic scientific steps for producing the material. In the fall of 1953, Drs. Ivy and Durovic saw a United Press announcement about a microbiology conference being held in Rome. At the conference, the Bayer research director reported that he had achieved "remarkable results" in human cancer patients with a fungus filtrate of actinomyces. Another researcher reported remarkable results against cancer cells in animals. However a later report stated that Actinomycin C, the substance being given to patients, was too toxic for general use.

Questioned on the Bayer statement at the Legislative Hearings, which were still going on in the fall of 1953. Dr. Ivy stated, "The German scientists are working on the basis of Dr. Durovic's theory. He was the first to use actinomyces in the treatment of cancer. However, instead of making the patient sick (with the German substance), Dr. Durovic makes the horse sick and thus induces it to produce the growth-regulating substance we call Krebiozen".

As the Hearings began to near the end, Dr. Ivy challenged the AMA to have a double-blind test carried out with Krebiozen, neither the doctor nor the patients knowing who is receiving the drug. The AMA aerily dismissed his challenge, stating that they had already satisfied themselves that the substance was worthless.

The Committee ran out of money and the Hearings finally ended in the spring of 1954, having gone on for nearly a year. The Committee's report held that all of Dr. Ivy's research had been done according to the highest scientific standards. They said that they did not find Dr. Moore or his colleagues involved in a conspiracy at the University of Illinois, their area of responsibility, and dropped the matter there.

What had been accomplished? The lurid charges against Dr. Moore had come out and he never denied even one of them, simply repeating that he was only trying to protect the American public.

Dr. Ivy's testimony left the AMA's Status Report on Krebiozen thoroughly discredited, but the Report was never withdrawn or corrected and remains the AMA's official position.

As a young student of podiatry in Chicago, Dr. Morton Walker (whose book on DMSO is a prime source for the next chapter), attended the Hearings. He confirms (personal communication) that the testimony he heard was exactly what Herbert Bailey wrote about the AMA Treasurer in *A Matter of Life and Death*.

When it was all over, did the Hearings make any difference? Even after the revelation in sworn testimony of what and who had been manipulating the various events that befell Dr. Ivy and Krebiozen, did it change things? Not to any discernible degree. The AMA had spoken, and for many, that was enough. It was like the little boy who was told where babies come from; he thought a moment and then exclaimed, "*My* parents would never do *that!*"

After the tumultuous years of 1951-53, the next few were somewhat anticlimactic. Herbert Bailey's first book *K-Krebiozen, Key to Cancer?* came out in 1955. He put an ad for it in the *New York Times*, but his request to place a second ad was turned down. An insurance broker wrote Bailey in September 1955 about asking for Bailey's book in the New York Public Library, the largest in the world. "The librarian-in-charge advised me that the library decided not to purchase your book...When I asked 'why?' she told me that in view of the fact that the author 'went against the AMA', it was decided that this book was to be 'taboo'".

The library finally relented and stocked the book a year later.

About the same time, Dr. Stoddard published a book blaming his firing from the University of Illinois on Krebiozen. Dr. Ivy found it so full of inaccuracies that he got over his aversion to lawsuits and sued Stoddard for $375,000 on 47 counts of libel.

In 1956, research on Krebiozen had been going on since 1951, so Dr. Ivy prepared a five-year report. One medical journal after another rejected it, explaining that they had been told by AMA headquarters that they would lose all their pharmaceutical advertising if they printed it. Finally, Ivy had his *Observations on Krebiozen in the Management of Cancer* published by Henry Regnery in Chicago and it was reviewed favorably in the *New York Times*.

In May 1956, the University of Prague reported success in lung cancer with Krebiozen. Of interest to those with eye problems, Drs. Ivy and Durovic were able to corroborate in several elderly people with both cancer and cataracts the same results which the first experiments with dogs in Buenos Aires had shown; when treated with Krebiozen, tumors diminished and cataracts disappeared.

Movie legend Gloria Swanson read Bailey's first book and called him to offer help. TV interviewer Mike Wallace had first Dr. Ivy and then Gloria Swanson on his 1957 version of *60 Minutes*. In 1956-57, *Pageant*, *Argosy*, and *Inside Story* all national magazines, carried articles on Krebiozen. In July 1957, United Press science editor Delos Smith did a series on Krebiozen. *Clubwoman* magazine invited Dr. Ivy to write an article, which it then rejected, Dr. Ivy learned, because of AMA pressure.

In 1957, Dr. J. J. Moore was voted back in as Treasurer of the AMA - as if nothing had happened. Ivy and Durovic began to receive reports of a rumor mill in operation; people had been told at Sloan Kettering in New York that Krebiozen had been tested there and found to be absolutely worthless - but not one single ampule of Krebiozen had ever been sent to Sloan Kettering. The same report came back from other hospitals. Ivy and Durovic felt that the depth of depravity had been reached when two doctors each reported a patient dead when in fact both patients had recovered and no longer needed Krebiozen.

Meanwhile, the Durovics filed for FDA approval, which would allow them to enter into agreements with pharmaceutical companies. At that time, both the FDA and the U.S. Public Health Service were under the Surgeon General. FDA regulations were much simpler then, mandating that licenses for distribution be granted within 90 days after non-toxicity had been established. Since that had long since been proven, there seemed to be no problem, but it didn't work out that way. While drugs were regulated by the FDA, serums were the responsibility of the Public Health Service. On the supposition that Krebiozen might be a serum, Surgeon General Scheele transferred the application to the Public Health Service, where there was no 90-day deadline. The law at that time permitted him to sit on it indefinitely, which he proceeded to do. The Durovics insisted on scientific grounds that Krebiozen was not a serum but a non-toxic drug, and there the matter sat for several years.

In May 1958, Dr. Ivy testified at hearings held by the California Cancer Commission. The *San Francisco Examiner* reported on May 8, 1958 that after extensive testimony on Krebiozen, Ivy surprised the committee by informing them that he had visited Harry Hoxsey's Dallas Clinic before it closed. He stated that among the ingredients of the tonic he noted several that might be effective against cancer, especially potassium iodide, and added that he had seen two or three patients whose cancer had disappeared apparently as a result of the Hoxsey treatment. Having once "exposed the cancer quackery of Harry Hoxsey", at least Dr. Ivy was willing to go and look.

In 1958, Bailey's second book *A Matter of Life and Death - The Incredible Story of Krebiozen*, came out to good reviews. In it Bailey reported the seven people living and cancer-free who had been declared dead or dying in the AMA Status Report, and he brought Gary Cathcart's case up to date. Gary had received no Krebiozen after December 1953 for two years but then collapsed and was taken to a hospital, where an intestinal obstruction was found. His parents called Dr. Pick, who quickly realized that the old nemesis was back. He gave Gary another massive dose of Krebiozen and for the third time, it "performed a miracle. Two days later, Gary was out of bed, rid of his 'intestinal obstruction', and walking around before the eyes of astonished doctors. With more shots, Gary's tumor again disappeared. He has received Krebiozen every week since then and there has been no recurrence. Today (1958) Gary is a strapping, healthy, six-foot college sophomore, active in sports and leads his class in scholarship, with no evidence of a tumor." In an audio tape of a radio broadcast, Dr. Ivy spoke of Gary Cathcart of Cheyenne, Wyoming, and recalled how Gary's tumor had shrunk from 8" to 1" after four weeks of Krebiozen shots. He referred to Gary as a mathematical genius who had gone on to be a Rhodes scholar. Age 16 in 1958, Gary Cathcart would be 58 in the year 2000. If he is still alive, it would be interesting to hear him tell his experiences with Krebiozen. Or did a tumor recur, this time with no Krebiozen around to help?

Dr. Ivy retired from the University of Illinois in 1961 and accepted a tenured professorship at Roosevelt University in Chicago. He continued his research in cancer and decided to try making Krebiozen on his own. Finding a farmer friend with horses, Ivy followed the Durovic process, tried what he produced in terminal cancer patients - and it worked. But the farmer began to have intensive problems with state regulatory agents who at one point even staked out his farm. Hearing Dr. Ivy's story, the farmer marched into Chicago and confronted AMA investigator Oliver Field, who admitted that he indeed had talked to the regulatory agencies. The agents then stopped their 24-hour vigil.

In 1960, Ivy and Durovic had negotiated with the National Cancer Institute for a test but, following the same pattern as the

Hoxsey therapy, the data of the Krebiozen Research Foundation was rejected. By 1961, over 3,000 doctors had treated more than 4,200 people with Krebiozen and Ivy and Durovic made a resubmission to NCI. Privately, high officials of NCI were beginning to wonder if NCI was not requiring more of Krebiozen than of hundreds of other compounds it tested.

Perhaps nothing would have been different even if it had not been for thalidomide, a drug not approved by the FDA which was found in the early 1960's to cause birth defects abroad. Since thalidomide could never have passed an adequate examination for toxicity (it caused such defects in animals), FDA safety regulations needed to be tightened up to require better animal testing. In the scare that followed, well-intentioned Senator Estes Kefauver was persuaded to get behind legislation, which he succeeded in enacting, to require the FDA to test for efficacy. But the issue with thalidomide was not efficacy but safety. (The efficacy requirement is what has been largely responsible for the FDA new drug approval process becoming extremely costly, complicated, and very time-consuming.) The Durovics tried without success to maintain that their application of several years earlier was enough to keep Krebiozen legal. Finally, they faced a deadline of June 7, 1963, the date the new FDA law would take effect. If they did not apply under the new rules, the FDA threatened to seize any Krebiozen shipped across state lines. This is why hundreds of Krebiozen patients and their relatives picketed the White House on June 5 and 6, 1963. At the last minute, the Durovics applied under the new rules, but there was no longer any 90-day deadline within which the FDA had to act. On June 7, Krebiozen could no longer be shipped across state lines until such time as it was approved by the FDA. It remained legal inside Illinois.

In July, Senator Paul Douglas and fifteen other senators introduced a resolution to force the National Cancer Institute to "test fairly" Krebiozen.

The Krebiozen patients organized a Citizens Committee for Cancer Survivors on Krebiozen. In August, they again picketed the White House, pleading for access to Krebiozen for those unable to travel to Illinois. On August 7, the *New York Daily News* reported, "A group of black-clad men and women began a 'death watch' in front of the White House today beseeching President Kennedy's aid in their fight for the 'anti-cancer' serum Krebiozen". On the same day, the *New York Telegram* reported, "About 200 of them, some en route to Chicago and many wearing the symbolic black of mourning, appeared before the White House yesterday in support of their plea. They also picketed the Health, Education, and Welfare Department. They sought an executive order which would guarantee that those now taking the serum could continue to do so until the National Cancer Institute has tested the drug. A group of Senators and Congressmen sought to get an appointment with the President for the cancer survivors. The tragic death of the President's infant son prevented such an interview from taking place".

In September, the FDA announced that it had submitted Krebiozen to spectrographic analysis - and had found that it was nothing more than creatine, (which is stored in the body as creatine phosphate and aids in energy production). Wouldn't it be nice if a simple injection of creatine would save the Gary Cathcarts of the world? The FDA published a picture of the spectrogram of Krebiozen superimposed on one of creatine, showing that they matched. The picture was published in *Life* magazine and elsewhere.

But what was Krebiozen? In 1950, the Durovics had sent some to a chemist who reported that Krebiozen was a unique substance he had never seen before, not related to proteins, but perhaps related to some hormones. It was Dr. Durovic's theory that the uncontrolled cell growth which we call cancer was caused by a deficiency in growth-regulating hormones. He considered Krebiozen to be a growth-regulating hormone which in effect would restore balance between growth-producing and growth-restraining activities in the patient's cells, thereby returning the cancerous cells to normal.

As if the creatine smear wasn't enough, shortly after that, the FDA announced plans to prosecute Drs. Ivy and Durovic under criminal charges. The FDA had twice tried to convict Dr. Koch under its pre-1963 rules, so dealing with cancer even then had not been without its perils, and after June 1963 it became even more dangerous under the new rules.

In October 1963, the National Cancer Institute announced that it would not test Krebiozen, since the FDA had found it to be only creatine. The NCI also stated that 24 independent experts had analyzed 504 cases submitted by Drs. Ivy and Durovic and found no evidence of Krebiozen's effectiveness in cancer. Senator Paul Douglas knew Krebiozen's track record first hand through personal acquaintance with many recovered patients and did not believe either the FDA or the NCI. Deciding to do his own investigation, he organized a team of experts with impeccable credentials.

A month later, the Douglas panel came back to the Senator with their report. They had found that the FDA had rigged the evidence, just as in the Koch trials in the 1940's when FDA claimed that glyoxylide was only distilled water. The Douglas team found that the NCI "experts" had dealt with Dr. Ivy's 504 cases along the same lines of the AMA Status Report and the Cole Commission report, twisting and omitting.

On December 6, 1963, Douglas took to the Senate floor to denounce what he had found: that U.S. government agencies had lied. He announced that the NCI "experts", meeting in secret, did not interview a single patient or a single doctor who had used Krebiozen, nor did it permit Dr. Ivy to testify. He also announced that the NCI "experts", who were not NCI employees but supposedly independent scientists, had all received NCI grants. He announced that the standards they had applied to review Dr. Ivy's cases were far more rigid that were used to judge other therapies.

The FDA had asserted that spectrographic analysis of Krebiozen and of creatine showed that the substances were identical. Senator Douglas announced that his team had found that in superimposing the two spectrograms, the FDA had moved one by 7%, just enough to make it appear that the two were identical; without this falsification, they clearly were not.

After detailing the NCI misrepresentations and the FDA fabrication, Senator Douglas told the Senate "It is a terrible thing that we cannot really trust either the Food and Drug Administration or the National Cancer Institute". His speech is in the Congressional Record of December 6, 1963.

Margaret Fuhro, retired in Florida, was one of the organizers of the Krebiozen Citizens Committee and writes, "Senator Paul Douglas' bill for a fair test of Krebiozen gained support of other senators. Picketing at the White House and sit-ins of cancer patients at the HEW building appeared to have a positive effect, but all this was shattered when President Kennedy was assassinated on November 22, 1963."

However, Senator Douglas' announcement and the sit-ins brought Krebiozen to the public attention once again. Jack Mabley of the Chicago *Herald-American* wrote:

I have interviewed 6 to 8 doctors who have treated hundreds of patients with Krebiozen and have spent hours talking with patients who have been in what physicians described as the last stages of cancer, but who have regained normal health after using Krebiozen. I simply cannot disregard this evidence... This drug Krebiozen must be tested. That is all Dr. Ivy has ever asked - a fair test for Krebiozen. The American Cancer Society and the National Cancer institute spend tens of millions of dollars testing every conceivable drug and potion that comes along. But here is a drug that has been used by physicians on 4,000 patients under the guidance of one of the most distinguished physiologists in the country, and they go to outlandish lengths to avoid formally testing it... It is admitted by all that Krebiozen is non-toxic, that it does no harm. Why is there such violent opposition to a formal test? (Cures for Cancer? by Barry Lynes, Sarasota Eco Report, Dec/Jan 1998).

An article in the *Boston Herald* on December 9, 1963 stated "The FDA's announcement that Krebiozen is merely creatine appears to be thoroughly disproved by the Douglas investigators... But the AMA remains aloof and arrogant - and meanwhile the ground fills up, every day, year after year, with bodies killed by cancer."

As if fulfilling the Boston Herald's prediction, the Citizens Committee for Cancer Survivors on Krebiozen announced on June 7, 1964, the names of cancer patients in the New York area who had died after they could no long obtain Krebiozen:

Herman Eschenauer
Helen Gewandter - Mother of 2
Mrs. Mandel
George Leon - 4 years old
Walter Luebker
Dr. Tobias Weiser - Father of 6 - oldest 13 years
Frank Cirone - Father of 5 - oldest 14 years
Sol Robinson

The Citizens Committee stated, "Other survivors who cannot take up residence in Illinois will similarly die unless the drug is made available to them across state lines". But the FDA did not budge.

Armed with its new authority to require that efficacy of a drug be proved, the FDA picked up the AMA line that Krebiozen was not effective for cancer and on November 17, 1964, secured a 49-count indictment against Drs. Ivy and Durovic, accusing them with conspiracy, fraud, and mail fraud, enough charges to send them to jail for over 100 years.

The Citizens Committee for Cancer Survivors on Krebiozen immediately staged another sit-in, this time outside the office of HEW Secretary Anthony Celebreeze. The Secretary refused to see them, most of whom were ill with cancer. An ultimatum was given; leave or be arrested and possibly jailed. Margaret Fuhro, their spokesman, was quoted in the *Hannibal Courier-Post*, "They have chosen to be arrested. They are not going to leave the building. They feel that they are going to die without Krebiozen, and they will die in jail." The demonstrators were arrested and carried out.

By this time, Dr. Ivy, a man of legendary stamina, was 72. It's not good to be indicted at any age, but at age 72 it must have been awful. The trial started in April 1965. Independent scientists forced FDA "experts" who had proclaimed Krebiozen nothing but creatine to admit their errors under oath. In January 1966, Drs. Ivy and Durovic were acquitted of all charges, and the jury declared that Krebiozen had merit and should be tested - just as had been stated by the Hoxsey jury in Dallas. The foreman of the jury wrote a letter to President Lyndon Johnson pointing out that the $1,000,000 the Federal Government spent on the trial could have more than paid for a double-blind test to prove once and for all the value of Krebiozen. But there were no tests.

Kirkpatrick Dilling, the attorney who defended Drs. Ivy and Durovich, states (personal communication): "Dr. Ivy was the most honored scientist in America". It was Dilling's father who had defended Dr. William Koch 20 years previously.

The trial broke up the Krebiozen team. In 1962, the IRS had given Dr. Durovic a letter accepting his 1961 return and confirming that he was $90,000 in debt; both the return and the letter are attached to Senator Douglas' speech in the *Congressional Record*. However, after his acquittal from the threat of years in prison requested by the FDA, Dr. Durovic learned that the IRS was about to file a tax lien on him. Apparently having had enough, or perhaps like Dr. Koch, unable to afford any more legal expenses, Dr. Durovic flew to Switzerland, where he lived until his death. Marko Durovic, however, remained in the Chicago suburb of Winnetka until his death in 1976.

The FDA announced that it did not consider the jury decision as a mandate to test Krebiozen. It could seize any Krebiozen shipped across state lines, but could not prohibit it from being produced and used within the state of Illinois.

Following on the Ivy-Durovic victory, the Krebiozen Citizens Committee organized another visit to Washington on March 28, 1966, requesting an appointment with Dr. James Goddard, head of the FDA. The *Washington Daily News* reported on March 29 that "Yesterday, more than 50 members of the group... jammed into Dr. Goddard's office, determined not to leave without seeing him. Some were terminal cancer patients and they say the FDA ban on interstate sales of Krebiozen... is killing them. Some wore buttons saying 'I need Krebiozen to live'. 'Some of us', a lady said softly, 'won't be around next year'... Mrs. Laine Friedman, the group's spokesman, said, 'All we want is for the FDA to allow cancer patients on Krebiozen to get the drug.'...Jacob Jabs of Cleveland, Ohio, said, 'Why don't they let us use it in hopeless cases?' Finally, an FDA man told them 'It would make your day in Washington worthwhile' if they would go to a conference room. They refused....'Your presence in no longer desired', said the FDA man. And the General Services police began carrying out members of the Krebiozen committee. 'I'll pray for you fellows.' said Mr. Jabs. 'And I'll tell you fellows' - and he broke down - 'don't ever get cancer. It's no joke'. A General Services guard said 'I've been here 18 years and I've never had to do a dirtier job'. 'This is one of the darkest days of the Food and Drug Administration', said Mrs. Friedman."

In early 1967, the Poster Girl of the National Committee for Cancer Survivors on Krebiozen died of cancer. Cathy Hodnett of Allenhurst, NJ, a bright, pretty 11-year old, had been kept alive with Krebiozen. "If Krebiozen had not been withdrawn from the market", said her mother, "Cathy would probably still be alive... Cathy was given no more than six months to live, and that was seven years ago... During the years we used Krebiozen, she was free of cancer... A year ago, she was denied the drug completely... I knew I couldn't get any more. I was screaming for help, but nobody was listening." Cathy's health began to fail as soon as she was withdrawn from the drug, her mother said. Eventually she was forced to enter the hospital, where she died. (*Butcher Workman*, May 1967).

In 1973, Krebiozen's opponents finally won enough votes to outlaw Krebiozen in the State of Illinois. Now Krebiozen began the gradual slippage to oblivion that overtook Koch, Hoxsey, and

Rife. Of the four, three faced extinction, only the Hoxsey treatment surviving because of the fortitude of the remarkable Mildred Nelson.

Dr. Ivy and his wife had five sons, four of whom became doctors. The fifth, Robert, dropped out of Northwestern Medical School during the Legislative Hearings, disgusted at hearing professors disparage his father as a quack. Going into the pharmaceutical business, as of 1998 he was working on a cancer vaccine, a worthy son of his father.

After what he had been through, Dr. Ivy became more sensitive to the plight of some of his predecessors on the slippery path of trying to bring forth medical breakthroughs. Mildred Nelson remembered well when he came to visit her clinic in Tijuana. "He was such a nice man", she recalls, "so kind, always a gentleman". Dr. Ivy died in 1978 at the age of 84 at his home in Oak Park, a suburb of Chicago.

L'Affaire Krebiozen was over but unlike l'Affaire Dreyfus (Dreyfus won), Krebiozen lost, or rather we lost. Once again, a remarkable medicine vanished.

DMSO -THE PERSECUTED DRUG

A *New York Times* editorial on April 3, 1965 called DMSO the closest thing to a wonder drug produced in the 1960's. There was a great deal of publicity and controversy about DMSO in the 1960's and 1970's. On March 23 and July 6, 1980, Mike Wallace had two *60 Minutes* programs on DMSO.

The Persecuted Drug - The Story of DMSO (from which the title of this chapter was borrowed) was written in 1972 by the late Pat McGrady Sr. In the opening of his book he wrote:

This is the story of a drug which was glorified briefly as having almost panacean properties for the ailments of man and beast and diseases of plant life and then was banished by high United States authorities (the FDA) as dangerous and without merit.

This is also the story of a mild-mannered scientist (Dr. Stanley Jacob) who challenged the law and defied the officials and their police in a soul-searing struggle to make the drug available wherever there is life.

The drug is known as DMSO, or dimethyl sulfoxide (a liquid). It has been championed by reputable physicians as capable of healing or palliating many ailments. It has been represented as a 'wonder drug' or a 'miracle drug'. It is abundant; it can be extracted from such sources as coal, oil, or most commonly, lignin, the material nature uses to cement cells together in trees; it is cheap; it is most often administered by simply dabbing it on the skin; and, alone or as a carrier for other drugs, which DMSO

*often potentiates, it penetrates the skin to enter the blood-
stream where it is borne to all parts of the body.*

*Scientists contend that the (thousands of) papers pub-
lished in professional journals refute virtually all the
FDA's charges.*

On July 31, 1980, Senator Mark Hatfield of Oregon testified[2]
at a hearing of Senator Edward Kennedy's sub-committee on
health:

> *I cannot make an absolute statement that DMSO is indeed
> the wonder drug of our century, but every bit of evidence
> I encounter reinforces the premise that it is. After 1,200
> scientific publications on the merits of DMSO, after inter-
> national symposia in Germany, the U.S., and Austria - all
> concluding that DMSO is safe and effective - after three
> separate pharmaceutical firms have submitted four new
> drug applications to the FDA (all rejected), DMSO is still
> not available to Americans, although it is available in
> many other countries. I have urged the Senate to support
> my legislation (to approve DMSO) on behalf of all
> Americans who are suffering from diseases untreatable by
> any other known substance and those who may have need
> of this drug in the future.*

Strokes are the third biggest killer in the U.S., causing over
150,000 deaths a year. They are also "the primary cause of serious disabilities", *U.S. News* reported on March 30, 1998, "leaving 3,000,000 people annually unable to work or take care of
themselves". If given soon after a stroke, DMSO, one of the
world's greatest solvents, has been shown to dissolve the clot that
causes the stroke, thus restoring circulation and avoiding paralysis. How soon? Dr. Stanley Jacob says within the first few hours
is best and intravenously is better than oral, but oral works too.
Once DMSO gets into the body either daubed on the skin, given
I.V., or by mouth, it permeates the body and crosses the blood-

brain barrier, so even taken orally it can improve circulation. One man who had a stroke at 7:30 AM refused to go to the hospital until after his wife had spoken with Dr. Stanley Jacob, which didn't happen until 6:30 PM. Starting at 7 PM the day of the stroke, she gave him one ounce of 50% DMSO in a little orange juice every 15 minutes for two hours and then every half hour for two hours. The next day, her husband was better and soon returned to normal. A substance that can stop a stroke as it's happening is something many might want in their home medicine chest.

Neurosurgeon Dr. Jack de la Torre is professor of physiology and neurosurgery at the University of New Mexico in Albuquerque. He and Dr. Jacob believe that DMSO should be in every ambulance and emergency room so as to start giving it intravenously to stroke victims in the ambulance as soon as picked up or, at the latest, as soon as the patient arrives at an emergency room. If such were the established practice, the number of people dying or incapacitated from strokes would plummet.

Not only would many lives be saved, but also the awful hardship of paralysis or loss of speech might be prevented. A stroke, even survived, can often bring a person's effective life to an abrupt halt. The savings to the medical system would be astronomical. The cost of the product: pharmaceutical grade DMSO retails at $30-40 a gallon.

DMSO's ability to stop strokes is only its most dramatic and unappreciated attribute, and the one which would save the most lives, the most suffering, and the most money.

A close second is DMSO's effectiveness with head and/or spinal cord injuries. Dr. de la Torre states there are around 1,000,000 head injuries each year. Of these about 500,000 are hospitalized with 50-80,000 being severe, another 50,000 moderate, and the rest less serious. Of the 50,000 severe, 60-70% either die or have severe continuing neurological problems (*i.e.*, paralysis), a multi-billion dollar a year expense.

Research in animals indicates to Dr. de la Torre that if Christopher Reeve had been given DMSO intravenously immediately after his accident, he might never have been paralyzed.

Dr. Jacob has given DMSO intravenously to people who were already paralyzed - paraplegics - and little by little they regained use of limbs. One man, quadraplegic, recovered enough to go through college and then to work in a bank.

A recent study in Turkey combined DMSO with fructose diphosphate. In 20 patients with head injuries, the combination proved very effective in decreasing intracranial pressure. De la Torre declares that in his experience, nothing reduces intracranial pressure faster than DMSO.

Animal tests in the 1960's and then human tests on prisoners in 1967 demonstrated that DMSO is non-toxic, indeed, less toxic than aspirin.

In Dr. de la Torre's tests on dogs, injuries that normally would have caused paralysis healed completely when DMSO was given. The mechanisms of action by DMSO are much the same in both strokes and spinal cord injuries. In *DMSO, Nature's Healer*, Dr. Morton Walker summarizes Dr. de la Torre's testimony to Congress in 1980 on DMSO's methodology, based on his research with the drug which began in 1971:

> ► *DMSO permits and promotes better blood flow by dilating blood vessels, thus increasing the delivery of oxygen and by reducing blood platelet stickiness.*

> ► *Because DMSO dilates blood vessels, carotid artery blood flow to the brain increases after DMSO is given intravenously.*

> ► *After I.V. administration of DMSO, there is an elevation in the amount of spinal cord blood flow to the region of trauma. One of the first things that happens after spinal cord trauma is that a reduction of oxygen and blood flow sets in, inasmuch as the blood vessels constrict or shut down... Without some treatment, the tissue swells. Eventually, this leads to paralysis. In*

cerebral stroke, the animal will either become comatose or lethargic or die. With DMSO infusion immediately after injury (or stroke) all this is prevented.

▶ *Thirty minutes after giving DMSO I.V., there is an increase in the flow of cortisone, a natural body substance which helps fight off effects of trauma, even though the animal being tested had already stopped secreting cortisone.*

▶ *DMSO crosses the blood-brain barrier, enters the brain, picks up water from an injury, and rushes it out of the system, thus relieving intracranial pressure.*

▶ *In animal tests, the animals are brought to a point where the electroencephalogram reading becomes flat, just preceding brain death... Ten minutes after injection of DMSO, the electroencephalogram returns and the brain becomes active again.*

Dr.Walker adds, "DMSO tends to protect nerve cells... following injury. It provides better protection than any other treatments. Scientists have verified this by observation with the electron microscope and the light microscope. Thus DMSO prevents the paralysis that may ensue following trauma; it alters the severe effects seen after a brain stroke".

Drs. Jacob and de la Torre believe that DMSO is the treatment of choice in strokes and note that de la Torre's work has been confirmed by at least three different groups of investigators in other parts of the country. They also believe that the combination of DMSO with fructose disphosphate should be the treatment of choice in spinal cord and closed head injuries, where the fructose diphosphate provides energy to help restore damaged tissue.

Dreaded Alzheimer's disease will also be another area, they expect, where the combination of DMSO and fructose diphosphate (patented by Dr. De La Torre) will become the treatment of choice, the fructose diphosphate being carried across the blood brain barrier by the DMSO to help restore energy to a deteriorating brain.

In experiments with rats, Dr. de la Torre has combined L-dopa with DMSO, which carries the L-dopa across the blood brain barrier into the brain where it becomes dopamine and turns off the part of the brain which causes the trembling and other symptoms of Parkinson's.

While strokes are the third largest killer in the US, heart attacks kill the most people - about 3/4 of a million per year. Remembering DMSO's ability to dilate blood vessels and improve blood flow, it is not surprising that South American research indicates that DMSO is effective in heart attacks and angina; prompt use of it in heart attacks has been credited with preventing damage to heart muscle. Reporting this in his book, Dr. Morton Walker says, "There is a crying need for research on the use of massive doses of DMSO (2 grams per kilogram of body weight) in the treatment of heart attacks".

If DMSO is that good, then where is it? Why can't we get it? Why isn't it used? That is another story, and a sad one when one thinks of the suffering that could have been relieved or avoided if research in DMSO had not been stifled by the FDA. But this story isn't over yet. DMSO, in addition to being a very safe and effective non-toxic drug, is also a commercial solvent used in many industrial processes. Unlike Koch, Rife, or Krebiozen, it cannot be stamped out since it can easily be bought in many hardware stores. Everyone involved in DMSO research is upset at private use of commercial grade DMSO for any medical purpose, and with good reason since it contains impurities. However, people suffering from arthritis or other pains have taken matters into their own hands. There is a large underground market in the substance, and pharmaceutical grade can frequently be found, not sold for healing purposes, of course. Cutting in half or less the time to heal sprains, many athletes count on it. It's legal for veterinarians to use in dogs, cats, and horses.

It should have been otherwise. DMSO should be a prescription drug available to doctors for general use, as it is in Europe. Instead, it is approved by the FDA for use in humans in just one rare disease, a painful bladder condition called interstitial cystitis. The health uses of DMSO make it one of the most versatile substances ever found - a wonder drug indeed. It was discovered in 1866 by Russian scientist Dr Alexander Saytzeff, who noted in a paper he published in a German medical journal the following year that it would dissolve virtually anything combined with it.

Entering the body either painted on the skin, taken orally, or via I.V., DMSO rapidly penetrates the cells and cleans them of toxins, a desirable mechanism which may explain much of its versatility.

Athletes still know about DMSO. June Jones, once quarterback and later coach of the Atlanta Falcons pro-football team, knows of DMSO. His career almost didn't happen, he told the House of Representatives Committee on Aging in 1980, which was investigating why the FDA was still telling people that DMSO was dangerous. With a bursitis calcification in his right shoulder, he could hardly lift his arm, let alone throw a football. From Oregon, he was aware of DMSO and of Dr. Stanley Jacob, and had used DMSO for sprains, like thousands of others. So he went to Dr. Jacob, who gave him a shot of DMSO in the shoulder and told him that the calcification might disappear if he used DMSO for 30 days straight. He followed instructions and it did disappear. The FDA still has not approved DMSO for sports medicine.

Former Oregon Governor Tom McCall knows about DMSO. Stricken suddenly by bursitis in 1963, two daubings of DMSO on his shoulder put an end to the problem as the DMSO dissolved the calcification that caused the painful condition.

A byproduct of wood pulp production, this "tree juice" as the late Pat McGrady called it, helps so many human problems that one is reminded of the Book of Genesis, where God said that He had placed on the Earth something for every human condition. It takes us awhile to figure some of them out, and then even longer to clear away the man-made obstacles to their use.

In 1960, Robert Herschler, chemist and chief of research at Crown Zellerbach, a huge paper and pulp manufacturer near Portland, found an inexpensive way to produce DMSO as a byproduct of the pulp industry. He noted that the chemical had a remarkable ability to penetrate the skin and spread throughout the body very quickly. By itself not toxic, Herschler learned that when DMSO is put together with something toxic, there can be problems if the combination is put on the skin or ingested. Since DMSO is a solvent, he and an assistant regularly washed their hands in it until the day he did so after having handled pesticides and became quite sick.

To this day, after many hundreds of thousands, probably even millions of people have been treated with DMSO and thousands of studies have been done, this is the only danger associated with DMSO; *beware of what you mix it with.*

Realizing there could be medical possibilities in DMSO, in 1961 Herschler got permission from his superiors to check with the University of Oregon Medical School in Portland, and was introduced to Stanley Jacob. The meeting made medical history. Dr. Stanley Jacob, brilliant graduate (in surgery) of Harvard Medical School and professor of surgery on the faculty of the University of Oregon Medical School, had published 40 papers in prestigious medical journals before he heard of DMSO. Holder of numerous academic and professional honors, he was already a pioneer. Heart transplants were still the stuff of science fiction in 1961, but even then Jacob and his associates were getting puppy hearts to beat in mature dogs for several days, and he was looking for ways to preserve them. He found it in DMSO, which is now used worldwide for storage of organ transplants.

After hearing about DMSO from Robert Herschler, Jacob painted some on his arm and within moments became aware of its oysterish taste in his mouth. He knew that this meant that the substance had not only quickly penetrated his skin but that it had gone into his bloodstream and permeated his entire system. He realized that this could mean an entirely new medical principle for delivering medicines. As Pat McGrady put it, DMSO "was to change Stanley Jacob's life and what he learned about it was to change the lives of many others and had the capacity to change many more".

Dr. Jacob and Herschler devised numerous experiments, one showing that mice which had sustained burns were more comfortable after being daubed with DMSO. Herschler soon profited from this knowledge. After an accidental chemical burn on his hands, arms, and forehead, he called Jacob. "Apply DMSO on one side and see what happens", Jacob told him. Herschler called him back in 15 minutes, "The pain stopped. Now I'm going to do the other side".[1] A few weeks later, one of Herschler's assistants sprained an ankle. In 15 minutes after DMSO was applied, the pain was gone and in 30 minutes the swelling as well.

Someone complained to Dr. Jacob of a splitting headache and gave him permission to apply some DMSO after hearing of its capabilities. The headache was gone in minutes, came back in four hours, and left for good after DMSO was applied a second time. Used for one purpose, sometimes it did another; put on a cold sore, within a few hours it cleared up a woman's sinusitis. A woman who had had a stroke found after DMSO was painted on her painful jaw that she could now write with her paralyzed hand and could walk better. Dr. Jacob found that it could also suppress inflammation.

The tree juice worked in trees, too. Withered old apple trees became youthful and full of leaves after DMSO was injected under the bark.

Applying DMSO where it hurt to a six-year-old wasted from rheumatoid arthritis, in a half hour the child could move her shoulder and turn her head for the first time in two years. Persuaded to try walking, she managed a few steps and then burst into tears. "Why are you crying?" Dr Jacob asked her. "Because it doesn't hurt anymore", she replied.[1]

DMSO was very cheap, Herschler told Jacob. "I could pipe it down here. You could have it by the barrel or the tank!"[1]

Impressed with what he was seeing but wanting someone

skeptical to play devil's advocate, Dr. Jacob sought out Dr. Edward Rosenbaum, a physician in private practice in Portland. Rosenbaum did not pay much attention until a patient with severe bursitis started laughing, proclaiming his pain gone 15 minutes after his shoulder was painted with DMSO. Another colleague poopooed DMSO until after one of his bursititis patients had recovered via the chemical. He then declared that obviously the case must have been misdiagnosed - and asked if he should buy some stock in Crown Zellerbach (which produced DMSO).

In 1963, Dr. Jacob and Robert Herschler submitted two papers on DMSO to medical journals. Before the articles were published, the press broke the DMSO story on December 10, 1963 when Crown Zellerbach and the University of Oregon filed at the state capital a contract in which they became partners in the patented uses of DMSO. The patents were requested in the names of Herschler and Jacob and spelled out the major results seen from DMSO research, so the news was now public. On December 18, the *New York Times* carried the story on its front page and Crown Zellerbach's stock jumped 10%.

The January and March 1964 issues of *Northwest Medicine* published articles by Jacob and Rosenbaum on bursitis and arthritis. This gave some legitimization to DMSO in scientific circles but stirred up animosity as well among those who resented hearing about DMSO first in the popular press. When Jacob presented his work to the University of Oregon Medical School faculty, there were a few jeers of "liar, charlatan, quack". It was hard for many to believe that something as versatile as DMSO could exist. Dr. Jacob sent a memo describing 20 of his cases to his immediate superior and friend, who replied with a note saying "This smacks of Andrew Ivy!" A few months later, the same friend told Jacob that he had dreamed the previous night that the DMSO affair had been turned over to the National Academy of Sciences. Then Stan Jacob remembered his father's dream. A week before he died, his father said he had dreamed that Stan would find some wonderful chemical from wood, and people all over the world would be holding out their hands for it!

That dream was coming true. It would be eight years before his colleague's dream came true, and a lot of fur would fly before then.

In 1965 Merck, Syntex, and Squibb Pharmaceutical all sub mitted New Drug Applications (NDA's) to the FDA, stating that DMSO was ready to be a prescription drug. The FDA turned all of them down. In July 1965, the first international symposium on DMSO was held in Berlin.

What happened to DMSO (and Krebiozen before it) is hard to understand without recalling the crisis atmosphere in the early 1960's surrounding the sleeping medication thalidomide. The request for approval of the drug was assigned to Dr. Frances Kelsey, Chief of the Investigational Drug Branch. She processed the application by doing nothing at all with it for about two years. During that time a number of babies were born in Europe without arms or other limbs and the cause was traced back to thalidomide. Since Dr. Kelsey had not processed the application and thus "saved" Americans from the drug, she got a medal from President Kennedy, (The truth, Dr. Morton Walker tells in *DMSO, Nature's Healer*, was somewhat different: 1,200 doctors in the U.S. had access to thalidomide through the FDA and there were thalido- mide babies in the U.S. Some were children of doctors.)

After Dr. Kelsey was honored, every other FDA bureaucrat was on the lookout for ways to show vigilance and for things to stop. On February 8, 1981, Robert Herschler appeared on David Hartmann's *Good Morning America* show and told his host about DMSO's reception at the FDA. "They complained bitterly in 1964 that DMSO was both a commercial solvent and a drug. They could not control it. Frances Kelsey raised her hands and said 'We simply cannot cope with a product like DMSO. We envision hundreds of (new drug) applications coming in and we simply don't have budget or staff'. After that, the FDA took a hard line on DMSO."[2]

Remembering thalidomide, the FDA apparently was looking for things to stop, and found its chance in late 1965. The FDA learned that tests in rabbits, dogs, and pigs (but not humans) had shown some problems. When quantities of DMSO equal to about ten times the maximum human dose (*i.e.*, equal to 350 grams a day for a 175 pound man) were given every day over a period of six months, slight changes in the lenses of the animals' eyes would result, enough to produce a slight nearsightedness. The lens changes were not enough to cause dogs difficulty when running - they didn't bump into things - and in some cases, the changes disappeared after the massive DMSO doses were stopped. In no test at that time or since has DMSO ever caused cataracts, either in animals or in humans.

The FDA decided that DMSO was the dangerous drug it was looking for. The first Dr. Jacob and his colleagues knew of the animal tests was on November 10, 1965. On that crucial date, the FDA sent notices to all the drug companies involved in DMSO research (Squibb, Syntex, Merck) that "administration of the drug must be discontinued and the drug recalled from all clinical investigation". In addition, the FDA put out a series of press releases carried by media all over the world warning of the blinding effects of DMSO, and leading people to believe that DMSO caused cataracts. But no animals were blinded, and the FDA knew that. The "spin" was designed to show that once again the FDA had "saved" us.

Thus research was stopped in its tracks on a drug which was stopping pain (when nothing else could) from bursitis, arthritis (including rheumatoid), and gout, which was cutting at least in half the time needed for recovery from athletic injuries, and which had even saved a boy's life when his neck was broken in an accident. DMSO prevents swelling and rapid injection of the chemical soon after the accident prevented the swelling which otherwise would have choked him to death.

Drs. Jacob and Rosenbaum and Robert Herschler had constantly been looking for any indication of DMSO toxicity and had found none. Learning of the animal data, as quickly as could be arranged they brought past and current patients to the ophthalmologists at the University of Oregon to look for lens changes of any sort. After months of testing, absolutely no lens problems were found. To the contrary, several reported they could see better after using DMSO (on other parts of the body). So the order to stop research had been based on an inaccurate pretext.

Informed of the tests by Dr. Jacob and others showing that humans were not experiencing the same lens changes as the three animal species, the FDA at first seemed to have second thoughts. Had they overreacted?

An FDA less eager to play "gotcha" might have handled the situation quite differently. Upon receiving the initial lens data, they might have immediately informed the drug companies and Dr. Jacob and asked them urgently to check if any humans were experiencing the same problems as the animals, which is what Jacob and his team did anyway, being responsible scientists.

Or, after its first release, the FDA could have announced that it was good to be vigilant but that DMSO was not causing the same results in humans as had been seen in some animals. It could then have said quietly to the researchers, "watch very carefully for human problems because if such occur, DMSO will have to be withdrawn". If the FDA had done that, everybody would have been happy. The FDA would have shown its vigilance for drug dangers, which is what it's supposed to do. And nobody would want to work with a medicine that caused eye problems.

Finally, FDA adopted an all too human attitude; they did not want to admit they had made a mistake. They apparently arrived at a decision that DMSO must be another thalidomide and that if FDA agents only looked hard enough, they would find the evidence and all would be heroes. If it had turned out that way, they would have been, but it didn't.

In 1965, the JAMA printed an article by Dr. Jacob on DMSO. Interestingly, his trouble has only been with the FDA, not the AMA. The JAMA has never turned down one of his articles, and he regularly writes its book reviews.

Before freedom in DMSO research was withdrawn, orthopedic surgeon Dr. Forrest Riordan saw DMSO save a frostbite patient's limbs. Arriving home after midnight on a -15 degree F night, a 59-year-old woman slipped on the ice outside her garage, hit her head, lost consciousness, and lay beside her car for six hours. By the time Dr. Riordan saw her, her feet and hands were purple, and her fingers were turning black. Having already treated 50 patients with DMSO and being aware of its use in preserving and restoring tissue, Dr. Riordan decided to give it a try. Pat McGrady describes what happened,[1] "The question was, would DMSO give new life to the lady's dying fingers and restore blood to her limbs? Ten minutes after Riordan had swabbed DMSO on the patient's hands and lower legs, the treated areas reddened with the return of blood. The DMSO odor was on her breath, showing that the drug was permeating the woman's system. On the second day, blisters had popped out on the frozen areas and that evening she regained consciousness...On the third day, sensation began returning to some of the toes and later the tips of the fingers began to have feeling again. By Day Seven, she was able to flex her joints. For an entire month, the patient was sloshed, swabbed, and dabbed with DMSO. Almost a gallon of it was used, but side effects amounted only to an occasional rash, a bit of burning and itching...By Day Fourteen, it was clear that all tissues were viable...Riordan concluded that the drug should be applied within 12 hours of freezing and that 24 hours may mark the critical point in reversing damage to the involved blood vessels."

This is the sort of experimentation that was going on before FDA halted DMSO research, a freedom to "try it since nothing else is working" approach, which in this case probably saved one lady her life and certainly her four limbs. How many others today might have saved limbs if the knowledge of this one case had been broadcast and DMSO's use encouraged instead of discouraged?

Planning had been going on for some time for a Symposium on DMSO to be held in March 1966 at the New York Academy of Sciences. On November 9, 1965, a top FDA official told Dr. Jacob that he had it on good authority that the Symposium would never be held, not explaining that he would announce the DMSO ban the next day.

He was wrong. Dr. Chauncey Leake of the University of California Medical Center, who had agreed to chair the Symposium, told Dean Baird, Dr. Jacob's superior at the Medical School, that he'd been asked to drop plans for the symposium on the grounds that it would be embarrassing for both the drug companies and the FDA. Baird replied "Chauncey, when have you and I as deans and educators ever let political or economic considerations compromise the search for scientific truth?"[1] Baird also told Jacob that Crown Zellerbach, unused to such controversy, had urged him to call off the symposium. The New York Academy of Sciences, a large, prestigious organization founded in 1828 with over 25,000 members, made their displeasure at political interference evident by putting up the $60,000 cost of the meeting when pharmaceutical companies refused to do so.

Undeterred by the FDA, over 1,000 people from the world scientific community were in attendance when the symposium opened at the Waldorf Astoria on March 14, 1966, to go on for three days. When one of the FDA officials spoke, stating "this symposium is a measure of the freedom of investigation... prevailing in this country"[1], people wondered if he was being ironic.

The papers presented showed great enthusiasm for DMSO and its unusual medical properties. Its ability to protect living cells from cold and radiation was discussed, and its lack of toxicity was stressed. Pat McGrady, who attended, wrote, "the studies covered a spectrum of diseases probably far greater than any ever before considered in relation to a single drug".

McGrady called special attention to an extraordinary paper presented by Dr. Eduardo Ramirez and Dr. Segisfredo Luza of the Ayetano Heredia University in Lima, Peru. After extensive tests on animals and then on normal humans, Dr. Ramirez reported "injecting 50% or 80% DMSO intramuscularly into patients with acute and chronic schizophrenia" and that "of the 14 acute cases, every single one was discharged from the hospital within 45 days after the start of DMSO treatment... He said that 4 of the 11 chronic cases, one of whom has been ill for 14 years, were discharged eventually, and the other 7 improved a great deal and were given occupational therapy... He observed rapid decrease in agitation... recession of persecution feeling, a relatively sudden tendency to communicate and to stay clean... the wane of obsessions, return to alertness, and a calmness where there had been restlessness and anxiety."[1] The only side effects were the characteristic garlic-like odor of DMSO.

At the end of the symposium, after an almost dazzling presentation of papers, McGrady reported[1] that "an FDA agent turned to Ann Sullivan of the Portland *Oregonian* and said 'DMSO is through'. Ann looked at the man in amazement and asked 'Where did you ever get that idea?' 'My boss told me', the agent answered."

Meanwhile, the drug companies who had been doing clinical trials were reexamining patients and gathering data regarding possible eye damage. Squibb collected 3,000 cases, Merck 17,000 cases, and Syntex 7,000. No eye changes or damage or any other sign of toxicity were found. By this time, DMSO had been used in 100,000 people, and there had been no complaints of eye problems anywhere. Additionally, sufficient animal tests had been carried out to make it clear that the lens changes that had been observed were "species specific", *i.e.*, they only occurred in dogs, rabbits, and pigs, and not in monkeys, other primates, or any other animals.

Neither the pharmaceutical reports or the new animal tests seemed to have much effect on the FDA's new commissioner, Dr. James Goddard. Goddard soon showed that he intended to use the police powers that Congress had given him to investigate scientists, who had never before been treated that way by federal regulators. Quickly adopting a tough line, he took the FDA into some surprising new areas. Speaking to an AMA convention, he announced that "the FDA is now a third party to the practice of medicine"[1], to the general consternation of the doctors. It began to look as though Dr. Goddard was out to prove he too could stop a thalidomide and that he suspected maybe DMSO was it.

DMSO patients, however, did not agree. Those who had found DMSO a veritable WD-40 for arthritis were furious when their pain returned after the FDA stopped DMSO. They talked to the press, they called their senators and congressmen, and wrote angry letters to the FDA. Pat McGrady provides a few samples[1]:

> *My brother has arthritis of the spine. He is in pain and bedridden more than half the time. When he is treated with DMSO, he is able to lead a normal, active life...Just ONE application of this cheap, safe DMSO changed my brother from a grimacing patient into an active, pain-free man in exactly 30 minutes! Multiply him and my family by thousands of times, then think what the FDA's Divine Right of Kings Law is doing to thousands and thousands of patients and their families.*

> *I had arthritis for four years, gradually getting worse until I was in such agony day and night I was almost at my wit's ends... I heard of Dr. Jacob and went to visit him...Almost from the first I began to get relief. Now I am on my feet, well and active... I have never in my life wished ill of anyone but experiencing the caliber of this agency (FDA) I wish every last one of them would suddenly have an attack of acute arthritis so painful that you could hear them yell from there to here and have to beg for the only drug discovered that could give them real help.*

FDA statements continued to refer to DMSO's dangerous side effects but gave no specifics, no who, when, where. Pat McGrady pressed four consecutive FDA commissioners for data on the "dangerous effects". They all replied that the information was in their files. He asked them to produce it - four times. They promised to send it to him - four times, but it never came.

While Official Medicine had stopped DMSO research in the U.S., at least it could go on freely elsewhere. A Third International Symposium on DMSO was held in Vienna in November 1966 and 250 scientists from 12 countries attended. Dr. Chauncey Leake, as keynoter, said, "Fortunately, members of the health professions throughout the world are not all bound by the bureaucratic regulations and judgments of the U.S. Food and Drug Administration".[1] Pat McGrady, who also attended, commented "It was strange hearing this statesman of science in this hall and this city, which less than a generation ago had been occupied by one of the bloodiest regimes in history, now apologize for regimentation in America".[1]

He also reported, "As at the Berlin and New York symposia, scientists said they had failed to induce eye damage with DMSO in any animal species close to the human, and they could find no evidence of eye troubles attributable to DMSO in any patient".[1]

Some of the interesting papers presented, McGrady wrote, showed that DMSO benefited 77% of patients with rheumatoid arthritis and 84% with osteoarthritis, controlled many kinds of pain, sped healing, offset injurious effects of radiation therapy, and proved superior to all other therapy for winter and sports injuries. Experiments in animals showed that when given to mice ten days before infection, DMSO prevented typhus, and that DMSO tended to stabilize collagen, a possible anti-aging effect. McGrady noted that "scores of scientists confirmed the majority of claims Jacob had made... Distinguished scientists clustered around him and congratulated him for what some called a classical contribution to science and medicine"[1]. It was learned at the conference that Germany quietly was restoring DMSO to drugstores as a prescription medicine.

Dr. Richard Brobyn, while a consultant for Merck, had devised a plan for human toxicity experiments in prisoners. After the FDA crackdown, Merck lost interest but Squibb liked his idea. Squibb proposed to the FDA that Squibb and FDA split the cost for Brobyn's plan and the FDA agreed. Arrangements were made for Dr. Brobyn to carry out the trials at the state prison in Vacaville California in the fall of 1967.

By this time, all research with prisoners was carried out in accordance with the ethical principles worked out by Dr. Andrew Ivy when he was the American medical ethics adviser at the Nuremberg trials. Years later, Dr. Brobyn told Pat McGrady that he himself took the amount of DMSO to be given to the prisoners "because I wouldn't expect a patient or experimental subject to do something I wouldn't do myself"[1].

Brobyn's plan was for 67 male prisoners to cover themselves with ten times the permissible human dose of DMSO every day for two weeks, after which they were closely examined. Finding no trace of any effects other than a rash (an occasional result of DMSO applied to the skin), the second, 90-day phase of the test started. Forty prisoners similarly doused themselves each day with DMSO, which quickly penetrated the skin. Regularly put to numerous exams with special attention to eyes, at the end of 90 days no evidence of toxicity had been seen in the prisoners and the attending ophthalmologist saw no effect at all on the prisoners' eyes. Dr. Morton Walker observed in *DMSO, Nature's Healer* that "if sugar, salt, coffee, or tea had been taken by the prisoners over three months in quantities equal to the DMSO they absorbed, it would have killed them". Pat McGrady later asked Dr. Brobyn what if he had given the prisoners ten times the permissible dose of aspirin ever day for three months. Brobyn replied, "You're asking …is aspirin more toxic than DMSO? My answer: Certainly."[1]

Brobyn was right. The classic test for toxicity is known as the LD-50 test, which measures the lethal dose (LD) at which half of a group of test animals is killed. The LD-50 tests for aspirin and DMSO show that aspirin is seven times as toxic as DMSO.

A year after the Vacaville tests, the FDA lifted its ban on clinical testing in humans and approved tests of DMSO in rheumatoid arthritis and scleroderma and, separately, in sprains, bursitis, and tendinitis. This did not release it to doctors for general use in these conditions, but only permitted drug companies to prepare complicated applications for testing in them.

In 1970, Dr. M. Brandsma of Los Angeles reported that a case of systemic lupus erythematosus, which had not responded to prednisone, had gone into remission for three years (at the time of reporting) from DMSO. The same year, British scientists found in two double-blind studies that DMSO combined with idoxyuridine stopped the suffering from painful shingles in from 2 to 9 days.

Various pieces of research had shown DMSO to be effective against viruses and an important clue as to why this happened was given in 1971 by Dr. M. Kunze and associates in Vienna. Their study checked the production of interferon in mice following infection of the mice by the scientists with certain viruses. They reported that when DMSO was injected 10 minutes after the mice were infected with viruses, "the animals produced anywhere from 2 to 16 times as much interferon as they would have had no DMSO been given after their being infected"[1].

The very significant fact that DMSO would cross the blood brain barrier had been evident from Dr. Jacob's early research. For those interested in "smart pills", the early 1970's work which John L. Brink and Donald G. Stein of Clark University published in Volume 158 of *Science* magazine is relevant. Magnesium pemoline (PMH) had already been noted to improve learning in rats and in humans. Brink and Stein reported that PMH dissolved in 100% DMSO greatly increased rats' learning abilities over what was achieved with pemoline alone. Injecting into rats (1) a solution of radioactive PMH or (2) a solution of radioactive PMH dissolved in DMSO, they noted that the DMSO/PMH solution was from 50%-100% more successful in crossing the blood-brain barrier than the PMH+water solution alone.[1]

Pat McGrady once asked Dr. Stanley Jacob who would gain the most from DMSO. Here is Dr. Jacob's answer[1], "Quadraplegia is the saddest thing that happens to people. It occurs most often to the young and healthy, to soldiers fighting our wars, to youngsters driving, to athletes in personal contact games. As a quadraplegic, you lie in bed, a total vegetable. Your mind functions but you cannot pass urine or have a bowel movement without help...So many of them eventually say to me 'Dr. Jacob, I couldn't even commit suicide'."[1] Jacob told McGrady about one such patient, a case where he was called in almost immediately following an accident. "A 16-year-old girl, a fine athlete, who dove off a board and landed on her neck on the bottom of the pool. Her doctor was pessimistic but willing to try almost anything that offered a glimmer of hope. She was a complete quadraplegic, utterly helpless. She was on DMSO for an entire year. Gradually - one by one, it seemed - her organs began to function again. Eventually, she walked. And now she is in college, doing very well."[1]

This was accomplished with the medicine on which FDA banned research in the U.S. in 1965. It was 13 years later before the FDA approved DMSO as a prescription drug for use in interstitial cystitis.

Grey Keinsley of Littleton, Colorado, is the one-time quadraplegic mentioned earlier by Dr. Jacob, who went on to college and to a job in a bank. But Keinsley did not start DMSO until February 1965, two years after his accident. By August 1965, he lifted both arms over his head and put on a T-shirt unassisted. A little later sensation began to return to his lower chest and his right hip. Then the FDA banned DMSO, and he was deprived of it for three years, starting again only in 1968. The next year, he received his bachelor of arts degree in economics. His mother told McGrady that Dr. Jacob not only did not charge for his services, but paid bills for extensive medical examinations which were done in Colorado. McGrady reported that as of 1973, Grey Keinsley could move both of his legs. Grey Keinsley is the only known case of a quadraplegic regaining movement of the lower limbs when therapy was started two years after the accident. Dr. Jacob has seen two quadraplegic patients recover completely when DMSO was started within one hour after the accident.

In 1971, Squibb Pharmaceutical again filed an NDA, stating once more that DMSO was ready to become a prescription drug, and again was turned down by the FDA.

In 1972, the prediction in 1964 of Stanley Jacob's colleague came true; the FDA asked the National Academy of Sciences (NAS), through its National Research Council to make an "independent review" of all information on the effectiveness and toxicity of DMSO. However, the NAS got much of its funding at that time from the FDA. An NAS officer told Pat McGrady "we have been asked to wash the FDA's dirty linen, and we have agreed".[1]

McGrady learned that the NAS intended to take 4 months just to plan how it would read the 1,200 papers (at that time) on DMSO, and then to take 18-24 months to do so. At a press conference, McGrady told the NAS president that, having read all the papers, he calculated that he, as a slow reader, could read them all in three weeks, or a fast reader could go through them all in two weeks.

Instead of taking two years to read the material, McGrady challenged, why not set three fast readers to go over the papers in two weeks and then free the drug for medical use if no reason was found to continue the ban. This would be preferable, he pointed out, to holding up research on DMSO, since the published studies seemed to show no toxicity to humans. He further suggested that the FDA be required to provide solid evidence of toxicity, if they had any, while Dr. Jacob and his colleagues be invited to provide all favorable and unfavorable reports.

These suggestions were apparently far too sensible to be taken seriously. When the report came out in 1974, it seemed as though the Official Medicine of the FDA was speaking through the mouth of the NAS. The report stated (despite 1,200 papers to the contrary) that "there was inadequate scientific evidence of effectiveness of DMSO for the treatment of any disease, and that the toxicity potential was sufficiently great that the drug should remain an investigational drug".[2] Thus DMSO would not be released for doctors to use in general practice, but would remain bottled up.

In 1974, another symposium on DMSO was held at the New York Academy of Sciences. In 1975, the universally liked Pat McGrady, once science advisor to the American Cancer Society, died of cancer. His *DMSO, the Persecuted Drug* is a classic on the early years of DMSO.

Meanwhile, in Houston, Dr. Eli Jordon Tucker, an elderly and highly respected orthopedic surgeon, was treating cancer with a combination of DMSO and hematoxylon, a non-toxic dye sometimes used as a medicine. In experiments in cancerous mice conducted by Thomas D. Rogers, PhD, under the supervision of Vernon Scholes MD at North Texas State University, the mixture was seen to go directly to tumors and nowhere else, where it effectively starved them. Hematoxylon without DMSO was found to have no effect at all on cancer. In 1972, Houston KHOU TV newsman Ron Stone did a documentary on Dr. Tucker's achievements in cancer. Dr. Tucker himself never published his DMSO-hematoxylon results after 1968 out of concern over losing his license for using an unapproved drug. Dr. Morton Walker devoted 30 pages of his *DMSO, Nature's Healer* to the fascinating story of Dr. Tucker. (With Dr. John Sessions, Dr. Walker has also written *Coping with Cancer*, a further discussion of DMSO therapy for cancer; both books are available from Freelance Communications, 484 High Ridge Road, Stamford, CT 06904-3095.)

Finding his DMSO-hematoxylon mix effective in large cell lymphosarcoma and adenocarcinoma in dogs, Dr. Tucker worked out a human dosage which he gave only to terminal patients.

One who remembers the DMSO combination and Dr. Tucker very well is Alva Ruth Wilson in the Houston area. She qualified for his treatment because when she sought him out (after hearing the TV program), she had been given six months to live from lymphosarcoma. Starting in January 1973, she took an intravenous drip of the DMSO-hematoxylon mixture five days a week. Before requesting Dr. Tucker's treatment, Mrs. Wilson had maximum amounts of chemotherapy and radiation, but neither helped - the tumors kept on spreading. Chemotherapy had to be stopped because its side effects were giving her leukopenia, a disease in which her white cells had dropped to way below normal, leaving her with almost no immunity. While she was on Dr. Tucker's program, her conventional doctor wanted to give her more radiation. Dr. Tucker told her that since she was on DMSO, the radiation would not hurt her, a fact well established by clinical studies in various countries and virtually ignored in the United States. Although no primary source of her cancer was ever found, some cloudiness in X-rays of the stomach aroused suspicion, so that was where the radiation was directed. Another woman (not one of Dr. Tucker's patients) who started radiation of the stomach the same day returned for the second treatment in a wheelchair, so ill had the radiation made her, and for the third on a stretcher as a patient in the hospital. But Mrs. Wilson, taking her daily DMSO I.V., took the same radiation and felt great. By January 1974, after a year on Dr. Tucker's program, no more tumors could be found and she continues in fine health in 2000.

As far as Dr. Jacob knows, DMSO was not used on those who suffered radiation damage at Chernobyl.

Another of Dr. Tucker's success stories, Joe Floyd of Spring, Texas, was 71 and in good health when interviewed by Dr. Walker in 1989. In 1974, Floyd was stricken with deadly adeno-carcinoma. By coincidence, his doctor's wife had the same kind of cancer and the doctor urged Floyd to take the chemotherapy his wife would take. Floyd demurred and sought out Dr. Tucker.

Six months later, he was back at work, but the doctor's wife was dead.

Clyde Robert Lindsay knows about DMSO. At 3 years of age, in 1966, he was given up for dead with cancer. Dr. Tucker gave his mother a dropper bottle of DMSO+hematoxylon and told her to give him 5 drops in distilled water every morning on an empty stomach. In 1992, Dr. Walker found him to be a big, strong young man of 29.

While researching for *DMSO, Nature's Healer*, Dr. Walker visited Dr. Tucker, who gave him his formula. Then, as Walker explains, "Dr. Tucker himself came down with a form of cancer that would have responded to his DMSO+hematoxylon treatment, but before he could administer it to himself, he fell into a coma." No one had access to the formula, and Dr. Walker did not know that Dr. Tucker needed it until after Dr. Tucker died.

To make sure Dr. Tucker's formula does not get lost, Dr. Walker printed it in *DMSO Nature's Healer* with complete instructions for preparation and dosage. Walker notes that the treatment solution can be taken orally (the way Clyde Robert Lindsay took it).

Dr. Tucker's remarkable work, as yet unnoticed by conventional medicine, should not be considered surprising since there have been numerous studies indicating that DMSO either by itself or in combination with other drugs can be helpful in cancer. As mentioned earlier, DMSO is known to stimulate the body's production of interferon which, synthesized, has been used in cancer treatment. DMSO has been found to potentiate certain chemotherapies while rendering them less toxic, and this has been reported in the medical literature. DMSO would permit safer and more effective use of radiation in cancer treatment, because of its protective action (as noted in Mrs. Wilson's case). This was originally reported in 1961. The March 1985 Russian radiological journal *Meditsinkaya Radiologia* reported on the use of DMSO with radiation in cancer treatment.[2]

Pat McGrady noted[1] that the late Dr. Florence Seibert, one of the researchers in pleomorphic organisms, observed that "organisms frequently found in cancer and leukemia patients suspected as a cause for cancer (the sort that Royal Rife and Dr. Gruner of Montreal saw) stopped growing when exposed to 25% DMSO... Dr. Robert Schrek and associates of the Veterans Hospital in Hines, Illinois, found that two per cent DMSO, which had no effect on normal cells after two days, killed 90% of the leukemic cells in a single day... Noted virologist Dr. Charlotte Friend of New York's Mount Sinai School of Medicine transformed leukemic cells back to normal, hemoglobin-manufacturing cells with a very weak concentration of (2%) DMSO added to the medium in which cells were growing... In April 1973, Drs. Etienne and Jennie Lasfargues of the Institute of Medical Research in Camden, NJ, reported that while DMSO increased the number of virus-infected mouse breast cancer cells sixfold for awhile, by the end of three months, DMSO had completely rid the cultures of infected cancer cells."

McGrady also noted that "Dr. Leo Stjernvall, a University of Helsinki pathologist, and his associate Dr. K. Setala... reported that cancer cells... build a protective 'cytoplasmic barrier' which prevents the poisons of (various cancer drugs) from seeping inside the cells and killing them or arresting their growth. Stjernvall dissolved the anti-cancer drug vinblastine sulfate in DMSO and dabbed it on cancer that he had induced with chemicals applied to a mouse's skin. The fibrous cytoplasmic barriers melted away and other structures changed so that the cancer cells took on the appearance of benignly overgrown but otherwise normal cells. Other common anti-cancer drugs became equally effective when dissolved in DMSO. The experiments showed that DMSO transported-drugs can alter the malignant cell toward normal." The fibrous barrier referred to by Dr. Stjernvall is the fibrin cover described in the Hoxsey chapter. Whatever will dissolve that cover opens up a cancer tumor to attack by the body's immune system - if it is healthy - or by cancer cell killing (cytotoxic) drugs so much in current use.

How did the National Cancer Institute's "War on Cancer" overlook the extensive research on DMSO and cancer?

Heart attack, cancer and stroke - the three greatest killers in the U.S. - and DMSO has relevance to them all, but how many people know this?

The FDA, at least, knew about Dr. Tucker. Invited to New York in 1978 by doctors wanting to learn about his cancer treatment, he asked Joe Floyd to go along. While planning the trip, Tucker received a call from Dr. K. C. Pani, the FDA official in charge of DMSO since 1968. Pani had heard of Tucker's work and invited him to stop in Washington en route to New York. Tucker visited Pani, showing him various patient records, X-rays, and slides. Dr. Morton Walker tells the story[2], "When they came to Floyd's record, Dr. Pani asked 'How long did this one last?' Tucker replied 'He's sitting down in the lobby'. Pani said 'I want to meet this dead man'. They sought out Mr. Floyd, who told his story. Then the FDA official, visibly impressed, said he would be in touch with Tucker soon. He also mentioned that he was in contact with Dr. Stanley Jacob of Oregon and that he was monitoring the use of DMSO."

About one week later, the FDA approved the use of DMSO in the treatment of interstitial cystitis. This 1978 action was the first time FDA had approved DMSO as a prescription drug for any human ailment. Considering that it had been 13 years since the crackdown, it was a major breakthrough, and it certainly seemed that Dr. Tucker had had something to do with precipitating it.

Unbelievably, as we enter the 21st century all these years later, it is still the only FDA-approved human use for DMSO. It is also approved for the preservation of frozen human tissues, the first use to which Stanley Jacob put DMSO. Ironic to think that surgeons soak in DMSO tissues such as the bone marrow which they will later place in human bodies. This chemical is famous for its penetrating abilities, so such transplants are obviously drenched in DMSO. It's considered safe enough to be approved for that, but not for general medical use, for doctors to use in any of the hundreds of ways where DMSO can be effective.

What does the FDA think it is saving us from?

The FDA used the bogus issue of eye damage for several decades to hold back DMSO. Dr. Walker points out that "adverse eye findings have been reported with all the arthritis drugs, such as Anaprox, Naprosyn, and Motrin (as per their package inserts) yet no one has suggested that these minimally effective drugs be taken off the market".[2]

As far as eyes are concerned, the evidence on DMSO is quite to the contrary. When several patients treated with DMSO for muscular problems reported to Dr. Jacob that their vision had improved, he sent them to Dr. Robert O. Hill, ophthalmologist at the University of Oregon Medical School. Confirming the favorable changes, Dr. Hill began his own experiments with DMSO (after it was known that the lens changes did not happen in humans). His research showed drops of 50% DMSO to be effective in retinitis pigmentosa and macular degeneration, and presented a report on this at the New York Academy of Sciences symposium in 1971.

In the 1970's, my late mother developed macular degeneration. Having read Dr. Hill's study, I called him. In addition to what he had written, he added that one should use cold compresses after using the drops. I relayed this to my mother and when she was at home one summer, her housekeeper put two drops of 50% DMSO in each eye twice a day. When my mother was getting ready to return to Florida for the winter, she said, "Those DMSO drops worked. When I came home in June, lying in bed I could not see the individual slats on the venetian blinds in my bedroom and now I can."

Deise, a friend from Brazil (where DMSO is legal), told me that a New York eye doctor had told her she was developing macular degeneration, so I told her the above story. A year later, she informed me that the same doctor had told her that her signs of macular degeneration had disappeared. The previous year, she had persistently put DMSO drops in her eyes several times a day.

Telling another friend with macular degeneration of Deise's experience, she looked for DMSO at a health food store and then balked. The bottle of DMSO, she pointed out, was clearly labeled "Do not get into the eyes. Do not touch the skin. If gets on skin, call a physician". The label also read "This is sold only as a solvent". Calling the 800 number on the label, I learned that the product was pure DMSO, not industrial grade. With that sort of warning on the label, how could anyone guess that the liquid in that bottle is used on the skin of many athletic teams when there are muscular injuries. Such is the result of FDA's policy of censoring truthful health claims, preventing Americans from learning what this and other products can do for them.

In 1978, Dr. Arthur Scherbel, then chief of Rheumatology at the Cleveland Clinic, carried out a study of the use of DMSO intravenously in scleroderma, a particularly miserable disease affecting around 150,000 Americans. Parts of the body increasingly calcify and become rigid, an eventually fatal condition for which there was then and still is no cure. Dr. Scherbel found clear evidence of DMSO's efficacy in scleroderma and submitted his trial with a New Drug Application (NDA) to the FDA, which turned him down. DMSO is approved for use in scleroderma in Canada.

Something else happened in 1978 that opened windows in the overregulated U.S. medical system. The chemical EDTA has long been on the "GRAS" list (Generally Regarded As Safe) and is FDA-approved for use intravenously for the removal of lead, in cases of lead poisoning. Reasoning that if EDTA could remove lead it might also remove calcium, certain medical pioneers tried EDTA to deal with calcified arteries, and saw patients' circulation improve. The late Dr. Ray Evers was one of the foremost of those pioneers. Soon the FDA came down on him for his "unapproved" use of EDTA. Instead of caving in, Dr. Evers sued the FDA in Federal Court, asking for an injunction to stop the agency from interfering in his practice of medicine. This was not their business, he declared, but rather making sure that drugs are safe. Since FDA had long since declared that EDTA was safe for use in humans, he told the court that as a licensed physician it was his right to use a safe drug in whatever way he found to be useful. The FDA's interpretation of current law was then and still is that it requires them to control every usage of every drug. To their chagrin, the Court agreed with Dr. Evers, stating, "Congress did not empower the FDA to interfere with medical practice by limiting the ability of physicians to prescribe according to their best judgment". The FDA appealed, and he won again. The FDA did not appeal a second time, letting the ruling stand.

The Evers Ruling thus makes it legal for a doctor to use an FDA-approved drug in any way he/she thinks fit. Combined with the FDA's 1978 approval for use in interstitial cystitis, this meant that since DMSO had been approved for one human use, doctors could now use it for other human uses, and many did.

In 1979, just to make sure the FDA didn't interfere, the Oregon legislature passed a bill protecting Dr. Jacob's right to use DMSO within the state.

In September 1979, the FDA published a regulation abolishing its 1965 regulation which had banned general research in DMSO, but its posture was still suspicious. The unbending bureaucracy was beginning to bend a bit, but it was a little late. FDA had said no so many times that drug companies were beginning to believe they meant it and medical studies began to slow down. It was taking the patience of Job to persist with DMSO against such opposition, a repeat of the pattern with Dr. Ivy. The FDA had put out so much static that the scientific community began to back off.

Still, the Evers Ruling had opened things up considerably, and certain bold doctors proceeded to use DMSO intravenously, often seeing dramatic results. One of those pioneers was Dr. William Campbell Douglass, a person used to making his own decisions. Mrs. Ruth Lewis of Sarasota, Florida, told Dr. Morton Walker of her experiences with Dr. Douglass. Rheumatoid arthritis caused her so much pain she could not walk without a cane. After a back injury, she was told she had to remain in bed for six months. Realizing that if she did so she might never walk again, even with canes, she decided to try something else. Her son and husband literally carried her into Dr. Douglass' office, then in Marietta, Georgia, "unable to put both feet on the ground"[2], she told Dr. Walker. "After 2 1/2 weeks of DMSO treatment, I walked out of that office without any help whatsoever or a cane. I had been unable to close my right hand completely for over a year. It kept me awake at night with pain. But after the I.V., topical, and oral treatments, I can now close my hand tightly. The arthritis has not returned."

In *DMSO Nature's Healer*, Dr. Walker explains DMSO's action in arthritis, "DMSO is a scavenger of hydroxy radicals, and this chemical ion is dominant in arthritis. Hydroxy radicals are responsible for breaking down the synovial fluid and the cartilage of the joints. [DMSO is] one of the few known substances responsible for detoxifying this radical...Neutralizing this highly toxic free radical causes the reduction of inflammation and the diminishing of pain in arthritis. It is probably the primary mechanism that allows DMSO to work effectively against arthritis."

Dr. Douglass told Dr. Walker of another startling case. Penelope Pappas of Sarasota, Florida, then six years old, put her index finger into a live light socket. Before she could withdrew it, it was "cooked through and burned ash white at the tip". Within 30 minutes, Dr. Douglass was able to have the finger soaking in full-strength DMSO as the child screamed with pain. By the end of 20 minutes immersion in the liquid, the child had stopped crying because she felt no more discomfort. She slept undisturbed all night and the next day showed a pink and healing index finger. At the time...it was felt that she would probably lose the tip of her finger from gangrene.[2] The finger healed completely.

In 1980, Mike Wallace featured DMSO on two programs, first on March 23, and then on July 6. Dr. Richard Crout of the FDA appeared on the March show, insisting that there could be no FDA approval of DMSO without double-blind studies. He knew as well as anybody that this is virtually impossible with DMSO because of its smell; anyone who takes DMSO either orally, topically, or via I.V., will soon exude a characteristic garlic-like odor, and if it is taken orally, it has an oyster-like taste. In a double-blind test, neither doctor nor patient is supposed to know who is getting the drug being tested, and who is getting a placebo. How could this be done with DMSO? And how could it be done with chemotherapy, with its sometimes burning and poisoning effects? For similar reasons, double-blind tests are impossible with many chemotherapies, but the FDA allows the use of these very costly drugs, which are so profitable to the pharmaceutical companies.

Mike Wallace presented Sandy Sherrick of Riverside, California, on the March show. She had lived for two years in constant pain following a whiplash injury from an auto accident. "The pain was extremely bad. I was to the point where I cried continuously. I did not cook meals. I did not clean. I barely got myself dressed."[2]

Learning of DMSO in November 1979, she flew to Portland and Mike Wallace filmed her treatment. Dr. Walker describes the program, "By the third day of I.V. and topical applications, the patient began to feel somewhat better, reported Wallace. *60 Minutes* followed her progress on videotape. Dr. Jacob showed her where and how to apply DMSO. The television camera then switched to Mrs. Sherrick in her Riverside home. She was taking no medicine for pain relief. She said 'The pain is totally, completely gone from my neck...I'm telling the honest-to-God truth'.

She could do her housework, drive a car, lift packages. 'I've not found anything I can't do'."

The *60 Minutes* show had an estimated 70 million viewers. Dr. Jacob's office was swamped with calls, begging for pain relief. Their calls might better have been directed to their congresspeople, demanding that the FDA get out of the way.

Wallace had scheduled his show on the eve of congressional hearings on DMSO, which began the next day. Dr. Crout testified at the hearings and immediately demonstrated that he did not understand the first thing about DMSO - its remarkable ability to penetrate the entire body no matter where applied. Explaining why he had not approved Dr. Scherbel's scleroderma application, Crout described Dr. Scherbel's test; a person with both hands affected by scleroderma would dip one in DMSO, the other serving as a control. Since both hands began to heal, not just the treated one, Crout said it was impossible to say if DMSO had worked or not. He ignored the fact that the hands had not healed before application of DMSO, and that DMSO had simply done what is in its nature to do; applied to one hand, it had gone through the system and reached the other one. Dr. Crout showed the same bias as Dr. Frances Kelsey had done 17 years before when he said, "DMSO is unorthodox. It would be far easier for a new drug to have its application approved if it was closer to something already in the marketplace, such as a new antibiotic or tranquilizer that duplicates an existing one."[2] So much for innovative breakthroughs. Dr. Kelsey had admitted years earlier that since aspirin has 38 indicated usages, it would have trouble being approved under present rules. And DMSO has been called the aspirin of the 20th century. Crout even told the Congress that the DMSO new drug applications for the previous 17 years had all been faulty, submitted by companies who did not know how to prepare a proper application. He was referring to Squibb, Merck, and Syntex, who all had had many drugs approved by the FDA. Dr. Crout had shown his underlying philosophy in 1976 when he stated that when investigational new drug applications come from institutions other than the NCI or top universities, "You want harsh regulations... sometimes we say it is proper to hinder research". One couldn't accuse the man of not practicing what he preached.

A year later, appearing with Robert Herschler on *Good Morning America*, Dr. Crout stated that "DMSO is not dramatically effective and a number of people have recognized that"[2]. Did he not see Sandy Sherrick and others on the very show on which he too appeared? Actually, Dr. Crout's own Bureau of Drugs, which he directed, contradicted his statement, Dr. Walker points out[2]. The FDA has a classification for new drugs in which 1A means a breakthrough discovery. Of 34 drugs within a certain period, only four were rated 1A by Dr. Crout's department and DMSO was one of those four.

Mrs. Jean Puccio of Washington, DC testified at hearings of Senator Edward Kennedy's sub-committee on health in 1980 on her recovery from scleroderma. Diagnosed in 1971, she was told that no medication would help, and that she would probably soon face a wheelchair and early death. By the time she found Dr. Jacob (through word of mouth), she told the Senators, "I was having difficulty breathing, walking, and eating"[2]. The disease "thickens the tissue and makes your skin so tight you cannot move. It was difficult for me to drive... to turn the ignition in my car or turn my body". Her dentist could not work on her for awhile because she could not open her mouth. "Now", she said, "I can open my mouth like anybody". After her sensitized skin burned from topical application of DMSO, Dr. Jacob suggested taking it orally. "Within six months", she testified, "my condition reversed almost immediately. I can do anything anybody else can do now."

In 1980, Senator Mark Hatfield of Oregon introduced legislation to approve DMSO, but the Senate did not pass his bill, and the FDA did not budge.

Following the March 1980 hearing of the House Committee on Aging, Lillie Forister of Artesia, NM, had written to Chairman Claude Pepper telling of her 19 year battle with scleroderma, during which she lost 3 toes to amputation from the disease. She wrote "you can't sleep for the pain. The pain is with you day after day until you don't think you can take it anymore...That's the bad side of scleroderma. Now for the good part, the only ray of hope I've had in 19 years. I went to Portland to see Dr. Stanley Jacob last July (1979). He started me on a treatment with DMSO. After the first week, I felt better than I had in 19 years. I could button my own clothes, reach behind my head. Four months later, I no longer had chest pains... I feel that now I might have a chance to see my children grown and to be able to enjoy my grandchildren. Please help us. We need you to help us fight for a better pain-free life."[2]

The Florida State Legislature passed legislation authorizing the use of DMSO given topically, orally, or intravenously. Shortly after, the Florida Medical Society (Florida branch of the AMA) put out an announcement that doctors who used DMSO for anything other than interstitial cystitis would be dropped from their malpractice insurance, which they obtained from the Society at favorable rates.

In 1980, the famous "PDR", the *Physician's Desk Reference*, listed DMSO for the first time, stating that there are "no known contraindications". With Americans dying from FDA-approved drugs in scandalous numbers, how many drugs can be described this way?

Compassionate Dr. Jacob, after a full day of surgery at the University of Oregon Medical School, would treat patients with a large variety of problems with DMSO - for free. Unlike many of his colleagues, he did not maintain a private practice in downtown Portland, and regularly overextended himself helping others. Generous to a fault, he would even borrow money to lend to those in need. In 1982, his generosity was seen as a fault. Dr. Pani, the FDA man handling DMSO, was losing his wife to cancer. Dr. Jacob had tried to help, but to no avail. Dr. Pani was having a hard time with astronomical medical bills, so Dr. Jacob loaned him money. This was done by personal check, and Dr. Pani repaid the loan by personal check. Unfortunately, the FDA got wind of it and decided that Dr. Jacob was trying to suborn a federal official. In 1982 the FDA secured the indictments of both Dr. Jacob and Dr. Pani. The first trial, like Dr. Koch's, ended in a mistrial. Dr. Pani then plea bargained to a misdemeanor and lost his job, but Dr. Jacob fought, certain he had done nothing wrong. The second trial started. When the FDA's Justice Department attorneys saw that the judge and jury were much more likely to believe in Dr. Jacob's well-known generosity than in his conspiring to bribe a federal official, they withdrew the charges. They stated, "We are dropping all charges against Dr. Jacob and we wish to take this opportunity to commend him for his good service to the community"[2]. Dr. Jacob was vindicated.

In 1993, thirteen years after Jean Puccio had testified at the Senate Hearing, the FDA finally approved a new drug application for scleroderma - but in 2000, it is still not approved as a prescription drug for this purpose, athough it is in Canada.

In 1992, the FDA approved an Investigational New Drug (IND) application to permit DMSO to be tested in severe closed head injuries. Drs. Jacob and de la Torre formed PHARMA-21 in Escondido, CA, to carry out the clinical tests and to develop their DMSO/fructose diphosphate product, patented in 1996. However, funds have been slow coming in to finance human trials. Meanwhile, a substance which might have prevented Christopher Reeve's paralysis, and that of other less famous paralyzed persons, is not approved by the FDA.

The FDA turned down three applications for clinical trials of DMSO in arthritis. How far off course have we gotten in our regulatory procedures? What is the FDA doing stopping research in non-toxic therapies for pain relief? As Dr. Morton Walker puts it[2], "if something is safe enough to use internally, why is it not safe enough to paint on sore joints?"

Dr. Stanley Jacob has said from the beginning that DMSO is not a new drug but a new therapeutic principle. Dr. Morton Walker quotes chemist Dr. Harry Szmant as explaining the principle in this way[2], "Cellular damage can be repaired and cells healed and restored to near normal by changing the water structure within a cell" - and DMSO can do this. Cell wall permeability, increased by DMSO, also "alters what normally goes into and comes out of a cell, permitting the flushing of toxins out of the cells". Dr Jacob points out that water bonds with DMSO one-third more tightly than with other water molecules; because it can flow through cell membranes, it can carry water into cells, replenishing and renewing them. DMSO can also carry other substances which normally would not move through cell membranes - *i.e.*, it is a new therapeutic principle, a new way of cleansing and supplying nutrition to cells. DMSO also boosts the immune system, increasing the production of white cells and macrophages, and facilitating their movement as they search the body for materials that should not be there (such as microorganisms), destroying them.

In an age where bacteria are becoming more resistant to standard antibiotics, a hugely significant aspect of DMSO's therapeutic principle is that it sensitizes bacteria to antibiotics and other drugs to which they have always been or have recently become resistant. Dr. Jacob told a convention of the American College for Advancement in Medicine (ACAM) "I would combine DMSO with antibiotics, since it will convert bacteria resistant to antibiotics to being sensitive to that antibiotic". Dr. Morton Walker comments[2], "This DMSO characteristic of resensitizing bacteria could possibly restore an entire group of obsolete antibiotics for the use of medical practitioners". In a 1968 test in Portland, DMSO accomplished this feat by dissolving part of the coating of a bacillus, or bacteria, thus allowing antibiotics to destroy it.

Has this aspect of DMSO been forgotten? At a time when we hear of outbreaks of "Strep A" carrying people off in three days, this long overlooked capability of DMSO needs to be remembered and used.

DMSO has anti-viral capabilities, and it is likely, Dr. Walker points out, that DMSO, the great solvent, "dissolves a virus organism's coating of protein and leaves it unprotected with only its core of nucleic acid exposed to the immune system"[2]. Could this be an approach to AIDS? Since DMSO functions systemically, it could dissolve the protein coating of the viruses throughout the body, leaving them exposed to whatever potent antiviral the DMSO had been combined with. Could the Hanta virus be attacked in the same way?

French scientists in 1988 reported improved dissolution of chloresterol gallstones when DMSO made up 30% of a solution containing methyl tert-butyl, a chemical frequently used for that purpose. A previous Japanese report indicated that DMSO helped to dissolve the calcium type of gallstones.

DMSO's vast range of applications is why Dr. Jacob thinks of DMSO as a new therapeutic concept rather than as a new drug. For those accustomed to thinking of one drug, one application, DMSO's variety of usages is almost unbelievable. But this is not the fault of DMSO but of our current licensing laws, which treat toxic and non-toxic substances exactly the same way. When something has been demonstrated to be absolutely non-toxic, as is the case with DMSO, why should the FDA be involved at all?

Why shouldn't the market in non-toxic therapies be freed so that doctor and patient together can decide how to use them?

Dr. Jacob wryly observed to Pat McGrady that he made a mistake right from the beginning, "If I'd shown that DMSO was good just for sprains, but only sprains of the left foot, DMSO would be on the market"[1].

Dr. Richard Brobyn (of the Vacaville tests) felt that DMSO would have fared better if only one condition had been highlighted. "Like hemorrhoids", he told Pat McGrady. "The clotted hemorrhoid is common - 15-20,000,000 Americans get it. DMSO is the ideal treatment; it reduces the pain, swelling, and inflammation. If DMSO had started with something like this, it would have been on the market in 1967."[1]

One of DMSO's most significant features is its ability to combine with other therapeutic substances, but after 1965, research in DMSO needed a freer atmosphere than that in the U.S. Nicolas Weinstein, PhD in chemistry and a pharmaceutical chemist by training, owned the Laboratorios Recalcine, the largest independent pharmaceutical company in Santiago, Chile. Intrigued by

Stanley Jacob's 1965 article in the JAMA, he acquired some
DMSO and began testing in rats and other animals. Confirming
Jacob's findings, he tested DMSO in humans. When the Winter
Olympics were held in Portillo (Chile), a woman skier recovered
overnight from a twisted knee and sprained wrist with Dr.
Weinstein's DMSO spray. The next day, she won a gold medal. In
1971, Weinstein visited New York, told Pat McGrady what he had
accomplished, and the following is excerpted from McGrady's
book.

Combining antibiotics and antivirals with DMSO, Weinstein
amazed veterinarians by curing hoof and mouth disease (aftosa).
With his combinations he saw shingles, asthma, peritonitis, and
burn wounds heal rapidly. Born in 1901, he was especially interested in working with the aging. Putting DMSO together with the
amino acids GABA, GABOB, acetylglutamine, acetylcholine,
and the memory enhancer centrophenoxine, he formulated a
product called Merinex. In another called P-92, he combined
DMSO with magnesium pemoline. In one called Ipran, DMSO
was combined with procaine, which Romanian Dr. Ana Aslan
made famous for combating senility.

Treating 84 elderly men and women suffering from various
psychological problems with Dr. Weinstein's products, Dr.
Gustavo Muinzaga, professor of neurology at the University of
Chile, reported that 95% showed favorable responses. Other neurologists found that Ipran produced benefits in 75 out of 100
senile persons with cerebrovascular diseases, and helped people
recover from strokes faster. In another study, neurologists treated
70 men and women with anxiety and depressive neuroses and
intellectual deterioration. Weinstein told McGrady, "More than
one half with various neuroses enjoyed excellent responses to
Merinex…Those with neuroses lost their anxiety, irritability, and
aggressiveness".

Dr. Morton Walker, too, checked on Weinstein's work and
found that Dr. Carlos Nasser, head of the Department of
Abandoned Children of the Chilean National Health Service, had
conducted a research project in 1969 on 44 school-age children

with learning disabilities. Some had been retarded in learning to walk or speak. Some had "unmotivated aggressiveness, rebellion, irritability, and convulsive attacks".[2] IQ's ranged from 35 to 85. The experiment with DMSO-based therapy (Merinex and Ipran given both by capsule and injection), went on for 6 to 10 months, with the IQ test repeated at 3, 6, and 10 months. Dr. Nasser saw "an increase in the IQ... an overall improvement in intellectual capacity, evident progress in reading, writing, and mathematics, and a decrease of behavioral problems... The doctor... observed the elimination of anger for no reason, a general reduction of irritability, and a lessening of disobedience."[2] And all without Ritalin.

In his *DMSO Nature's Healer*, Dr. Walker explains what could cause these results. "The amino acids in (Weinstein's) products are agents for the resupply of the nervous cells and are considered indispensable for the biochemical process that controls the cerebral metabolism. The products have been used for the treatment of depressive neuroses, anxiety, psychic disorders connected with menopause, apathy and fatigue of geriatrics, and poor intellectual performance in children. With assistance of DMSO, the amino acids penetrate the brain and activate the neuronal function, which is suppressed in many syndromes of mental retardation. In children, the earlier this treatment is begun, the greater the possibility of achieving patient improvement."

At the 1974 symposium at the New York Academy of Sciences, five prominent doctors from Chilean hospitals and universities presented a very extraordinary study of the use of the DMSO-amino acid Merinex therapy in the severe mental retardation known as Down's Syndrome. Taking a group of 55 children with the syndrome, holding 24 as controls, 31 were treated over one year with Merinex given by intramuscular injection. In the treated group, all measurements improved and the doctors declared that the DMSO-based medicine offered "an evident advance in the therapy of this syndrome"[2]. In later work, they mentioned that they gave higher doses and saw better results.

This was no surprise to Dr. Jacob, who had seen similar

improvements with Down's Syndrome children brought to him for treatment. To check on the reports of the Chilean doctors, he flew to Santiago and was given a hero's welcome.

Dr. Weinstein was so enthusiastic about his DMSO-based products that, with an eye to distributing them in the U.S., he invited the FDA to come to Chile to look into the research. FDA sent representatives to visit Weinstein and for awhile even permitted Merinex to be sent into the U.S. for clinical studies. However, Weinstein and his sons found that the FDA was always asking for more and more data. After Nicholas Weinstein died in 1980, sales of the DMSO-based products dropped off, and they were eventually discontinued.

After Mike Wallace's two *60 Minutes* shows on DMSO in 1980, a number of clinics opened in Tijuana to treat arthritis with DMSO given intravenously for three days. The characteristic DMSO odor was the worst problem. This was easily resolved by staying an extra two days and enjoying the beach, after which the smell disappeared.

As we enter the 21st Century, use of DMSO in Brazil is second only to the United States. Dr. Efraim Olszewer of Sao Paulo, one of the leaders of the "orthomolecular" movement, as non-conventional medicine is called in Brazil, estimates that he has successfully treated around 6,000 people for arthritis with DMSO.

By 1991, over 3,000 clinical studies had been carried out with DMSO involving over 500,000 patients. DMSO has the widest range of therapeutic applications of any single chemical.

The FDA never was able to document its earlier concern over human vision problems from DMSO, since they only occurred in certain animals. These concerns seemed particularly strange in 1998 with the advent of the male potency pill Viagra. On May 11, 1998, *Business Week* reported that "The FDA has issued plenty of material on (Viagra's) risks, which include headaches, blackouts, and vision problems" - yet it approved Viagra as a prescription drug.

The persecution of DMSO - and Pat McGrady chose the right

word - teaches us a great deal about what's wrong with our therapy regulatory process. It has been known since 1967 that it is almost impossible to give a human enough DMSO to do harm. It is seven times safer than aspirin, safer than penicillin, and safer than arthritis drugs. The Vacaville trials proved DMSO was non-toxic in 1967, and it should have gone on the market then. Considering all the people who have suffered - and are suffering - from pain, from arthritis, bursitis, traumatic injuries, strokes, scleroderma, and from unnamed other conditions where DMSO would help either alone or in some combination, the FDA is light years late in approving DMSO for general medical use. FDA has no business having jurisdiction over non-toxic therapies at all.

Once he was convinced that it was non-toxic, Dr. Stanley Jacob has taken an ounce of DMSO orally every day; as of the Year 2000, that is 40 years. He says that he decided that if long-term use was going to have a harmful effect on a human body, he preferred it would be his. Effects? He hasn't been ill in years. Considering all those many attributes of DMSO, that's not surprising. And its versatility continues to amaze him. He even found and patented a method to use DMSO as a spray to solve one of mankind's oldest problems - snoring!

In the best of all worlds, Stanley Jacob would already be a Nobel Laureate for having discovered the healing properties of DMSO. With the patience of a saint and the persistence of a bull-dog, he is still dedicated to bringing to the world the benefits of one of the most versatile and extraordinary compounds the Almighty ever put here. For DMSO is not a concocted, man-made chemical; this "tree juice" is a gift of God. And many people would be a lot better off if more use were made of it.

Why are we being "protected" from DMSO?

1. *The Persecuted Drug*, by Pat McGrady
2. *DMSO, Nature's Healer*, by Dr. Morton Walker

THE COLOSTRUM STORY
Antibodies, not Antibiotics

Berkley Bedell is an American success story. Growing up in northwest Iowa, he became an avid fisherman and early on displayed an ingenuity for making better fishing tackle. Encouraged by local merchants and his family, at age 15 with $50 of savings from his newspaper route, he founded the Berkley Company to produce and market the equipment he had devised. A few years later, he fitted out a car with a bed in the back, set out on a sales trip, and came home with $20,000 in orders - a lot of money in the 1930's. World War II interrupted what was becoming a fine business, and Berk became a flight instructor in the Air Force. After the war, he again threw his energies into the business. Marrying his college sweetheart, they launched a family of three children as the business began to take off. By 1964, the Berkley Co. was doing so well that Berkley Bedell was selected as the first National Small Businessman of the Year and then elected to the Young Presidents' Club. By 1974, the company had become world-class. Very well known and very well liked, Berk Bedell ran for Congress that year and became the second Democrat ever to hold that seat. Always unruffled, with a great sense of humor, he and his gracious wife Elinor were very well regarded in Washington. His calm deliberation but willingness to act when action was required won him so much respect in Congress that there's no telling how far he might have gone, but his career was cut short. On a fishing trip (still his favorite sport) at Quantico Naval Base in 1985, he was bitten by a tick and developed Lyme disease. As a congressman, he had access to the best medicine in the country, but intravenous antibiotics did not stop the disease. Gradually, he became sicker and by February 1986 realized that he would not have enough energy to take care of his constituents.

So Berk and Elinor Bedell arrived at the sad decision that, after 12 great years, it was time to leave Washington. Accordingly, he announced that he would not run for reelection.

A few days later, some constituents called, told him about someone they felt sure could help, and took him to see a farmer named Herb Saunders just north of the Iowa border in Minnesota. Learning the Congressman's problem, Saunders told him to get hold of some killed Lyme disease spirochetes. "Once you have them," he told Bedell, "they will be injected into the udder of a cow two or three weeks before she is to have her calf. After she gives birth, I'll make whey from the colostrum (the first two days' milk), and you'll sip some of that every hour and a half for a month or two."

With the best doctors and the best medicine in the U.S. not having been able to help him, Berk Bedell couldn't see what he had to lose. He followed Saunders' suggestions, and what happened next was to change the direction of his life. A month or so after he started sipping the specially prepared colostrum, his Lyme disease symptoms disappeared completely and never returned. He had been healed by a mechanism as old as mammals - the ability of a mother to create antibodies to whatever she has been exposed to, a process all of 20th century science has not been able to equal.

Bedell could hardly wait to announce his cure to all the others suffering from Lyme disease, he told Saunders. But the farmer begged him not to do so, telling Bedell "They might throw me in jail for practicing medicine without a license". Bedell was shocked to learn that the distribution to humans of colostrum thus prepared, *i.e.*, against a specific target, was illegal. It was his first exposure to the prohibition of the use of many non-patentable, non-toxic treatments by Food and Drug Administration rules and regulations.

Saunders explained what had caused the healing. "The cow prepares antibodies to fight any illness, bacteria, virus, or fungus to which it is exposed. The cow that produced the colostrum you drank was exposed to the spirochetes that cause Lyme disease, so she prepared in her udder exactly the right antibodies to get rid of those organisms".

Antibodies are protein particles made by the immune system of any mammal (human, cow, goat, etc.). Their purpose is to fight what science calls an antigen, which is any substance (virus, bacteria, pollen) which threatens the body enough to cause the immune system to go to work. If the famous HIV test measures positive, that means that the body has produced antibodies against the HIV virus, which in that case would be the antigen. If the body thus affected were able to produce a sufficient quantity of the anti-HIV antibodies, theoretically, they should eliminate the virus; presumably this is why some who test positive are not sick. Antibodies created by an immune system in sufficient strength against, say, the staphylococcus bacteria will kill the staph. The colostrum approach to healing uses naturally created antibodies targeted against specific antigens as non-toxic medicine.

Harvesting antibodies from an animal is not a new idea; that was how Krebiozen was produced, with a fungus being the antigen which caused a horse to produce specific immune particles. It was relatively easy to bleed horses, a process from which they recovered. In the 1930's, several pharmaceutical companies, notably Merck and Lederle, were producing a variety of horse serums aimed at fighting diseases, particularly pneumonia. Penicillin put an end to the horse serum business.

The colostrum story really starts with Dr. Paul Erlich of the Koch Institute in Berlin, who is generally regarded as the father of immunology. In 1892, Erlich published a paper demonstrating that through the milk, a mother transfers to her offspring immunity to whatever illnesses to which she has been exposed, a principle common to all mammals. It was Dr. Erlich who coined the term "magic bullets" to describe antibodies.

Progress in the field was slow until 1946, when Dr. William Petersen, professor of dairy science at the University of Minnesota, demonstrated that a cow's udder could produce antibodies to bacteria. Widely respected and of Scandinavian origin, his work won attention in dairy-conscious Denmark, whose king bestowed an honorary knighthood on Petersen in 1952.

Dr. Berry Campbell, a professor at the University's medical school, discovered that antibodies are created by plasma cells. Learning of each other's work in 1950, Petersen and Campbell joined forces and did an experiment. They examined tissue from a cow's udder and found it rich in plasma cells. They discovered, in effect, that a cow's udder is a veritable antibody factory.

Until then, following horse serum techniques, cows were immunized intramuscularly (IM). In 1951, one of Petersen's graduate students, R.M. Porter, wrote a PhD thesis proposing the then novel idea of immunizing a cow not IM but in the udder. Porter went on to a career abroad but Petersen and Campbell developed the idea.

Because of the horse serum work, it had been assumed that the antibodies a cow passed on to her calf were produced in the blood. Some, indeed, were, but through a series of experiments, Petersen and Campbell showed that far more of the only kind of antibodies known at that time was produced in the udder. As an antigen to stimulate the immune system, the professors prepared a vaccine of nine common disease-causing organisms affecting calves and injected it into a cow's udder. This produced an immune milk with antibodies targeted against the nine organisms, one of which was E coli bacteria. Fourteen 3-to-5-week-old calves selected for having no antibodies to E coli were divided into two groups. Group 1 was given normal milk and Group 2 was given the immune milk Petersen and Campbell had produced. Then both groups were "challenged" with E coli, i.e., they were given massive amounts of it. All the calves in Group 1 died, while all but one in Group 2 survived. Most of Petersen and Campbell's tests involved milk given orally, but one experiment was done differently. Calves were given E coli and all went through the symptoms of what is usually a highly fatal disease called "white scours". When pneumonia developed, immune protein derived from the immune milk was given to the calves intravenously. When it was given slowly enough to avoid shock, all recovered dramatically. In another experiment, just to see what would happen, as scientists do, Petersen injected colostrum into the peritoneal cavity of a mouse (the space around the stomach). Things did happen; a large quantity of antibodies quickly appeared in the mouse's blood.

It was evident to Petersen and Campbell that their method could produce antibodies against any disease-causing organism they injected into a cow's udder. In effect, they could produce colostrum targeted to any antigen; staph, strep, whatever. But could the antibodies (protein substances) pass through the assorted digestive enzymes and trypsins of the gut without being digested and therefore destroyed? Conventional wisdom held that they could not. Petersen and Campbell felt that if immune milk were taken in sufficient quantities, the enzymes would be overwhelmed and some antibodies would get through. Petersen decided to do a test on himself. He injected a cow with chicken typhoid bacteria, eventually obtaining milk containing antibodies against the disease. On January 18, 1955, he drank a quart of the milk and did the same for three days. Examining a sample of his blood, he saw strong activity of chicken typhoid antibodies. He had thus shown that humans can absorb antibodies through the gastrointestinal tract if taken in sufficient quantities. In addition, Dr. Petersen found that colostrum contains antitrypsins, which would tend to help them get past the trypsin digestive enzymes. Petersen and Campbell later pointed out in an article entitled "Immune Milk", published in the *Journal of Immune Milk* of June 1964, that Strasbourg researcher Felix Klemperer had addressed this question in a study done in 1893. Klemperer's study showed that when milk from a goat injected with salmonella bacteria was given for seven days to a nursing mother, salmonella antibodies would show up in her milk by the eighth day.

In July 1955, Petersen proved, as had Klemperer, that antibodies produced in cows can cross species , *i.e.*, they are as effective in humans as in cows. After ten days of drinking milk from a cow immunized against four strains of streptococcus, he noticed that the pain from his medically diagnosed rheumatoid arthritis had disappeared. A colleague with the same disease also soon had remission, plus ten friends and relatives. In his article "Immunity from Milk", published in the June 1964 *Journal of Immune Milk*, Petersen describes one of the cases, "Mrs. A. P. drank the milk in September 1955 for three weeks, with complete remission (from arthritis), only to have symptoms return in December. On December 28, she went on 1½ quarts of milk daily through February 5. During the first week of January 1956, pains had completely left, and there has been no sign of return in more than four years."

In the same article, Dr. Petersen discussed research with viruses, which when used as antigens were not killed, since it was thought that they must multiply in the cow's mammary gland in order to produce antibodies. Petersen reported on the work of Canadian veterinarian researcher Dr. Charles A. Mitchell, which had been published in the *Canadian Journal of Comparative Medicine* of January 1971. Mitchell had found that after injecting viruses in the udder, they grew rapidly for a few days and then disappeared "precipitously" as soon as the cow started producing antibodies to them.

Petersen learned that goats can produce the same immune phenomenon as cows. A California forest ranger found that many residents of his area who were immune to poison ivy were drinking goats' milk. The goats had developed a preference for poison ivy and built up antibodies against it, which they passed on in their milk.

Petersen and Campbell produced an immune milk from cows immunized with pollen and found it remarkably effective. After drinking the milk, 96 out of 107 "difficult" cases of hay fever saw their symptoms disappear. Of the remaining 11, eight had partial relief, leaving only three cases as failures. Dr. Herb Struss, Petersen's assistant, later observed that the best results were obtained when the antigens used for immunization contained molds as well as ragweed.

Petersen and Campbell's research turned up a curious fact, which they called "dithelial immunity". In cows, humans, or other mammals, if the offspring gets sick during the nursing peri-od, the microbes causing the illness will be passed to the mother, who rapidly prepares antibodies which she passes back to her infant - a good argument for mothers to nurse their babies as long as possible.

The cows used by Petersen and Campbell never showed any signs of damage from the numerous immune "challenges" put to them, appearing to produce both antibodies and milk with equal contentedness.

Petersen and Campbell were granted Canadian Patent #587,849 on December 1, 1959. Their U.S. patent, #3,376,198, was filed the same year and granted on April 2, 1968. This cov-ered their method for producing milk and colostrum targeted against specific microbes.

The significance of Petersen and Campbell's work attracted several first-rate graduate students. Among them were Herb Struss, who took his PhD in milk secretion, R. M. Porter, Dr. Sarwar, and Jim Collins. It would have seemed that the ground-breaking research would have been received with open arms in dairy-conscious Minnesota, but petty politics got in the way. Herb Struss recalls what happened (personal communication). Dr. H.S. Diehl, dean of the University of Minnesota Medical School, invit-ed one of his best friends to lecture. During the question period, Dr. Berry Campbell, brilliant but not very diplomatic, asked sev-eral piercing and embarrassing questions which exposed errors made by the lecturer. In 1960, learning of Campbell's research with Petersen, Diehl got back at Campbell by ordering it stopped. When their research came to a halt, the Petersen-Campbell team broke up and Campbell went to Loma Linda University in California. Jim Collins, joined by his sister Mary and his brother Bob, offered assistance and finally Petersen asked them to take over the work. Buying his patents, they founded the IMPRO Co. (IMmune PROtein) in Waukon, Iowa. After first joining the Collinses for a few years, Dr. Sarwar was lured to Cincinnati by Ralph Stolle, a wealthy businessman, who set up Stolle Milk Biologics.

Dr. Herb Struss, upset at the action of the University, bought a dairy farm and set up a company called Immune Milk. He collected the first ten days of milk produced in a manner he had worked under Petersen to develop. Distributing his immune milk first in liquid form and later frozen, with instructions to drink two pints a day, he supplied sufferers from arthritis and hay fever who had letters of approval from their doctors. In June 1961, Dr. Cyril Smith, a Duluth, Minnesota physician, conducted a survey of consumers of the milk who had responded to questionnaires. Dr. Smith found that 72% reported improvement after taking the immune milk. Of these, 28% stated that they first experienced more pain and then in the second to fourth weeks, they enjoyed marked improvement. Distribution of the milk was first in Minnesota, then in surrounding states, and eventually even abroad.

As a tribute to his mentor, Dr. Struss set up the W. E. Petersen Research Foundation. He also founded the *Journal of Immune Milk*, gathering research from all over the world.

Focusing on health applications and believing that doctors would not be willing to prescribe milk, Struss decided to change to capsules. After he had immunized cows with ten strains of streptococcus, two strains of staphylococcus, and one strain of diplococcus, Struss gathered colostrum from just the first four days after birth of a calf. He reduced that to a solid which he placed in 250 mg capsules, and he called the product "Specific Serum Protein". With his capsules, Dr. Struss conducted a test which proved, again, that the "protective principle" (as Petersen called it) of colostrum could pass the digestive system. In a skin test for allergies, after three weeks of taking the capsules, the skin of allergic people was no longer sensitive to allergens.

Herb Struss had been in contact with a man in the Minneapolis office of the FDA who had seemed friendly. Struss had given him copies of reports such as the Cyril Smith study. After Struss developed the capsules, in cooperation with the Borden Co. he applied for designation of the product as an IND (investigational new drug), which was granted in early 1965.

Then the friendly FDA man was transferred.

His replacement wasn't so friendly and notified Struss that the IND had been canceled. The agent never suggested that Struss had broken any FDA rules and never offered any reason whatsoever for the action. With the IND canceled, Herb Struss' shipments across state lines suddenly became illegal. Struss' first plan was to distribute only within Minnesota, thus avoiding FDA jurisdiction. This idea crashed when, three weeks after the FDA bombshell, he received notification from the Minnesota Board of Pharmacology that his products were illegal in the State of Minnesota. As if to rub in the message, two weeks after that, he learned that the IRS planned to investigate him. The FDA agent then told Struss to shut down his business, or else the FDA would prosecute him and send him to the Sandstone federal penitentiary in Minnesota. With a wife, two children, and a mortgage, Herb Struss didn't have too many options, so the Immune Milk Co. closed down. Unfortunately, the FDA action also killed off the *Journal of Immune Milk*, for Struss estimated that each issue was costing the equivalent of a new car. Without income from sales of immune milk, he could not afford to continue the journal. His fourth issue was to feature Dr. Charles Mitchell's work with viruses and Soviet research with colostrum. The three issues he published are collectors' items.

After the Immune Milk Co. closed around 1965, a reporter from *Mother Jones* magazine asked the FDA if it had observed the company's products to have any adverse effects on health. The answer was no. Had there been any complaints? No.

In 1967, Herb Struss took a job as chief chemist at the Minnesota Department of Agriculture. In 1970, Dr. Andrew Ivy's former chemist came to work for him; this was when Krebiozen, too, had been beaten down. "She wouldn't talk about Krebiozen", Herb says, "but she worshiped Dr. Ivy".

Herb Struss talks about the past without bitterness, but with difficulty. He'd been privileged to work for Petersen, and felt that Petersen and Campbell should have had the Nobel Prize. They were onto something big. He'd seen the results; he'd known a lot of people who were relieved of suffering from arthritis and hay fever. "Milk secretion was the field in which I took my doctorate," he remarked. "It's hard to lose a love."

At IMPRO, Mary, Jim, and Bob Collins had a tiger by the tail. Taking advantage of the capability of targeting colostrum to specific culprits, they quickly produced a line of products for veterinary medicine equal to their slogan, "Antibodies not Antibiotics". The Collins' original game plan was to use profits from sales in veterinary medicine to finance going through the FDA approval process for use in humans. However, there were speed bumps along the way. Just as one bad apple can spoil a barrel, a tangle with a disgruntled U.S. Department of Agriculture (USDA) extension service veterinarian cost IMPRO a lot of momentum. At first enthusiastic about their products, he turned against the company when the Collinses refused to take him in on a sort of partnership which he proposed. Mischief with the USDA went on for years.

The first case occurred when the Collinses applied to USDA (which has authority over veterinary medical products) for a license to ship products in interstate commerce. The application was turned down. The extension agent was overheard in a private conversation at an extension meeting saying "we don't want IMPRO licensed - for the time being."

If the use of targeted colostrum products were to take off, sales of antibiotics to farmers (and to humans if FDA-approval were obtained) might fall, so potentially there was opposition from more than just one disgruntled USDA employee.

IMPRO's Mary Collins was a very persistent person, and the USDA announced in November 1965 that the company would receive a two-year license the following spring. When the license came, it was only for six months. It also contained the proviso that the USDA facility at Beltsville, Maryland, would carry out its own tests, rather than relying on the company's own data. Fair enough on the surface, but that isn't how the USDA (or the FDA) treats pharmaceutical companies, who submit data which USDA (or FDA) then evaluates. The Beltsville tests would be on whether IMPRO's product called, "MBA" could boost production in dairy cows.

Mary Collins smelled a rat. Still, when the preliminary results came in, they were outstanding; MBA caused increased production of 4,000 pounds of milk per cow per year. In 1998 dollars, at $10 per 100 pounds (a conservative average), this would mean $400 per cow per year; if a farmer had 100 cows, that would bring in an extra $40,000. a year.

Then USDA announced the final results of the Beltsville tests, stating that they found no benefit at all from the IMPRO product in increased production. Enlisting the help of Iowa Congressman H. R. Gross, Mary Collins went to Washington, raised hell, and smoked out what had happened. Another herd which had not been treated with the test material, and whose milk production had not increased, was added to the number of cows treated, thus lowering the average increase to practically nothing. Mary tracked down the USDA employee responsible for the untreated herd, who was in Africa, and called him. In a recorded conversation, he told her "My cows were not treated with your product; they told me they just needed to include the numbers in some statistics they were putting together".

To add insult to injury, the USDA published in the 1970 issue of the *American Journal of Veterinary Research* their version of the 1966-67 Beltsville tests. The Collinses sued, but it took 12 years to get satisfaction. On September 2, 1982, the U.S. District Court for the District of Columbia ordered the USDA to cease releasing the offending article. The Court said that it was all right for the USDA to release the results of the tests so long as it told the whole truth about the test, which would have showed how the numbers had been doctored. USDA could have said it made a mistake and apologized. It did not.

During the 1970's, IMPRO obtained from FDA an IND (permit to test an investigational new drug) to test products prepared in the manner of Petersen in arthritis and allergies, using staph and strep to immunize. They eventually let the IND lapse, but while it was valid, they corroborated Petersen's and Struss' results.

In 1985, Congressman Berkley Bedell, by then chairman of the Operations Sub-Committee of the House Agriculture Committee, learned that someone, somewhere, had inserted into the USDA appropriations bill a provision that would put IMPRO out of business. Bedell announced that he would not move the vital appropriation bill through his committee until the problem was resolved. USDA wrote Congressman Bedell a letter guaranteeing that as long as no therapeutic claims were made, IMPRO's products could continue to be sold as before. The company stayed in business.

However, farmers are unlikely to learn, for example, of the successful results in raising milk production other than by word of mouth unless they are psychic. They have no trouble learning about rBGH (recombinant bovine growth hormone), which was approved by the FDA in the 1990's despite consumer concern over being subjected, in effect, to a long term test of its effect on humans. If the USDA ever admitted that a harmless, nontoxic whey product actually does increase milk production, what would have been the excuse for approving rBGH?

In the 1960's and 1970's, there was little criticism of widespread use of antibiotics, and rare is the person who has not profited from them. However, their overuse has become a notorious problem in the 1990's. Their presence in milk and beef from cows treated with antibiotics has made American beef unwelcome and suspect in Europe. There is no drug carry-over in milk or beef from cows treated with targeted colostrum products, since antibodies, not antibiotics, are the natural products used to restore and maintain health.

At the other offshoot from Dr. Petersen's work, Stolle Milk Biologics in Cincinnati, Dr. Sarwar helped Ralph Stolle to set up an operation similar to that of Dr. Herb Struss. There is one major difference: the Stolle company has only marketed its product outside the United States, and from production facilities outside the country. The Stolle immune milk product is collected from cows immunized with 26 antigens.

Ralph Stolle put a good deal of his wealth into research. Of considerable significance is a Stolle study which showed that "milk from hyperimmunized cows", as Stolle liked to call it, blocked the formation of arterial plaques in rabbits put on a high fat diet. Further, a certain line of rabbits bred to develop high cholesterol did not do so when fed immune milk. Ralph Stolle died in 1996 at the age of 94, active until the end, and the company was sold. It may be that the new owners will try to market their product inside the U.S. Widely sold in Japan and Taiwan, it is offered as a substitute for mothers' milk.

Ralph Stolle's pride and joy was his "Ohio Survey", in which he gave away immune milk in the Cincinnati area, which extends into northern Kentucky. In exchange, he asked recipients to report if and how it helped them. Results in order of the most reports received about any condition helped are as follows:

► arthritis	75-80% reported improvement	
► muscle cramps	75%	" "
► lack of energy	75%	" "
► cholesterol	73%	" "
► high blood pressure	70%	" "
► heart ailments	(exact percentage unavailable)	
► sleep problems	(exact percentage unavailable)	

Muscle cramps or spasms are a frequent indicator of a magnesium deficiency, and their correction may have resulted from the presence of magnesium in Stolle immune milk. While calcium helps muscles to contract, magnesium helps them to relax. Studies have shown that many heart attacks and strokes are caused not by blockages in blood vessels but by spasms causing momentary contractions in them. A British study reported that 40% of heart attack victims suffer from magnesium deficiency. A spasm in a leg muscle is called a "charlie horse", but a spasm in a blood vessel supplying the heart can bring on a heart attack, or, in a vessel supplying the brain, a stroke. Thus the magnesium in immune milk could have been responsible for the improvements noted by Ohio Survey respondents not just in muscle cramps, but in heart ailments and blood pressure problems as well.

The Ohio Survey lasted from 1960 to 1995, when the FDA asked Stolle to close it down. The FDA asserted that since Stolle asked people to fill out a questionnaire, his gift of immune milk across state lines was in effect on a quid pro quo basis, a kind of barter. Therefore, reasoned the FDA, this was interstate commerce, which was their jurisdiction. Since by that time the Stolle company had a wealth of information on the effects of immune milk and didn't really need more, there seemed no point in resisting.

Thus the FDA would not permit Herb Struss to market immune milk and would not even let Ralph Stolle give it away. In both cases, the major beneficiaries of the product were arthritics. In contrast with its hostility to immune milk as a remarkably healthy, non-toxic, and effective help for arthritis, the FDA licensed an arthritic drug called Oraflex, produced by Eli Lilly Co., in April 1982. By the time it was licensed, it was known to have been related to 81 deaths overseas (where it was distributed by a Lilly subsidiary) and to have had 3500 adverse reactions. After 14 Americans died of the drug soon after its release, the FDA withdrew it from the market in July 1982.

Another company, GalaGen, once a division of Land O'Lakes Dairy, also is involved with immune milk and colostrum. However, their policies have been guided by the belief that very few antibodies pass the digestive system. Therefore, they have been pursuing FDA approval of an injectable product.

In the early 1960's, Herb Saunders suddenly began losing cattle - seven or eight were dying every night. A vet determined that chlamydia was the cause, but could not stem the outbreak with antibiotics. After losing 100 cows, Saunders tried a colostrum targeted at chlamydia and saved the rest of his herd in two days. Impressed, he learned how to immunize cows and decided to experiment on himself. A childhood accident had injured Herb so severely that his wife had to tie his shoes. He began to improve and gradually, most of his infirmities left him. Neighbors noticed the improvement, and heard how he'd stopped the chlamydia epidemic. Occasionally, someone would ask him for help. In the 19th century, the Hoxsey family used their herbal formulas first on their animals and their neighbors' and then on their family and friends. In the same way, Herb Saunders would help his family and neighbors. He never advertised his targeted colostrums, but was willing to assist those who asked for help.

Maggie Hunt's husband was one who asked for help, not for himself but for his wife. Maggie was diagnosed with multiple sclerosis (MS) in 1982. By 1985, she could no longer climb stairs, and her husband insisted they go to Herb Saunders. Maggie didn't want to go and on the way complained that he was taking her to a quack. When they arrived, unable to walk unassisted, she had to be helped to where Herb kept his colostrums. Mixing several kinds together, he offered them to her to drink. She and her husband were at Saunders' for about four hours. She particularly remembers that when they got up to leave, she could walk unassisted. Amazed, she walked alone the entire length of the barn. Returning home with three bottles of a special colostrum mix, she took two or three tablespoons four or five times a day. Improving steadily, after three months she could again climb stairs and even ride a bike. There seems little doubt about the validity of her diagnosis, since she had begun to deteriorate in the manner typical of MS. Reflecting on Herb Saunders, Maggie Hunt came to the conclusion that he definitely was not a quack. Generally a quack advertises, and Herb never did. In addition, a quack's remedies usually don't work. Herb's did, and that, Maggie decided, made him not a quack but a healer.

Lee Ross, a clinical laboratory scientist who did not live far from Saunders, went to him for what she presumed was chronic fatigue syndrome. Things turned around quickly for her, within a day. Impressed, she asked if, in connection with her research, she could take before and after blood samples of people who came to him. She was again impressed, regularly seeing in the blood an almost immediate response in a broad spectrum of immune measurements. She saw white cells increasing in number and engulfing microbes. Large monocytes (immune particles) increased in number and in vigorous activity. Clumped blood platelets would loosen up. The almost gelatinous nature of many sick persons' blood would lessen as the treatment progressed.

Years earlier, someone had told Herb, "If I had cancer, I'd inject some of my blood into the udder of a cow and drink the colostrum". Later, in a case where his standard colostrums weren't getting results, Herb remembered the suggestion, tried it, and it worked. No designer drug could ever be more perfectly tailored to a patient than this; a cow dutifully organizing the correct antibodies against whatever its antibody factory sees as potentially harmful in the person's blood.

Saunders had a schedule for having his cows bred so that at almost any time there would be a cow about two or three weeks from "freshening" (farm language for having her calf). Thus special colostrums tailored to someone's blood could be ready in less than a month.

Lee saw another MS case that was quite dramatic. Beth Grings had been diagnosed with MS but was still active. One day she was riding her three-wheeler through fields with her boyfriend. That evening, she asked her mother to look at her legs, which were covered with large bumps; something apparently had bitten her. Within a few days, she became very sick, developed a high fever, and was almost comatose. Lee Ross saw her blood before and on several occasions after Beth started taking Herb Saunders' special colostrum, some of which was prepared with her blood. Beth improved rapidly, especially her mental condition, did not totally recover, but went on to college and holds a job.

Nothing always works, of course, but from what Lee Ross saw, most people were helped by Herb Saunders' colostrums.

Berk Bedell returned to Herb Saunders on two occasions for arthritis, once in the knee and later in the shoulder. Fifteen minutes after Saunders gave the congressman some colostrum which was on hand, the pain in his knee vanished and never returned. The pain in the shoulder took a little longer, a day.

One case brought a lot of complications. A cancer victim went to Herb, lived five months more than doctors had predicted, but then died. Despite this five-month reprieve, her sister wrote a complaint to then Minnesota Attorney General (AG) Hubert H. Humphrey III. The Bureau of Criminal Apprehension then opened an undercover investigation, which was joined by a drug enforcement agent. The AG asked the FDA to investigate. FDA could find no evidence of interstate commerce and dropped the case as being outside its jurisdiction.

So it happened that in June 1993, at the AG's request, County Attorney Daniel Birkholz of Watonwan County, Minnesota, had the sheriff arrest Herb Saunders on charges of practicing medicine without a license, fraud, and cruelty to animals.

Calvin Johnson, Public Defender for a 15-county district, was assigned to help Herb, who was not getting rich from his colostrum activities and couldn't afford a lawyer. Ironically, some years earlier, when Johnson's wife was dying of cancer, Birkholz had urged him to take her to Herb Saunders, explaining Herb's method. Considering the idea bizarre, Johnson put it out of his mind. In 1993, Cal Johnson was defending Herb and Birkholz was prosecuting him for activities of which the County Attorney had been aware for years.

Preparing for the trial, Johnson was joined by Diane Miller, a lawyer who also had studied immunology. Diane offered her services "pro bono", *i.e.*, without fees, out of deep interest in the case. Berk Bedell put up money for their expenses, providing around $20,000 before the matter ended.

In May 1994, Cal Johnson joined Diane Miller in working pro bono on the Saunders case. He had become so fascinated by its implications and had spent so much time on it that he was fired as Public Defender.

By this time, former Congressman Bedell had become a spokesman for alternative medicine, having used alternative treatments to recover not only from Lyme disease but also from prostate cancer. Working with his longtime friend and colleague Iowa Senator Tom Harkin, the two had conceived of, and Harkin had succeeded in legislating, the creation of an Office of Alternative Medicine (OAM) within the National Institutes of Health (NIH). Because of his role in setting up the widely heralded OAM, Berkley Bedell had become a lightning rod for innovative medical breakthroughs and was in touch with cutting edge researchers all over the U.S. and abroad.

One whose work had fascinated Bedell was Dr. Hugh Fudenberg, MD, of Spartanburg, South Carolina. In conjunction with Dr. Giancarlo Pizza of the Orsola-Malpighi Hospital in Bologna, Italy, the two researchers had been studying something they called "Transfer Factor"(TF). TF, they found, is a family of ribonucleic acid (RNA) peptides capable of stimulating or transferring immunity and which works across species. Thus TF made in a cow is just as effective in a human as in a cow, and Fudenberg had found TF in bovine colostrum. Fudenberg had reported some success with TF in Alzheimer's, autistic children, and AIDS. Fudenberg and Pizza published "Transfer Factor 1993; New Frontiers" and "Transfer Factor in Malignancy", which appeared in 1994 in *Progress in Drug Research*, a Basel, Switzerland, medical journal.

After Berkley Bedell called their attention to the work of Fudenberg, Cal Johnson, Diane Miller, and Herb Saunders traveled by train to South Carolina in October 1994 to meet the scientist. The lawyers were well aware that truth is the best defense for fraud, with which Saunders was charged. By bringing back a statement from Fudenberg, they planned to show that the latest science supports the use of targeted colostrum, since it contains Transfer Factor.

Anxious to stretch Berk Bedell's funding of their trip, the trio dispensed with hiring a taxi and decided to walk the mile or so from the Spartanburg station to Fudenberg's house. Along the way, a car stopped beside them, and it was the Minnesota homicide expert assigned to the case, whom Johnson had informed of their trip. "Hop in", he said, "I know where you're going and I'll take you". So when the group arrived at Dr. Fudenberg's, it contained the accused, the defense lawyers, and an assistant to the prosecution. The latter was quite friendly, offered to videotape the entire four hours of the interview with Fudenberg, and provided copies of the tapes to the lawyers.

Just before the trial got underway in February 1994, the prosecution threw out all charges except the practice of medicine without a license. This reduced Saunders' maximum potential penalty from twenty-five years (fraud) to two years. The trial lasted for three weeks, the longest in the history of Watonwan County. Berkley Bedell testified. Maggie Hunt testified. Beth Grings' father testified in her behalf, as well as others more than satisfied with Herb Saunders' colostrum treatments. Lee Ross was called by the prosecution, but felt that her answers were helpful to Saunders. Dr. Fudenberg came and testified about Transfer Factor in colostrum. Noted medical researcher Dr. William Regelson of Richmond, Virginia, testified that colostrum contains pyrrol quinoline quinone (PQQ), a new vitamin and growth factor.

Immunologist Walter Clifford of Colorado Springs had come to Minnesota to testify for Saunders at a pre-trial "omnibus" hearing in late 1993. However, when the trial date rolled around, Clifford was laid low with an infection. Undaunted, Cal Johnson and Herb Saunders drove all one night to Colorado Springs to take Clifford's testimony on videotape. It was worth the trip. Clifford told the jury via video that what Saunders was doing is in fact old American folk medicine. He explained that Indians near where Clifford grew up knew that when someone was sick, they should look for a cow or a horse that had just given birth and drink the colostrum. Clifford took some of Saunders' colostrum for his infection. Highly experienced in live blood analysis, he then examined his own blood. Some of the favorable changes he observed were so rapid as to defy explanation.

One of the six jurors had lost her mother to a painful death from cancer shortly before the trial. Only hearing of people helped and not hurt, she remembered her mother's suffering from chemotherapy. She found it impossible to vote for conviction, so the trial ended with a five to one hung jury in March 1995.

The prosecution quickly announced that it would seek a new trial. Johnson and Miller prepared an appeal, partially based on the Minnesota Constitution's "Farmers' Amendment". Unique to Minnesota, it guarantees farmers the right to sell what they produce. The lawyers also cited the 9th Amendment to the U.S. Bill of Rights, sometimes called the Forgotten Amendment, since it has never been used. It states, "The enumeration in the Constitution of certain rights shall not be construed to deny or disparage others retained by the people". It did not occur to the Framers of the Constitution to enumerate a right to privacy, since it was taken for granted as retained by the people. It did not occur to the Framers to list the right to take whatever medical treatment one chooses, either from a recognized doctor (there were no licensed doctors in 1787), or even from a farmer. It did not occur to them that they needed to list such rights, since the Framers considered them to be retained by the people. That was the sense behind the 9th Amendment.

The appeals court rejected the Johnson-Miller appeal.

The second trial, in May 1996, lasted less than a week. Split three to three, the second jury was more hung than the first. Shortly after, County Attorney Birkholz, who had recommended Saunders to Johnson years before, gave up and dismissed the indictment.

English common law, the basis of the British and American legal systems, developed over centuries out of the accumulated decisions of judges and juries pronouncing their opinions on what was right and what was wrong. In 1926, deciding charges against Harry Hoxsey, a grand jury ruled that "It's not against the law to save people's lives; indictment not warranted". It may be that the Hoxsey and Herb Saunders decisions, among others, suggest that a new consensus is forming, in the long tradition of English common law. Just as it has long been recognized that war is too important to be left to the generals, perhaps the new consensus is that healing is too important to be left only to the doctors. Maybe a new consensus is forming to the effect that what is wrong is to hurt someone and that there is no wrong if people are helped, not hurt, whatever the credentials of the healer.

Founding Father Dr. Benjamin Rusk would probably have been pleased with the Herb Saunders decisions (and fascinated by the science). He might have said that such cases were exactly what he had in mind when he advocated placing in the Constitution a prohibition against any monopoly in the arts of healing.

Perhaps Herb Saunders' widely publicized trials, covered in the Nov/Dec 1996 issue of *The Sciences*, may raise public awareness of targeted colostrum as a particularly useful instrument of the healing arts. The awareness of ordinary colostrum is not new; in his later years, the first John D. Rockefeller drank only mother's milk.

In the 1974/75 *Nestle Research News*, an article concluded that "where breast feeding is not possible, supplementation with colostrum whey from hyperimmuinized cows is very desirable". Specially targeted colostrum products can quickly immunize babies from diarrhea-causing bacteria, which often do not respond to antibiotics.

In a book called *The Food Pharmacy*, author Jean Carpel cites the research of Dr. Robert H. Yolken, director of pediatric infectious diseases at Johns Hopkins Medical School. Yolken indicates that the same principle used to create colostrums targeted against specific microbes can be used in chickens to create similarly immunized eggs. Dr. Yolken points out that we can acquire immunity in two ways; active immunity, when our own bodies create the antibodies against antigens such as vaccines. (The effectiveness of vaccine-induced antibodies is generally thought to wear off after seven to ten years.) The second way, passive immunity, occurs when we take in antibodies created by other living creatures. Passive immunity does not last as long as active immunity, but it works. Dr. Yolken notes that in the 19th century, before antibiotics, passive immune therapy was widely used.

An article in the July 20, 1998 issue of *Business Week* reported on the millions of dollars being spent by genetic engineering companies to develop drug-producing rabbits, goats, cows, etc. Unfortunately, the best drugs which they could have such animals produce are unlikely to compare in effectiveness with targeted colostrums.

With new viruses and bacteria resistant to antibiotics, aren't the healing arts missing a bet? The Defense Department immunizes soldiers against anthrax, and some accept discharge rather than take the vaccine. It would be quick and inexpensive research to see if the targeted colostrum method could prepare a weapon against anthrax. Killed anthrax viruses could be injected into the udder of a cow about to "freshen", and three weeks later, a colostrum targeted specifically against anthrax would be available. Its effectiveness could quickly be tested in mice. The mice would be fed the colostrum and then "challenged" with anthrax, *i.e.*, exposed to the virus. Would they live? Would they die? Also, mice could be first "challenged" with the anthrax virus and then given the anthrax colostrum. Would they live? Would they die? It would be easy to find out.

The same procedure could be used with Strep A, a form of which caused a number of fatalities in Texas in 1998. The method could be used to provide colostrum targeted against variant E coli 0157:H7, a killer bacteria described in the August 3, 1998 issue of *Time* magazine's cover article "Anatomy of an Outbreak". The same mechanism could be used to develop a colostrum against new strains of tuberculosis resistant to antibiotics.

Lyme disease is caused by an organism called a spirochete, a different version of which causes syphilis. If a cow can produce antibodies effective against the Lyme spirochete, could it do the same for the type that causes syphilis? If the antibody factory from a cow's udder can provide a way to get rid of spirochetes, how about the parasites that cause malaria? Malaria is one of the greatest scourges on the planet, killing an estimated 2.7 million people a year (*Business Week*, September 21, 1998).

Targeted colostrums have been successfully tested by independent researchers against pseudomonas, salmonella, and cryptospiridium, the parasite that killed over a hundred people in

Milwaukee in 1993. *Medical Microbiology and Immunology* published a paper by T. Ebina and others in 1984 reporting that an anti-measles colostrum had produced significant improvement in 5 out of 7 multiple sclerosis patients. The herpes 6 virus has recently been implicated in MS, having been found in affected (but not in normal) brain tissue of deceased MS patients. Research with a colostrum targeted against herpes 6 as well as measles might offer hope for those suffering from this disease.

Making popcorn in her pajamas, Peggy Waldron leaned over the stove, her pajamas caught fire, and she was burned very badly. A pseudomonas infection set in which antibiotics were unable to control. Finally, the doctor told her family she only had about three days to live. Her father got hold of a colostrum targeted to contain antibodies against pseudomonas and gave it to her orally. Within 72 hours, instead of dying, Peggy rallied and had no more pseudomonas in her blood. She recovered completely.

With cancer fast becoming an epidemic, one of the most intriguing leads in the colostrum story was published in The *American Farm* magazine of March 1964 in an article by James O. Niess entitled "Immune Milk". Niess reported on a paper presented at an International Cancer Society meeting by Dr. B. Sekla of Charles University, Prague, Czechoslovakia. In his paper, one of a series of four, Dr. Sekla described injecting rat cancer tissue as an antigen into a cow. When the immune milk from the cow was fed to other rats, it was found to be impossible to give them cancer. Around 1970, Norman Shealy, MD, PhD, of the Shealy Institute in Springfield, Missouri, replicated Sekla's work.

Does the Prague research point the way to building immunity against cancer? This is simple research which the National Cancer Institute with its billions could pursue. Using tissues from various types of cancers as antigens to produce colostrums targeted against those cancers, would it be possible to create immunity to cancer via antibodies, Transfer Factor, or something else in colostrum as yet undiscovered? The 500,000 Americans due to die of cancer each year would like to know, and very likely don't care so much about how it works as, just does it work? If it does, then an intensive program over a decade could render Americans immune to cancer. Success in such a program would render the NCI obsolete, so such research should better be conducted at a private institution not involved in cancer, with no conflict of interest.

A study by the Stolle Co. showed that their immune milk blocked the formation of arterial plaque in rabbits on a high fat diet. Does the Stolle study point the way for a simple way to prevent vascular disease, America's biggest killer?

Canadian researcher Dr. Charles Mitchell found that Petersen's mechanism of udder immunization produced just as good results against viruses as against bacteria. Does this mean that targeted colostrums against the HIV virus, the Hanta virus, the Ebola, or the latest flu virus could be developed? The mechanism is rapid, the tests simple, and the product inexpensive.

The targeted colostrum method is revolutionary. How big is this revolution, potentially? What are the limits to the method? So far, no bacteria, viruses, or fungi have yet been found that are immune to the antibodies in colostrums targeted at them. No side effects have ever been reported from any targeted colostrum products, which apparently could replace many medicines.

It may be that the time has come for the general use of targeted colostrums to treat human illnesses, or to keep people well. Imagine that the U.S. had a really free market in non-toxic health products, both for humans and animals. Who would want to take increasingly ineffective antibiotics for a staph infection if there were the alternative of a product with antibodies against staph already prepared, courtesy of a friendly cow?

It may be that the Colostrum Story is just beginning. The method for creating targeted colostrums offers a simple way to cure diseases or, better still, to head them off. That would lower healthcare costs drastically by creating the "magic bullets" Dr. Paul Erlich talked about a century ago.

As Dr. Herb Struss puts it, "it may be that the greatest contribution of the cow to the human race has not yet been realized".

GASTON NAESSENS
The New Biology

When Congressman Berkley Bedell was healed from Lyme disease by a colostrum product, it was a great victory. However, his problems were far from over, since he had also been diagnosed with prostate cancer. In 1987, he underwent an operation to remove his prostate, as recommended by the cancer doctors. Hopefully, that would be the end of the problem.

In 1990, Bedell told a friend about his colostrum adventure and the prostate surgery. He added, "Some days I get awfully tired. I wonder if the cancer could be returning". "It's easy to find out", his friend replied. "You just need to go to Quebec and visit a French-born scientist named Gaston Naessens. He can tell the answer to your question by looking at your blood. He designed a microscope which is the best since Royal Rife's, and which enables him to perceive a great deal about what's going on inside our bodies. Naessens can observe certain live particles in everybody's blood which other researchers can't see, not having that good a microscope. He calls these particles 'somatids' and finds that they change form according to conditions inside the body. He has observed that certain somatid forms give an early warning signal for cancer by appearing in the blood months or even years before cancer actually shows up in the body. So Naessens' blood exam could tell you if the cancer is returning. The electron microscope only sees dead material, so it does not see somatids, which are alive. Naessens' technology is exciting because it permits observation of live blood, magnified enough so that you can see the action in the blood while it's taking place. He also has a product called '714-X' which strengthens the immune system, thus heading off the cancer. Then the threatening patterns in the blood reverse."

Berkley Bedell did not build the Berkley Corporation or get to be the first National Small Businessman of the Year or win six terms in Congress by letting grass grow under his feet. He asked his friend, "How soon could you set up an appointment?"

Two weeks later, Bedell visited Gaston Naessens at Rock Forest, a suburb of Sherbrooke, Quebec, two hours drive east of Montreal. Before flying to Quebec, Bedell read *The Life and Trials of Gaston Naessens, Galileo of the Microscope*, by Christopher Bird. The book is a dramatic story of Naessens and his discoveries presented in the context of a trial brought at the instigation of the Quebec Medical Corporation (Quebec's equivalent of the AMA).

The tall, courtly Naessens showed Bedell his "Somatoscope", as he calls his powerful microscope, and described the "somatids", the discovery it permits him to see. The blood of every healthy mammal contains three basic forms of somatids, he told Bedell. The three appear to be indispensable to the life process since they produce a particle responsible for cell division, a kind of growth hormone. Naessens has found that cell division is only possible in the presence of the three basic somatids, and ceases in their absence. In effect, they trigger life, since life depends on cell division. Nobel Laureate Alexis Carrel also found the same growth hormone, which he called a "trephone". In a healthy person, inhibitors in the blood regulate the trephones. However, in conditions of stress, trauma, or toxicity, the inhibitors diminish and excessive numbers of growth hormones appear. Then the normal somatid cycle of three begins to expand, evolving from one stage to the next, changing forms "pleomorphically", without going through the regular process of cell division. The cycle may thus expand to as many as sixteen, depending on the degree and nature of the stress to the body. "Years of clinical experience have shown me", Naessens told Bedell, "that in healthy people, there is a strong 'gate control' to keep the somatid cycle from expanding beyond the normal three. Presence of the advanced somatidian forms indicates that gate control is weak - *i.e.*, the gate is open, permitting disease to develop. Five factors can damage gate control: (1) toxic products, such as chemotherapy, or nicotine and tar; (2) physical shock or trauma: broken bones, surgery, radiation, bruises; (3) psychological shocks; (4) being in a bad relationship; (5) feeling hopeless; (6) some belief systems; as you think, so you are."

"I presented these discoveries, which I call Somatidian Orthobiology, to the Academy of Sciences in Paris in 1963, but my presentation was ignored. When the macrocycle includes all of the thirteen additional somatids", Naessens explained, "it is certain that the immune system is in a seriously weakened condition. It is highly likely that a person with the somatid macrocycle will develop a degenerative disease such as cancer within two years unless preventive steps are taken. Indeed, it could be said that when the macrocycle occurs, the body is trying to die; the environment inside the body has changed so drastically that cells can no longer divide normally and maintain life. If your somatid cycle is out of balance, the reasons could be food, spiritual, or emotional. The blood is the only place where one can see all these elements; if they are in balance, conditions in your body are such that cancer cannot occur. Everything in the blood has a purpose, and the somatids have a purpose, whether we understand them or not."

"It takes 90 hours for the macrocycle to complete", Naessens explained. "I found it before time-lapsed photography was invented, so I stayed at my microscope for 90 hours in order to observe the complete cycle." (This is even longer than Royal Rife stayed glued to his microscope.)

"These are the particles which the Somatoscope has permitted me to see", said the biochemist, "I have captured them in photos and in time-lapsed photography, and here is a chart I have prepared to illustrate them:"

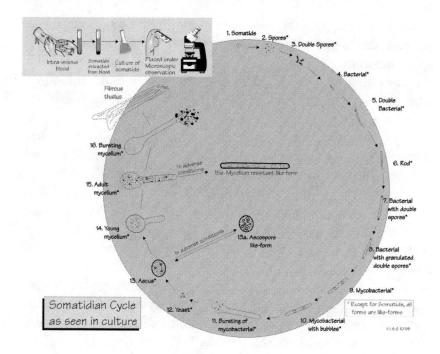

Somatidian Cycle as seen in culture

Describing the complete somatid cycle to his visitor, Naessens indicated the three normal ones: 1) basic somatids; 2) spores; 3) double spores. Then he showed the macrocycle, each one pleomorphically evolving out of the one immediately previous; 4) bacteria; 5) double bacteria; 6) little rods; 7) double spore bacteria; 8) granulated double spore bacteria; 9) and 10) mycobacteria with "bubbles"; 11) a bursting phase after which 12) yeast are produced which evolve into 13) ascospores which become 14) asci, which in turn put forth 15) filamentous thalli that after 16) bursting, dump back into the bloodstream a huge quantity of new somatids, which go on to produce an excess of growth hormones. The last three forms are fungal.

"My observation of this new particle revealed an unexpected phenomenon", said Naessens, "the capacity of a live particle to change its form in reaction to the immediate environment without going through the regular process of cellular division. This was a new vision of life. It was the true demonstration of polymorphism, a biological theory, proposed long before by various researchers, concerning this possibility of life to change form depending on the nature of the environment."

Naessens told Bedell, "Somatids are very curious entities, and can be seen under my microscope crossing the membrane of red blood cells. They are electrical in nature, they carry a negative charge, thus repelling each other, and are always in motion. It took me four years of experimentation before I finally found ways to extract them from the blood (of any mammal) and to culture them - *i.e.*, they can live independently outside the body in culture. I wondered what would happen if I added certain things to the culture. I started with an ideal environment in terms of nutrients, amino acids, and temperature. Then I changed the environment. When I created adverse conditions, I saw that the somatids developed into a resistant form which only occurs in culture, not in the blood. I have not yet found ways to destroy the resistant form, even after subjecting it to 50,000 rads of radiation, the equal of what you'd find at the heart of a nuclear reactor. Many years later, we looked at these resistant forms of somatids through an electron microscope at Sherbrooke University. After the liquid of the culture was drained away, these resistant somatids had become like a hard, red rock. The people at the University used up seven diamond drills before they could slice the material for viewing.

Somatids are carriers of some genetic information; in his book on Naessens, Christopher Bird called them precursors to DNA. In one of his experiments, Naessens explained to the Congressman, he took somatids from the blood of a white rabbit and injected them into the blood of a black rabbit. One-half of the black rabbit's fur then turned white, making it appear gray. Conversely, after he injected somatids from the black rabbit into the blood of the white rabbit, half of the latter's hair turned black, making it too appear gray. Still using the same rabbits, each containing the other's somatids, he took a patch of skin from the white rabbit and grafted it onto the back of the black rabbit. It was not rejected, as such a graft normally would be.

"Wait", Bedell interrupted, "wouldn't that be very important for organ transplants?" "Exactly", Naessens responded, "and now I'll tell you about another experiment. I injected a concentration of rat somatids into a cube of fresh rat meat, put it into a sterilized jar under vacuum and set it over there in my lab window - in 1978. Not only does the meat not rot", he told Bedell, "but it has continued to grow."

Existing in the liquids of all living organisms, both animal and vegetable, somatids are even found in mineral deposits, Naessens continued. Some geologists have called them nannobacteria. Naessens stated that he suspects somatids are a bridge between energy and matter, acting as transducers, condensing various forms of energy into matter. In effect, they appear to be the first materialization of energy. They almost seem eternal. "Indeed", he added, "the somatids from our bodies continue their work after our death, bringing our bodies to the decay stage. They transform our flesh, eventually reducing our remains into basic mineral elements. Present at the moment of conception, they last until our bodies have returned to their basic original elements. The somatids are essential at all stages of our life cycle - from dust to dust. In the dust from our bones or ashes after we die are somatids which were swimming around in our bloodstreams while we were alive."

Bedell asked "How long have you been studying somatids?" "Since I put together the Somatoscope in 1949", the scientist replied.

"I have been studying blood for more than fifty years", Naessens continued, "I was always fascinated by blood. In 1945, after receiving a degree in biological engineering, I opened a private laboratory in fundamental research. I was then performing conventional blood tests and doing intensive research in biology. Curious by nature, I wanted to explore the world of microscopy. At first, this was only a hobby, a challenge. Soon it became a passion, to the extent that some years later, I designed a light microscope that could achieve a magnification of 30,000 times and, even more important, a resolution in the range of 150 angstroms.

"With the incredible sharpness of detail provided by this new capability, I began examining all sorts of live samples - maple sap, dragonflies, and, of course, human blood. To my surprise, I noticed in the blood of all mammals a tiny brilliant particle, moving around in a very particular fashion. This particle was unknown at that time, nowhere mentioned in the scientific literature. As I suspected, the particle was alive, but I found that its growth pattern was altogether different. From a tiny particle, it evolved systematically from one step to another, as I've already explained, repeatedly reproducing a constant cycle, within a 90-hour time frame. To be quite sure of what I was seeing, I repeated the experiment over and over, hundreds of times. Each time, the same pattern, the same cycle. And that is how I discovered the somatids. When I first saw them, I realized that some of them were forms I had seen over the years in the blood of very sick people. Those trained in the Pasteur concept of looking for a specific microbe for each disease might have seized on some of these somatidian forms, thinking 'Here is the cause of (x) disease'. But these were not true external bacteria; they were coming from within the body and kept evolving pleomorphically from one form into another.

"From the beginning," Naessens told Bedell, "my work has been focused on the functioning of the human organism as a whole, especially on the organism's 'terrain', in other words, its internal environment. My research has not won acceptance because the medical establishment and I speak entirely different languages. Their cancer treatments have concentrated on the destruction of the cancer cell, yet cancer is the direct result of disequilibrium in the organism as a whole; repression has no long-term effect on cancer cells. Since 1949, I have defined cancer not as a localized disease which spreads but a generalized disease which becomes localized, a very important distinction. In some circles, my work has been called the New Biology.

"Every day", Naessens explained, "the body produces cancer cells. If a person is healthy, the immune system - the macrophages, phagocytes, lymphocytes, leucocytes, cytokines such as interleukin and interferon, and the NK (natural killer) cells - all these parts of the immune system dispose of the cancer cells we routinely make every day as a matter of course. However, if conditions have changed the internal environment and weakened the immune system, cancer cells may succeed in proliferating and forming a critical mass, a tumor. After its transition from a normal cell, a cancer cell behaves like a nitrogen trap, drawing nitrogen from healthy cells. While doing this, it simultaneously produces a Co-Carcinogenic K Factor (CCKF) which has the unfortunate capability of interfering with, and even paralyzing the immune system's work. At that point, once the CCKF has been produced, the somatid cycle goes into 16 stages and the growth hormones it produces (the trephones) are found in far greater quantities in the blood. They then stimulate cell division and specifically the proliferation of cancer cells.

"The concept of the CCKF did not originate with me", said Naessens, "but with Dr. Paul Nenoix, a distinguished 19th century French scientist. This factor has not been identified chemically, but is believed to be responsible for virtually paralyzing the immune system." Observing white blood cells, the immune system's first line of defense, Naessens sees them unable to move in the blood of cancer victims.

"When life was first triggered," Nacssens continued, "nitrogen was basic, so I wanted to introduce more nitrogen. Even if there is no cancer, the body needs nitrogen. So, I thought, if I can supply nitrogen to the body and combine it with some other product having a greater affinity for cancer cells than for normal ones, I might be able to arrest the production of this toxic CCKF that paralyzes the natural defenses and thus I might halt the evolution of cancerous cells in their tracks. Through research, I found that camphor is more attracted to cancer cells than to healthy ones. Then my challenge was to combine a molecule of nitrogen with one of camphor. I succeeded and that was how 714-X was born.

"My theory was that the camphor-nitrogen molecules would be attracted to cancer cells and over-supply them with nitrogen. Then, I hoped, those cells would no longer draw nitrogen from healthy cells, and would become so 'drunk' on nitrogen that they would relax and stop producing CCKF. During the 21-day cycle when 714-X is given every day, the malevolent influence of the CCKF is cancelled. The immune system is reinvigorated and returns to its regular business of getting rid of cancer and other abnormal cells. Incidentally, DNA, too, needs nitrogen, and I have found that 714-X repairs DNA.

"I injected 714-X into the lymph system of cats stricken with lymphoma. In less than two weeks, their cancers were all absorbed. In confirmation, their somatid cycles (which were at the 16-stage) returned to the normal 3-stage. In 1978, tests were carried out establishing the non-toxicity of 714-X. A patent was granted in 1980, with the product baptized as camphorminium chloride.

"The lymph system is the body's drainage and sewer system and is the optimal conduit for cancer metastases. Therefore I have used that route for the injection of 714-X, which is done through a lymph node in the groin for 21 days. During that period, any cancer cells travelling through the lymph system, seeking another place to establish themselves, are destroyed by the body's reestablished immune system. Thus all organs not already afflicted with cancer are protected from further metastases. In sick people, the lymph tends to clog up like jelly. Then, progressively, its drainage stops, just as a vacuum cleaner won't clean if it's clogged. The lymph liquefies and starts moving and draining again within one hour after injection of 714-X, which is like a drano for the lymph. Also, many toxins lurk in the lymph. 714-X, which could be called a deep cellular cleanser, flushes them out by bringing them into the circulating blood, which in turn carries them to the elimination organs. Only small doses are given (.5 cc/day). This dosage was arrived at after clinical experimentation. More is not better; larger doses could dump toxins out of the lymph too rapidly and overwhelm the liver and the organs of elimination. Happily, the product is completely non-toxic and causes no negative side effects. If 714-X is used before a cancerous mass appears, it acts as an inhibitor of the trephones, or growth hormones, which are produced in excessive quantities in the unbalanced body.

"The lymph channels operate with the blood vessels. Thus when the lymph is restored to normalcy by 714-X, it depends on the blood vessels to carry the lymph (and the immune particles it carries) to the tumor, flooding it with immune cells. Since shark cartilage operates on the principle of inhibiting the very blood cells upon which 714-X depends, shark cartilage cannot be taken with 714-X.

"But", Naessens cautioned, "714-X is not a panacea. Strictly speaking, it cures nothing. It has no direct effect at all on cancerous growths themselves (this is why orthodox medicine disdains it, for they seek something that kills cancer cells). What this medicine does is to reestablish the body's natural immune system, so that it can go back to its normal function of killing cancer cells. Like any medicine, it works better when given early. Sometimes it works at a late stage - and sometimes not, if the immune system has been destroyed (as after chemotherapy) and the disease process has become irreversible.

"After many years of hard research", Naessens summed up, "it was possible to find a statistical correlation between the state of degenerative disease and the presence of such-and-such somatidian forms. This research gave rise to my present test in live blood analysis. Subtle biological changes which are precursors to cancer and other degenerative diseases are visible only in fresh, live blood. When these are detected early, then it is possible to deal with the problem. Thus I think of my test not as diagnosis, but as an early screening for unfavorable conditions. We could call it an early warning system.

"Now", said Naessens, "if you would like, I will take a drop of your blood and we shall see the condition of your somatids. This test can only be done with fresh blood", he explained. "One day I hope to develop a compound which will preserve blood in its fresh state so that anyone anywhere can send in a blood sample for examination."

Placing a drop of Berkley Bedell's blood on a slide, Naessens projected the image from the Somatoscope onto a video screen. "I don't like what I see", he said. "There are too many forms of somatids; your 'gate control' is down. You are well into the macrocycle. Look, here are the ascus and the mycelium somatid forms. According to my research, this would indicate that your immune system is quite weak and that there could indeed be a danger of the cancer returning."

Berk Bedell decided to take Gaston Naessens' 714-X. Expecting that his doctor in Iowa could do the injections, he found, to the contrary, that his doctor had never heard of intra-lymphatic injection. In fact, he didn't know anybody who had, since it is not taught in medical schools. Bedell located a doctor who knew the procedure, boarded another plane, and learned how to find the exact place in the groin where injection into the lymph system is done. He then proceeded to inject himself for two series of 714-X: once a day for twenty-one days, a week off, and then the second twenty-one day series.

Six months after his first visit, he returned to Naessens for a follow-up blood exam. When Gaston Naessens again looked at Bedell's blood, he said "Regardez" (as his wife translated from the French in which he is more comfortable). "Your somatid cycle has returned to normal."

The tiredness (which had suggested to Bedell that he might have a problem) was gone, along with those threatening additional 13 stages of the somatid cycle. He felt fine, played tennis and golf regularly, and maintained a vigorous schedule. Until a member of his family learned the Naessens method of live blood analysis, Berkley Bedell returned to Rock Forest, Quebec, every six months for Naessens to look at his blood. A few years later, at a time when the Office of Alternative Medicine, his "baby", was not going at all well, the dangerous macrocycle again reappeared.

Bedell immediately took another 21-day course of 714-X and his somatid pattern again returned to normal.

Convinced that 714-X had averted a recurrence of prostate cancer, Bedell told his story in Washington and persuaded several officials to visit Naessens. On his next trip, he was accompanied by Dr. William Robb, acting head of the National Institutes of Health (NIH), one of Robb's colleagues, and a member of Iowa Senator Tom Harkin's staff. They saw the Somatoscope, saw the somatids and their cycles, heard of their significance, and learned about 714-X.

"Do other microbiologists see some of these particle that you see?" Bedell asked. "Only a few", Naessens replied, "since their microscopes are not able to look at live material. However, the main problem is that they have not been taught about life forms changing 'pleomorphically' according to the internal environment of the body. Accordingly, what they do see they dismiss as fibrin formation or 'artifacts', which to them means 'just stuff'. No one has ever explained where all these 'artifacts' come from on carefully prepared sterile slides", Naessens commented dryly.

Medically speaking, Naessens explained, people with the 16-stage somatid cycle cannot be called sick because a degenerative illness may not yet have manifested in the body. But if the cycle is not brought back to normal, after 12 to 18 months the body becomes more and more exhausted to the point where any additional stress can lead to the development of abnormal cells, with the ultimate consequence of a cancerous mass. "Remember", he told the Washington visitors, "somatidian forms are never the cause of a disease, but only an indicator, a witness. Just as a red light doesn't cause an accident unless you don't stop, somatids are an indication of danger; slow down, take precautions."

After their return to Washington, nothing further was heard from the NIH. Their reluctance to investigate further might have been based on the fact that his 714-X has long been on the American Cancer Society's blacklist of "unproven" therapies. Or perhaps the concept was too new, or too "far-out" from the way they had been trained.

How did Gaston Naessens develop what may be the world's most powerful microscope and several new pharmaceuticals? Born in 1924 to a well-to-do family in northern France, he showed an inventive streak early on that amazed and sometimes even alarmed his family. When very young, he built his own motorcycle and then an airplane just large enough to carry him. His mother thought it sensible to burn it before the young Gaston could make his maiden flight.

On the eve of World War II, Naessens was intensively study-ing physics, chemistry, and biology at the University of Lille. When the war broke out and the northern part of France was occupied, professors and students were evacuated to the south of France, where Naessens' education continued. In 1945, he was awarded a degree in biological engineering from the Union Nationale Scientifique Francaise, the provisional organization under which his education had been conducted. With the same attitude toward degrees as Royal Rife, Naessens never bothered to obtain an "equivalence", or diploma, from the de Gaulle gov-ernment after the war. Similarly, Rife never bothered to write a letter which would have won him an honorary doctorate from the University of Southern California. For both, knowledge and dis-coveries were more important than certificates.

As a science student, Naessens was bothered by the low res-olution power of light microscopes. In an article entitled "Blood Feud", which appeared in the December 1992 issue of the *Toronto Star's* newsmagazine *Saturday Night*, Paul William Roberts tells of how Naessens came across the idea which led to his unusual microscope:

> *Searching the literature for research on blood and microscopy, Naessens learned of a nineteenth century French biologist now best known as the 'noon lunatic'. Emile Doyen claimed to have observed through an ordi-nary microscope particles in human blood which were visible only around noon during the months of May and June. Naessens...began to wonder whether there was any scientific explanation of Doyen's findings. There was; during May and June in the south of France and at around noon, the natural light available to anyone using a microscope contained far more ultraviolet light than at any other time of the year.*

The work of the noon lunatic became the basis of the microscope Naessens went on to develop in the late 1940's, working in a lab funded by his mother at the family home in Lyons... Naessens' microscope, which identified particles with light refraction instead of staining, could approach 30,000 X magnification with living tissue at a resolution of 150 angstroms (one angstrom is one-hundred-millionth of a centimeter).

Once he had conceived the idea of using ultraviolet light, inspired by the "noon lunatic", Naessens consulted with German artisans who had worked for the Leitz optical company before the war. They helped him with arrangements of lenses and mirrors. However, electronic manipulation of the light, the key to the microscope, was the idea of Gaston Naessens, who has been called an electronics genius.

In a speech at Sherbrooke, Quebec in September 1989, Naessens described his microscope:

Through various electromagnetic procedures of my own devising, I was able to decrease the wavelength of light, which, in turn, permitted me to achieve a microscopic resolution of 150 angstroms. Consequently, I was able to see particles with dimensions as small as 150 angstroms. In so doing, I achieved a resolution 14 times superior to that attainable with the best optical microscopes currently utilized in laboratories. With my new microscope, I was able to see in fresh blood extremely tiny living organisms, smaller than viruses, measuring 150 angstroms in size. These entities I have christened somatids, based on the Greek for 'essential bodies'.

In *Galileo of the Microscope*, Christopher Bird quotes an article which appeared in a Quebec journal, *Guides Ressources*, which describes the Naessens microscope:

Two light sources, the first an incandescent one with a wave-length of about 3600 angstroms, the second an ultra-violet one with a wave-length of about 2200 angstroms, beat against each other to produce a third wave-length which passes through a monochromatic filter to produce a monochromatic ray. This ray is next exposed to magnetic fields - Zeeman effect - that divide it to produce numerous parallel rays that, in turn, pass through a Kerr cell that increases the frequency. It is this light source, invisible to the naked eye, that strikes the specimen slides. The image is reconstituted by the microscope. The principle of Naessens' microscope is that the shorter the luminous wavelength, the greater is the possibility of observing infinitely small detail. M. Naessens estimates it would cost $100,000 or more to make a similar microscope.

Without their extraordinary microscopes, neither Royal Rife nor Gaston Naessens could have made their discoveries. Medical science pays a high cost for not being able to see the tiniest of microorganisms in their live state, instead of after they're dead, which is the limitation of the electron microscope. Current researchers in microbiology are stuck in a false understanding of the nature of microorganisms, and people die as a result.

Naessens' super-scope permits him to see the pleomorphism of the somatid cycle, one form changing into another as the result of internal conditions in the body. Similarly Royal Rife wrote in 1953, "This BX virus (which he had determined in animal experiments to be capable of causing cancer) can be readily changed into different forms of its life cycle by the media (or broth) in which it is grown". Rife stated that a variation of as little as two parts per million in the media was sufficient to trigger the change.

Thus the somatid cycle can be changed from normal to abnormal by tiny variations within the body, caused by toxins, stress, or even emotions such as anxiety.

After first constructing his microscope, Naessens noted that the blood of healthy people was radically different from the blood of sick people. He found sixteen somatids in the blood of cancer victims, as compared with three in normal people. Then his challenge was to find some pharmaceutical which could return the somatid cycle to normal. His first product was called GN-24. It was capable of transforming lecithin within the body to something capable of destroying cells in states of extreme fragility - specifically, cancer cells - and it helped to boost the immune system. This was distributed by a Swiss laboratory from 1950 to 1960.

In 1950 he tried another tack and combined cultures of cancerous blood taken from people with both positive and negative A, B, and O blood types. Injecting the cultures into horses, after 45 days he recovered anti-cancer antibodies, which caused cancer to disappear in cancerous mice. This product, called Anablast, was patented in France in 1961 and sold by Swiss and German pharmacies. Naessens found his second anti-cancer medicinal to have more generalized effects than GN-24, restoring the somatid cycle to normal and even reversing certain types of leukemia. Commercial success permitted him to realize the dream of any young Frenchman, a move to Paris. However, this put him more in the spotlight. To his dismay, Naessens found that his discoveries were not greeted with open arms. To the contrary, he was charged with practicing medicine without a license and forced to pay a heavy fine. Much equipment was confiscated and his lab was sealed. He moved to the island of Corsica, a corner of France in the Mediterranean which he hoped would be quieter. Soon his patients followed him there, and the medical authorities were not far behind.

While in Paris, Naessens had saved from cancer the wife of an officer of the French police (the Surete). In 1965, the officer told Naessens that the sole purpose of an upcoming investigation was to put him out of circulation. He took the officer's advice and immediately moved to Quebec, leaving everything behind except critical parts of his microscope.

Working for several years in various aspects of electronics,

Naessens got back on track in 1971 when he was befriended by David Stewart, heir to a large tobacco fortune and head of the Stewart-McDonald Foundation in Montreal. Stewart was determined to find a cure for cancer, but thus far had only funded orthodox research, *i.e.*, the search for ways to kill cancer cells. Stewart was intrigued by Naessens' somatid cycle and his concept of strengthening the immune system and letting it kill the cancer cells. However, the Quebec medical authorities had heard from their French counterparts and warned Stewart against Naessens. Stewart decided to fund Naessens anyway but suggested he do his research away from Montreal. Marrying Francoise Bonin, a lab technician, Naessens and his wife moved to her family's house on the banks of the Magog river in Rock Forest, installing a lab in the basement for his research.

In 1972, David Stewart asked the McMaster University Medical School in Hamilton, Ontario, to undertake a project to confirm Naessens' somatid findings. The project got off to a problematic start when Dr. Peter Dent, representing the University, learned of Naessens' problems in France. However, it was not Dent but Dr. Daniel Perey, a young assistant professor of pathology and surgery, who was to conduct the research. At Perey's recommendation, the Foundation purchased special equipment which allowed Naessens to make a photographic record of what he was seeing through his microscope. Paul Roberts in his 1992 article quoted a letter Perey wrote in 1972 in support of Naessens, "The scope and insight which Mr. Naessens has brought to this area of research potentially stand to benefit mankind and may be a source of pride for Canada". In a September 1972 report to David Stewart, Dr. Perey wrote (as quoted in Christopher Bird's *Galileo of the Microscope*), "that he had been struck almost 'dumb' by the somatid cycle and its tremendous pleomorphism... Perey noted 'beyond the shadow of a doubt' that whereas 'normal bugs' (the first three stages of the somatid cycle) had appeared in the blood of 'normal' rats unafflicted with cancer, 'abnormal bugs' (the successive thirteen more stages in the cycle) had appeared in the blood of rats which had received transplantable cancer tumors. Even more striking was Perey's astonishment that 'while each of the separate forms showed some characteristics of organisms well-known in standard microbiology - bacteria, fungi, and viruses - the big difference was that, far from living independently from one another, they had all seemed to derive from one bug.'" Perey confirmed Gaston Naessens' findings that the thirteen additional members of the somatid macrocycle all evolve from the one immediately before it - pleomorphically.

After Perey's appreciative review of Naessen's work, he was sidelined from the project and other researchers with their own agenda were put in charge. McMaster University Medical School eventually wrote Stewart a very negative report. Curiously and unexpectedly, Perey died soon after, following a tennis game.

In *Blood Feud*, Paul Roberts reported that:

> *In 1974...Dr. Raymond Keith Brown, consultant to the Memorial Sloan Kettering Cancer Center in New York, visited Rock Forest. Brown wrote a memo to his directors stating, 'What I have seen is a microscope that reveals with spectacular clarity the motion and multiplicity of pleomorphic organisms in the blood which are intimately associated with disease states. The implications... are staggering... It is imperative that what its inventor, a dedicated biological scientist, is doing be totally reviewed. I am convinced that he is an authentic genius and that his achievements cut across and illumine some of the most pertinent areas of medical science. If the review of his work is confirmatory, this man should be brought to New York and given unlimited support and facilities to continue his research.'*
>
> *Dr. Brown returned to Rock Forest with an oncologist and a microscopist from Sloan Kettering. The three eventually drafted and signed a second and longer memorandum that reiterated the first. These two memos generated much*

excitement among the hierarchy at the celebrated center until someone noticed that Naessens' name appeared on the American Cancer Society's blacklist. Immediately, the memoranda were rejected, the concerns of cancer bureaucrats outweighing the first-hand observations of expert scientists.

In 1978, Christopher Bird, best-selling co-author of the *Secret Life of Plants*, heard of Gaston Naessens from Dr. Eva Reich, daughter of the late Dr. Wilhelm Reich. Already having researched Royal Rife, Bird had a solid background in biology and was fascinated by Naessens, his microscope, and his somatids. Bird's wife, Lois, was then convalescing from a brain tumor operation, After meeting Naessens, Bird flew with his wife to Rock Forest. Examining her blood, Naessens found the somatid macrocyle. The operation hadn't "gotten it all"; Lois still had cancer. After taking several courses of 714-X, her blood cleared and she began to regain her strength. Then one morning at breakfast, she collapsed. She died a day later from a massive brain hemorrhage caused by after-effects of the operation to remove the tumor. An autopsy showed no signs of cancer.

Chris Bird introduced many of his scientist friends to Naessens. One was Jan Merta de Velehrad, PhD, then living in Scotland. Merta had escaped from Prague, Czechoslovakia in 1968 a few jumps ahead of the Soviet tanks which put an end to the "Prague Spring", a momentary thaw in the Cold War. Brilliantly educated, Merta had studied not only Dr. William Koch and his work, but Royal Rife's as well. The Wellcome Museum in London has a Rife microscope, apparently the one Rife sold to Dr. B. Winter Gonin, physician to the Royal Family. Jan Merta has in his files a letter from the Wellcome Museum authorizing him to do research with its Rife microscope whenever he wishes.

Merta was visiting Naessens' lab one day when David Stewart was displaying immense frustration at finding so little interest in Gaston Naessens' work in any academic institution. He told Merta, "When I bring up the name Naessens, the atmosphere becomes frigid... I can say categorically that most scientific researchers with whom I have had to deal are highly opinionated, arrogant, condescending, and have built-in, insurmountable prejudices. While showing not the slightest desire to learn Naessens' techniques, they were nevertheless not loathe to brush aside his findings without having any knowledge whatsoever about them." (Christopher Bird)

On another occasion at Naessens' lab, Merta met a man who had brought his son. The boy had bone cancer and an appointment to have a leg amputated. The boy took 21 days of 714-X and the cancer was going away. Merta later learned that the boy's mother did not believe in "alternative" treatments and snatched the boy away, taking him to California. A doctor there said that since the cancer was in remission, it was a good time to amputate, and did so.

From the start, David Stewart was a staunch supporter of Naessens. Then in 1984, David Stewart returned from a trip to Switzerland quite ill, entered a hospital and died quickly from a rare viral infection. However, funding from his foundation continued. Because of David Stewart's wealth, prestige, and his support of Naessens, the Quebec Medical Corporation held back while Stewart was alive. Once Stewart was gone, it was a different matter. On December 13, 1984, Quebec Surete police and agents of the Quebec Medical Corporation raided Naessens' lab, seizing vials of 714-X and numerous patients' files.

With the help of his wife, Francoise, Naessens was then operating a low-profile clinic in his home, providing daily treatments of 714-X to numerous patients. Naessens thus had constant access to their blood tests, which allowed him to study their progress and the somatid pattern that accompanied it. He did not charge a fee, but would accept voluntary donations when patients wished to make them. He regarded the clinic more as an opportunity to do research than a way to earn a living. Naessens recalls this period as one of the happiest of his life.

It took the Quebec Medical Corporation until 1989 to act.

One day in late May of that year, Naessens arrived home to find his yard filled with journalists, tipped off that Gaston Naessens was to be arrested. Hustled off to jail, he was thrown into a filthy cell for 24 hours until released the next day on $10,000 bail. The charge against Naessens was for being an accessory to murder, with a potential penalty of 25 years. Naessens was 65 in 1989, so that would be a veritable death sentence. What had happened was that a Mme. Langlais had come to him with very advanced breast cancer after emphatically refusing breast removal, chemotherapy, and radiation. Unfortunately, it was too late and she died. Discovering her file among those seized in the 1985 raid, the Quebec Medical Corporation persuaded her husband to file charges against Naessens even though he knew that his late wife was totally unwilling to take conventional treatments. The Medical Corporation alleged that Naessens had promised Mme. Langlais a cure and had dissuaded her from taking orthodox treatments, which, it asserted, might have cured her. Therefore, the Medical Corporation reasoned, that meant he had contributed to her death and was an accessory to murder.

A Committee for the Support of Gaston Naessens was quickly formed under the leadership of Ralph Ireland, a local sculptor. When Naessens was arraigned at Sherbrooke courthouse on June 27, over a hundred demonstrators gave him an ovation. They carried signs reading "Freedom of Speech, Freedom of Medical Choice, Freedom in Canada"; "Long Live Real Medicine; Down with Medical Power"; "Cancer and AIDS Research in Shackles While a True Discoverer is Jailed!"; and "Thank You, Gaston, for Saving My Life".

Chris Bird described in his *Galileo of the Microscope* how for the next two hours, over a dozen former cancer patients, given up for dead by their doctors, told about their lives being saved by Gaston Naessens. Roland Caty told of having developed adenosarcoma of the prostate while in Africa, and of being advised to have all his sexual organs removed. When he refused, the surgeon told him he was crazy and would be dead in three months. Caty already knew Naessens, got hold of 714-X, learned to inject himself in the groin, and returned to his job in Africa. "And here I am testifying to you", he told the press, "eleven years after I got well!" Jean-Hubert Eggerman, a Belgian, told how intestinal cancer had spread to his liver. Chemotherapy made him so sick he decided to give up and die, but then he met Naessens.

Starting 714-X in February 1989, he said, "Now I feel fine". Then he described how undercover agents he presumed to be hired by the Medical Corporation visited him and insisted on entering his house without a search warrant, looking for vials of 714-X. "How the hell did those goons get my name or my confidential medical file?" Eggerman demanded. "When am I and the rest of us going to win the right to be treated as we see fit?"

Next, Bird wrote, was Bernard Baril, a Quebec catering consultant who had tested positive for AIDS. Cancerous growths began to fill his mouth and doctors at Montreal General Hospital said he was too far gone to be worth treating, his weight declining from 155 to 115. He met Gaston Naessens in April 1988 and started 714-X. Within three months, his lesions began to disappear. "Look at me", he told the press conference, "I now weigh 170 pounds! I feel entirely fit! Don't I look in the pink of health?"

On July 8, a second demonstration was held in Sherbrooke, and the *Sherbrooke Tribune* reported that Naessens was gathering impressive scientific, medical, and international support in his battle. A doctor told how she had flown from Belgium for the rally because 714-X had helped her patients. Dr. Ray Brown, who had urged Sloan Kettering to support Naessens, came to testify. He told about a patient he had treated with 714-X who had recovered from pancreatic cancer that had resisted all other treatments. Bacteriological expert Walter Clifford summed things up by stating, "Sad as it is, my scientific colleagues and I have found to our bitter dismay that if you don't 'toe the company line', medical pundits don't even want to know about your medical discoveries, no matter what they might be." At the press conference, Conrad Chapdelaine, Naessens' attorney, read a letter from Reynaud Vignal, former French Consul General in Quebec, to his old friend, the Quebec Minister of Justice. Vignal wrote how his wife, Anne, had been diagnosed with leukemia and given not more than five years to live. Then they had the fortune to meet Gaston Naessens. Now, wrote Vignal, "five years later, Anne is well and we have a healthy baby son which we were told she could never have after the chemotherapy she took." (*op. cit.*)

Finally, Gaston Naessens addressed the group. "As I go over the last forty years", he said, "I believe I can say without boastfulness and looking you all straight in the eye, 'Mission accomplished!' For if there were in this room or anywhere a single patient whose life was extended for one, two, five, or ten years due to my treatment, I would be prepared to go on the long and difficult trek I have made all over again." (*op. cit.*)

Because of the effectiveness of 714-X against AIDS, Naessens was invited to speak at a Montreal gay organization on September 21. He declared that "A state of necessity justifies urgent measures, even if they do not conform to existing regulations. Would you allow someone to drown, even if you had to pass through and trespass upon 'off limits' property to save the person?" (*op. cit.*)

The Naessens told Chris Bird that on the day before the trial began in November, 1989, a Quebec Surete detective appeared at their door. He handed them his card, and asked Naessens to get in touch with a colleague's relative to tell her how to obtain 714-X.

Commented Bird, "So while the whole of the Quebec legal system was doing its best to send Naessens to jail, one of its representatives was pleading for a cure the prosecutor was trying to uphold as phoney! This was like foxes, intent on raiding a chicken coop, deciding instead to consult King Rooster about their problems!" (*op. cit.*)

Chris Bird moved to Sherbrooke for the trial. Completely fluent in French (as well as Russian and Serbo-Croatian), Bird sat at the press table every day of the trial, taking copious notes.

At first the situation looked black for Naessens, Bird wrote in his book. The press headlined "714-X Shown to be Ineffective" after a doctor reported it had no effect in dogs. Then it turned out that he had not injected into the lymph but directly into the tumor, as though it was a cancer cell killer. Prosecution witness Dr. Lorenzo Hache, a cancer surgeon, stated that he was most surprised when Mme. Langlais failed to show up for a scheduled mastectomy. He added "We often send out police to locate such reluctant patients." Discussing Naessens' blood test, Hache stated that "we don't even know what kind of examination M. Naessens is making here". Chris Bird commented, "If the doctors don't know, why don't they find out?" Conrad Chapdelaine got Hache to admit that Mme. Langlais was in an extremely advanced stage of cancer. The prosecution's case depended on showing that Mme. Langlais was not already a hopeless case before she sought Naessens; he could not be held guilty of her death if she was already terminal.

At the Naessens' house, wrote Bird (*op. cit.*), "the scene was unimaginable. Cancer and AIDS victims calling from Quebec, from the United States, calls from sufferers who needed no attendance at any medical school to know that the whole orthodox medicine system might send them to their grave, after having preliminarily reached into their pockets, or into the tills of their insurance companies, for the average $50,000 it is estimated that a cancer patient must spend on fruitless treatments before his or her eventual demise."

The opening remarks of Dr. Boivin, representing the Stewart-McDonald Foundation, were, "I am orthodox and therefore biased." He remarked that when he had first looked into Naessens microscope ten years earlier, "I saw a whole new world". Bird noted that Boivin never bothered to take a second look. Boivin told the court that he had advised Stewart against renewing Naessens' grants.

Then it was the turn of the defense. Conrad Chapdelaine's first witness was Dr. Michel Fabre, a handsome young doctor who had flown over from France to testify. Fabre presented a particularly graphic analogy on the Naessens treatment. Wrote Bird (*op. cit.*):

Likening the appearance of cancer cells in the body to the appearance of a swarm of mosquitoes in an outdoor locale, the doctor said that traditional medicine sought only to destroy offending cells - through surgery, radiation, or chemotherapy - just as one might attempt to get rid of the mosquito swarm by spraying it with insecticides.

A hopeless task, Fabre continued, because just as mosquitoes come out of a swamp favorable to their breeding and generation, so cancerous cells develop in a bodily milieu, or terrain, favoring such development. It was therefore Naessens' aim not to seek to annihilate the mosquitoes (the cancer cells) one by one, but to eradicate the swampy conditions that had led them to develop in the first place. Chronic disease was closely linked to a morass-like condition in the body.

As for Naessens' principle discovery of the somatid and its many forms, all made possible by the invention of a unique microscope, the physician stated that he believed that this discovery was more important than any made by Pasteur in the past century.

The jurors, who had looked wooden during most of the prosecution's case, began to come alive, Bird noted.

Fabre told the jury what had led him to Naessens. A Parisian woman in her forties developed melanoma of the eye. Doctors in Paris, London, and San Francisco advised her to have the eye removed, but she refused. Hearing of Naessens, she visited him, started 714-X, and within a year her cancer disappeared. One of Fabre's own patients, he testified, "came down with lung cancer in 1988, refused to be operated, and instead took the 714-X. He's now in perfect shape". Fabre also reported that he was seeing steady progress in a patient with multiple sclerosis who had the disease for ten years.

Chapdelaine's next witness, Gerald Godin, was already well-known to everyone in the courtroom. He had served as minister in the Quebec government and also as a member of its provincial parliament. His fight against cancer had been featured just a week before in *7 Jours*, a popular Montreal news magazine. Operated on for a brain tumor in 1984, he was left unable to speak. After learning to talk again, the original tumor returned and he was operated a second time in July 1989. He took extensive radiation and chemotherapy from August 9 to September 28, but neither those nor the operation did any good. Then he electrified the courtroom by announcing what *7 Jours* did not know when it went to press: he "decided, as a last resort, to put himself in the hands of Gaston Naessens and take the 714-X treatment... From the end of September to October 20, Godin received intralymphatic injections of 714-X in the groin... 'I felt much more energetic and vigorous', he testified. So vigorous, in fact, that he was able to undertake an arduous election campaign and go on to win. On October 23, Godin's blood was examined... Naessens was able to tell him that his blood picture had returned to normal. Furthermore, Godin revealed that tests with a scanner had shown that a cancerous mass which doctors had been unable to remove had shrunk by 60%." (Bird, *op. cit.*)

Another defense witness was Helmuth Walleczek from Austria. Diagnosed in 1978 with a hopeless case of kidney cancer which had spread to his liver, he learned of Naessens, flew to Quebec, took 714-X, and regained his health. Austrian cancer experts declared him cancer-free.

Chapdelaine's next witness was a mechanic from Valcourt, Quebec, home of the snowmobile. At age 39, Jacques Vieu was sent home in June 1989 to die from cancer after having 7/8 of his stomach removed. On June 30, he started 714-X. In November, he returned to work.

Chris Bird wrote (*ibid.*), "Throughout today's testimony, the jurors were on the edge of their seats, hanging on every word. Quite the opposite from the bored looks they wore last week when forced to hear... the cancer experts."

Conrad Chapdelaine's next witness, Marcel Caron, looked like a movie star. He told of having been diagnosed with cancerous polyps of the intestines in 1981 and advised to have a section of intestine removed. He refused, recalling that his younger brother had the same condition in 1970, accepted the surgery, and died painfully six months later. Seeking out Naessens but not mentioning his diagnosis, Caron was told that he had a "deteriorated blood picture (Naessens did not mention cancer) that suggested a serious weakening of the immune system which could be reinforced by 714-X" (*ibid.*) Caron told the jury that Naessens had never once promised a cure or attempted to dissuade him from other treatments. Caron gave himself three 21-day series of 714-X. Then he went for a thorough checkup and was told that he had no cancer in his body. That, Caron told the jury, was in 1982. He also told the jury, "I am not here to defend alternative medicine against traditional medicine but to say that I and all other people should be granted the right to choose the treatment we see fit". The prosecution did not cross-examine.

The next witness was Suzanne Berthiaume, who had been diagnosed with breast cancer in December 1988. She was advised to have her breast removed, to be followed by radiation and chemotherapy. Recalling that her father had accepted similar advice, which had not saved him from dying of cancer, she refused all treatment. Recommended to Naessens, she took three sets of 21 injections of 714-X from December 12, 1988 to the end of April 1989. "Since then", she told the court, "I have had a tremendous feeling of well-being, even a renewed 'lust for life'. And when at my own initiative I went back to the clinic where I had first been diagnosed, I was told that I had no trace of cancer left in my body." The prosecution did not cross-examine.

The next witness was Reynaud Vignal, former French Consul General in Quebec. Now an ambassador, he had attended the July 8 press conference. Vignal told the court that what had first won him to Gaston Naessens were three things: 1) Naessens' complete humility; 2) the fact that Naessens had advised Mme. Vignal to keep up her chemotherapy, so as not to "burn any bridges"; and 3) Naessens never once asked the Vignals for a single dollar in fees. (*ibid.*)

To conclude the defense, "Maitre" Chapdelaine (as attorneys are called in the French language) sprang a mystery witness. After being sworn, Francois Wilhemy identified himself as a judge of the court of the Province of Quebec, *i.e.* a member of the very judicial system which was trying to send Naessens to jail. As Chris Bird put it (*ibid.*), "one could have imagined that a bolt of lightning had struck the tiny courtroom". The judge testified that he had taken his wife, diagnosed with cancer, to consult Naessens after his arrest. "The judge said it was not a 'charlatan' he had gone to see, but a true scientist. First treated for cancer in 1979, Mme. Wilhelmy's cancer began to recur in 1985; by 1989, they were told nothing more could be done. 'Mme. Wilhelmy has now got much of her strength back', declared the judge, 'and since getting 714-X, she has been able to take up all her various activities.'" The judge then concluded his testimony "with what may have been the trial's strongest statement, 'That such treatments as Naessens 714-X are not publicly available is more than distressing. Why do they have to be hidden? After all, in our society, any of us would make any and all attempts to rescue, to save, a drowning man, woman, or child... so why not a victim of cancer?'" (*ibid.*)

In his closing argument, Conrad Chapdelaine told the jurors, "You see, there are approaches in medicine other than the orthodox ones, approaches discovered by geniuses such as a Gaston Naessens. Dr. Fabre has clearly shown you that Naessens' approach is not one of spraying a few mosquitoes with pesticides, but of getting rid of the whole swamp which continues to proliferate them... The key is not to eradicate cancer cells artificially, as is everywhere attempted by cancerology, but to assist the immune cells to do so naturally... What we are dealing with here may be as fundamentally good an approach as seen in this century. Do we have to wait until the next century to see it approved? There's something totally incomprehensible going on here. Incomprehensibly inhumane! Thousands and thousands of terminal cases have been told things are 'hopeless'. Gaston Naessens can, and has, provided that salvation. And now he's not in his laboratory but in a courtroom. It's just hard to fathom how our society can brook such intolerance! I ask you for acquittal on all counts. In reaching such a decision, you may be helping thousands who believe that a new approach in medicine is necessary." (*ibid.*)

The jury deliberated from 4 PM to 9 PM on December 1 and then broke for the night. Gaston Naessens had some trouble sleeping that evening. His entire career was in the hands of twelve unknown people. He was risking imprisonment at 65 years of age. He prayed, asking for courage. His mind was at peace. He had only tried to help sick people. The rest was in God's hands. He went to sleep.

The next morning at 10 AM, the jury filed in to the packed courtroom. The chairman of the jury rose and delivered the same verdict on each of five counts: *Non Coupable! - Not Guilty!* Francoise Naessens sat silently weeping with joy. Conrad Chapdelaine was heard to let out a sigh of relief. Gaston Naessens said he "felt as if five heavy stones placed on top of my head were, one by one, being removed".

Quebec papers headlined, "Naessens Acquitted!" Suddenly a hero to the Quebecois, his smiling face appeared on every front page. Dr. Augustin Roy, who had precipitated the trial as president of the Quebec Medical Corporation, gave a press conference full of sour grapes. He attacked the prosecutor, saying the latter should have "savagely cross-examined" the patients who testified in Naessens' behalf, and that he had not sufficiently frightened them. Dr. Roy said, "All of them should stand at attention or, more properly, get down on their knees to thank orthodox medicine for having kept them alive". He overlooked the fact that those who testified for Naessens had been given up for dead by orthodox medicine. When called a medical czar by the editor of the Sherbrooke Tribune, Roy retorted "He should have kept his trap shut" (*op. cit.*).

At the office of the Committee for the Support of Gaston Naessens, calls came in from all over the world, congratulating Naessens - and wanting 714-X.

While no longer facing possible life in prison, Naessens still had legal problems - 82 counts of practicing medicine without a license put forward by the Quebec Medical Corporation, with trial set for June 1990. If found guilty, he would be fined anywhere from $25,000 to $400,000.

Faced with the continued vituperative attacks from Augustin Roy (like AMA head Morris Fishbein against Harry Hoxsey in the 1930's), Naessens sued Roy and the Quebec Medical Corporation for $300,000 for libel and moral damages. The suit accused Roy of having been motivated by a "hatred surpassing any normal limit" (*ibid.*) and went after the Medical Corporation for having done nothing to restrain its president. Faced with subpoenas, the Medical Corporation dropped most of the counts. Naessens paid a $5,000 fine and claimed a moral victory.

The day after his acquittal, Naessens had lunch with Chris Bird and asked if he planned to turn his voluminous notes from the trial into a book, hopefully to come out quickly. Chris obliged and his *Gaston Naessens, Galileo of the Microscope* was published in less than a year in English and French. Written in his elegant style, Bird portrayed Naessens as a Statesman of Science. Included in the second edition was the fact that the Virginia Beach psychic, Edgar Cayce, had predicted in one of his "readings" in the 1930's that a cancer cure would be found which involved camphor (which is part of 714-X).

Two months before the trial, Naessens had written to then Prime Minister Brian Mulroney proposing a pilot project using 714-X in cancer and AIDS. That didn't happen. What did happen, after the trial, was the de facto legalization of 714-X through its acceptance under Canada's Emergency Drug Release Act. This compassionate law permits unapproved drugs to be acquired by patients with life-threatening illnesses. Doctors began pushing Ottawa bureaucrats who, after initial footdragging, routinely approved requests for 714-X in 48 hours. In 1990, 28 doctors were using 714-X.

Gaston Naessens' story reflects history. After Galileo invented the telescope, a Roman Catholic cardinal looked through it but refused to look a second time. Later, the Church prosecuted

Galileo for his heresy and forced him to recant his observations, that the earth revolves around the sun and not vice versa. The latter day equivalent of the cardinal, in the person of the Quebec Medical Corporation, took the ostrich approach, refused to look through Gaston Naessens' microscope even once and had him prosecuted. But four hundred and some years after Galileo, we're making some progress; the Medical Corporation lost, and lost spectacularly. The result was to give Naessens not just notoriety but fame, gradual, growing acceptance, and, most important, legalization.

While news of Naessens' New Biology was spreading, it was limited by the fact that there was only one Somatoscope. To improve the situation, Naessens designed a condenser which can be fitted onto any light microscope, rendering it powerful enough to see the somatids and their cycle. Priced at around $1,800, it was accessible to most researchers. He announced the condenser in June, 1991, at a symposium in Sherbrooke held to expand knowledge of his science. Chris Bird recalled a high spot of the meeting when blood samples were projected onto a screen. Naessens, with no idea from whom each sample had been drawn, proceeded to describe what he saw. After his analysis, several people, forewarned of when their blood sample would be shown, commented on his startling accuracy.

By 1992, 200 doctors were using 714-X. But the year before, Gaston Naessens suffered a cruel blow when his wife and helpmate, Francoise, died from the side-effects of an "approved" drug.

With Christopher Bird's book came a spate of favorable publicity, such as Paul William Roberts' "Blood Feud" in the December 1992 issue of the *Toronto Star's Saturday Night*. This article greatly increased awareness of Naessens' work among Canada's English-speaking community. As part of a far-reaching article, Roberts wrote of the visit to Naessens in 1991 of Dr. Dietmar Schildwaechter, MD and PhD, and former member of the faculty of the University of Pennsylvania Medical School. The doctor had been working with a relative of George Bush who had a particularly severe lung cancer metastasized to the brain. He had been monitoring her with a series of computerized immune system profile tests developed by Hungarian-born Dr. Emile Schandl. At the end of 1989, Dr. Schildwaechter received the woman's Schandl tests and noted that her level of cancer activity, which had been kept low, was now at zero; coincidentally, her immune system values had improved dramatically. Calling her to see what she had been doing, the doctor learned that she and her husband had been to see Gaston Naessens, who had taught them how to inject the 714-X.

When he met Naessens in 1991, Schildwaechter warmly accepted Naessens' concepts. At a medical school in Europe, he told Paul Roberts, "We'd learned about Bechamps and others basically excluded from medical schools over here. I realized that there was something in the blood we'd not been able to diagnose, and that Naessens had discovered... what others had only partially seen". "Combining, as he now can do, Schandl's tests with Naessens' somatoscopic monitoring", Roberts wrote, "Schildwaechter... claims tremendous success with his German practice in detecting and correcting the imbalances that would lead to degenerative disease. He hesitates to practice in the U.S. for fear of Naessens-style persecution."

Schildwaechter told Roberts that, "cancer has become a truly preventable disease if we would only employ these blood tests". He is convinced that Naessens' day is coming and adds, "Szent Gyorgy, discoverer of ascorbic acid and one of the great Nobel Laureates, remarked that whenever you pioneer something, you first have to realize you may be called a quack. But the Establishment will check you out, and if they find your discovery useful, it will be accepted through the back door - certainly without giving any credit to the pioneer."

Roberts brought a Toronto microbiologist to see Naessens. Telling Roberts her reactions after they left, she said "It's never been possible to see these particular entities before, and I call them entities because they do appear to be living...yet the exciting thing for me is the extraordinary power of that microscope...

There has to be something to it (Naessens' work) and it certainly warrants further study. But it's so foreign to the accepted dogma, you know, that it's going to be a hard sell."

In 1995, Naessens had the good fortune to find and marry another wonderful helpmate, Dr. Jacinte Levesque, owner of an acupuncture clinic in Montreal. Completely bilingual in French and English, Mme. Jacinte thus helps to fill in for Naessens in English, is thoroughly familiar with his work and science, and is an excellent manager. Together, in 1995, they created the International Academy of Somatidian Orthobiology, a private institution where Naessens' theory and the use of 714-X are taught to health professionals.

In 1995, the Naessens invited interested parties to join the Academy's first class to learn live blood analysis and the use of 714-X. Among the students was Berkley Bedell's daughter, Joanne Quinn, who is trained as a lab technician. Dr. Eva Reich, who had told Chris Bird about Naessens, was also in the class. One of the participants had a first-hand experience which demonstrated the importance of finding the exact spot in the groin for injecting into the lymph. With his wife in poor health (not cancer), he started giving her 714-X injections and she improved significantly. Needing to be out of town for awhile, he taught the injection method to a friend who was a very competent nurse. Returning three weeks later, he found his wife had relapsed. Checking where the nurse had injected, it turned out she was two inches off the appropriate point. When he resumed injections in the correct spot, his wife again improved.

Diana Stewart, daughter of David Stewart, was stricken with fibromyalgia. She decided to take 714-X to see if it would help, and it did.

In the summer of 1997, Naessens lost one of his strongest supporters when Christopher Bird tragically died of a stroke.

By 1998, in no small part due to the publicity brought by Chris Bird's book, 2000 Canadian doctors were giving 714-X. This was made possible through the Canadian law previously mentioned, the Emergency Drug Release Act, later renamed the

Special Access Program. This permits patients with terminal diseases to obtain on compassionate grounds products going through the approval process. Meanwhile, the use of 714-X had spread to 45 countries.

In 1998, Gaston Naessens developed a Mark II condenser, much more powerful than the 1991 version. This will permit biology courses everywhere to see some of that whole new world various people have spoken of, after looking in the Somatoscope. While only the Somatoscope has two light sources and modulation of light frequency, the second generation of Naessens' condenser will open up Somatidian Orthobiology to many. Priced lower than the 1991 model, it became available in 1999.

In the best of all worlds, thousands will have learned Naessens' method of blood analysis, and be able to warn of degenerative disease approaching as much as two years in advance. In the best of all worlds, Naessens will have found a process or additive to preserve the integrity of the somatid cycle in a freshly drawn drop of blood. In that way, anyone anywhere will be able to send a drop of blood to a blood analysis center to do an annual or semiannual check for signs of degenerative disease. If the macrocycle is there in the blood, preventive action can be taken to restore a normal somatid cycle, in effect, to clean up the swamp.

Looking back, Royal Rife's story is seen as a tragedy, with his work and technology all but forgotten. The films of what he discovered are lost, but those of Gaston Naessens still very much exist. What Royal Rife saw is most likely what Gaston Naessens sees, simply using a different tool to look at the same reality in the live blood of sick people. So, in a way, we have a second chance. Will we do a better job this time around? Will we learn the New Somatidian Orthobiology and save tens of thousands of lives by preventing illness? Will we take advantage of Gaston Naessens' genius while he is still alive, as we did not do with Rife? How many times do these discoveries have to come around before they catch on? In computers and telecommunication, we don't seem to hesitate, but march resolutely on with staggering, breathtaking progress. Why should it be any different in biology and medicine? Lack of progress in computers would slow but not sink our civilization. Failure, yes, refusal to make use of healing breakthroughs could do so.

If disinterest in Gaston Naessens' New Biology prevails in the U.S., Canada, Europe, and Japan, there's another possibility. Third World countries such as China and Brazil or even Cuba might adopt his science in order to lower their health care costs. All they need to realize is that the pronouncements of Official Medicine in the U.S. are shaped by political pressures and concerns which they almost certainly do not share.

Toward the end of his book, Chris Bird quotes Dr. Jan Merta, "Because Gaston Naessens has offered - and offers - good health for a tiny fraction of the cost which people are forced to pay for bad health, he is simply not wanted, together with what he has discovered... As a single individual, Gaston Naessens has achieved more than dozens of institutes full of PhD's that have been supported, year after year, by billions of dollars."

Microbiologist Walter Clifford echoed Merta's remarks. "There are a few gentle giants who mold the age in which they live; Gaston Naessens is such a man... None of Naessens' detractors...have ever bothered to work with him in his laboratory. I have many times taken researchers into my lab to demonstrate...from their own blood, things they had never before seen, things Naessens has been reporting for years. Do you think that made any difference? Many of them unblinkingly told me that, because what they had seen was not approved by any professional society or governmental agency, they simply would not believe it - that is, believe their own eyes!"

"The very simplicity (of substantiating Naessens' work) mitigates against it", Clifford continued. "Naessens' investigations require no mega-bucks, irradiation machines, scanners, or other costly or complex equipment. And his findings will certainly not sell billions of dollars worth of toxic drugs."

Pointing to the ease of replicating all of Naessens' techniques and findings, Clifford told Bird, "His work can be learned with no great difficulty by any reasonably skilled technician. His products can be made in laboratories containing the most modest facilities, and be administered by virtually any family physician. As a professional in the field, I can further say that Naessens' microbiology can be duplicated by any researcher willing to accept a body of new knowledge of vast importance that has never been taught in a university or medical school."

The German philosopher Schopenhauer once stated, "Truth passes through three distinct phases; first a theory is created and introduced. Second, it is violently ridiculed. Third, it is accepted as truth."

With his second generation condenser coming out, with more seminars and more people learning his methods, and with increasing interest in his work, it may well be Schopenhauer's third phase for Gaston Naessens. In the 1990's he has been repeatedly nominated for the Nobel Prize. In Japan, the tradition would be to name one such as Gaston Naessens a "Living National Treasure".

On June 24, 1999, CBS' *48 Hours* included eight minutes on Gaston Naessens in a show entitled "Desperate Measures". One of Naessens' cases was a teenager who had run away from home at age eight to escape being given chemotherapy for his Hodgkins lymphoma, confirmed by biopsy. Instead, he took 714-X. He appeared on the show, well and happy. Also on the show was a small girl who was healed of sinus cancer with 714-X. Gaston Naessens was asked to answer just one question, "If 714-X were given early enough, would it cure a body of cancer?" His succinct, one-word response, "Certainly". CBS also put on the show a Dr. Batiste, a Montreal doctor who had only negative things to say. CBS did not make it clear that Dr. Batiste had no recent knowledge of Naessens, having visited Naessens' lab only once, in 1990, right after the trial. During that one visit, Dr. Batiste did not even look through the Somatoscope.

No matter. There is a saying in politics, "Don't worry if people spell your name wrong as long as they're talking about you". CBS was talking about Gaston Naessens, and Canadian CBC/TV quickly picked up clips of the cured patients. Since the program and CBC replays, the Naessens' phones have been ringing off the hook with calls from desperate people. CBS added to Naessens' credibility.

The inclusion of Naessens on the CBS program sends a strong signal that at long last some segments of the media are beginning to look at the medical revolution taking place outside their windows. They should have tuned in sooner, but better late than never, since 10,000 Americans die of cancer every week.

"The man who may well be recognized as a Galileo or an Einstein", wrote Paul Roberts, "continues the work to which he has devoted a half century, seemingly unconcerned by the fuss, the orthodox hostility. Gaston Naessens works in silence and concentration in his laboratory, his windows on the Magog River showing a landscape scarcely changed since the glaciers retreated. Others have begun to praise him, but he himself might be content to live by a line from Paracelsus, 'I pleased nobody except the people I cured'".

THE MIRACLE OF ELECTROMEDICINE

"We'd have had regeneration 15-20 years ago if it hadn't been for the government! Nobody knew how the salamander regenerated its limbs until Dr. Becker came along", exclaimed Ruth Harvey. A private researcher in alternative medicine, it was she who first put me onto the story of Dr. William F. Koch. (Chapter 3) Ruth was referring to Dr. Robert O. Becker, a world-renowned orthopedic surgeon and pioneering scientist in electromedicine - the kind of person who wants to know what makes living things "alive".

From 1958 to 1980, Dr. Becker was chief of orthopedic research at the Veterans Administration (VA) Hospital in Syracuse, NY. During those years, he published 150 papers in medical journals and was twice nominated for the Nobel Prize. Unfortunately, even in electromedicine, political decisions intruded and hampered his research. Almost all of his funds came from the VA. In 1980, all funds were cut off because of Department of Defense (DoD) irritation over Becker's warnings of danger from unlimited exposure to electromagnetic (EM) fields. Friends in Washington had told him that opposition to his VA funding was coming from the DoD; their people were saying, 'How do we shut this guy up?'" However, cutting off his funds did not shut up Bob Becker. Retiring to the foothills of the Adirondacks, he wrote *The Body Electric* (1985) and *Cross Currents* (1990). The first is a fascinating and highly readable description of his electromedical discoveries. All of them had been published in technical language in medical journals, but in *Body Electric*, assisted by writer Gary Selden, Becker presents them in laymen's language. In *Cross Currents*, Becker contrasts the marvelous promise of electromedicine with the perils of electromagnetic pollution - the potential dangers of careless and indiscriminate exposure to electromagnetic (EM) fields.

In the late 19th century, Sears & Roebuck listed in their catalog an "electric corset" for alleviation of arthritis pain. It sold well, which usually doesn't happen when things don't work. Many doctors used electrical treatments of one sort or another but there was no underlying theory of why they worked. The field of biochemistry, on the other hand, was constantly producing new discoveries. As the 20th Century dawned, there was a growing sense that the human body was a chemical creation, that "life was just an array of chemical reactions" (*Body Electric*), and that "modern" medicine, then, must be chemical in nature. This understanding laid the foundations for the great pharmaceutical companies, which deal in chemical drugs, some excellent, some dangerous. The acceptance of chemicals as the basis of medical treatment has become so ingrained that a cousin's reaction may be typical. As I was explaining the Rife device, he interrupted me to say, "It never occurred to me that medicine could be other than a drug." This perception of the taken-for-granted chemical nature of medicine was set off by the Flexner report of 1910, a study commissioned by the Rockefeller and Carnegie Foundations to bring medicine up to date. The study's director, Abraham Flexner, decreed that there was no scientific basis for electromedicine, which then gradually vanished. In the 1930's, Dr. Morris Fishbein warned in his JAMA editorials against the quackery of electromedicine. Electric corsets disappeared from the Sears catalog. That was the end of the first wave of electromedical research.

By the 1940's, the accepted scientific paradigm limited the effect of EM currents or fields on living organisms to electroshock and thermal effects - for instance electric blankets - or the electric chair. That was where things stood until Dr. Robert Becker came along. He is regarded as the creator of the field known as Bioelectromagnetics, in which he showed the profound biological effects of very minute electric currents and very low strength electromagnetic fields on living tissues. The rebirth of electromedicine as a recognized and respected field of medical study is largely due to his work.

Even in college, Robert Becker was fascinated by the salamander's ability to regenerate lost limbs. As an orthopedic surgeon, he had done enough amputations and dreamed of discovering how to replicate this feat in humans.

It has long been known that a "current of injury" exists at any wound, human or animal, and even in plants where a stem or branch is removed. The conventional view was that this current was simply ions (electric particles) leaking from dying cells, and that the current would eventually taper off and disappear. Becker didn't believe this, and suspected that the current of injury was somehow related to regeneration - in those animals capable of that feat. Curiously, nobody had ever bothered to measure how long this current lasted. As his first research project in 1958, Becker proposed to do just that. He would make such measurements in salamanders, which regenerate, and in frogs, which don't, and compare the currents in regenerating and non-regenerating limbs.

At that time, Becker was in charge of orthopedic surgery at the VA Hospital in Syracuse, which was closely associated with the State University of NY Medical School. Two months after he presented his proposal, he was summoned to a special meeting in the hospital director's office of the committee that governed research at the two institutions. As Becker tells it in *Body Electric*, "Now that was really strange. The director almost never paid any attention to the research program. Besides, his office was big enough to hold a barbeque in. It was a barbeque, all right, and I was the one being grilled". The committee chair came right to the point, "We have a very grave basic concern over your proposal. This notion that electricity has anything to do with living things was totally discredited some time ago. It has absolutely no validity, and the new scientific evidence you're citing is worthless. The whole idea was based on its appeal to quacks and the gullible public. I will not stand idly by and see this medical school associated with such a charlatanistic, unscientific project".

Becker replied that "I was sorry if it flew in the face of

dogma", but that "I didn't intend to withdraw the proposal, so they would have to act upon it" (*ibid*). After the meeting, one of the committee members took Becker aside to give him some kindly advice. "Go back to school and get your PhD, Becker. Then you'll learn all this stuff is nonsense" (*ibid*).

Two days later, Dr. Robert Becker got a break; the committee referred his proposal to Professor Chester Yntema, who had studied the regrowth of ears in salamanders. Yntema approved his project, observing, however, "I don't believe for one minute that it will work, but I think you should do it anyway. We need to encourage young researchers".

That was how Robert Becker's historic research got started. His first step was to measure current at the tip of the limbs of each of his 14 frogs and 14 salamanders, finding a negative charge of 8-10 millivolts in each. The experiment didn't take long to produce results. After anesthetizing the animals, Becker amputated the right forelegs of each of the animals. He noticed that the polarity at the stumps reversed to positive right after the injury. By the second day, the current climbed to 20 millivolts in both species. The salamanders' current dropped rapidly, however, vanishing to zero on the third day. Becker was almost ready to drop the project. Meanwhile, the frogs were holding at the original 20 millivolts, so at least their current of injury hadn't vanished. Then, between the sixth and the tenth days, the salamanders' electric potential returned, changed back to negative, and climbed to a peak of 30 millivolts (negative). At that point, blastemas formed. A blastema is a little ball of primitive or undifferentiated cells able to "differentiate" into all the various cells needed to reconstitute the missing limb. The blastema always forms at the stump of an animal about to regenerate a missing limb. The frogs' positive voltage began to decline as their stumps healed over (not regenerating), and the salamanders began to regrow their missing forelegs. When the frogs' wounds had completely healed, and the salamanders' limbs had completely regrown, both again measured the original 10 millivolts (negative).

In his very first experiment, Robert Becker thus had the

excitement of seeing something nobody had ever seen before. He had proved beyond question that the current of injury was not due to dying cells, which were long gone by the time the salamanders' electric charge had changed to negative. Moreover, the opposite polarities displayed by frogs and salamanders indicated a profound difference in the electrical properties of the two species. The negative potential seemed to bring forth the all-important blastema, without which regeneration did not happen.

Then Becker decided to apply negative current - which he'd seen the salamanders use to such good effect - to the stumps of frogs after amputating a foreleg. He dreamed of being the first to produce regrowth in a normally non-regenerating animal. Writes Becker in *Body Electric*, "The frogs were less interested in my glory. They had to hold still for up to half an hour with electrodes attached. They refused, so I anesthetized them each day, which they tolerated poorly. Within a week, my Nobel Prize had turned into a collection of dead frogs."

Writing up his research results, Becker submitted it to the *Journal of Bone and Joint Surgery*, the most prestigious orthopedic journal in the world, and hit paydirt - his study was accepted. He was launched and recognized as a pioneer in the vanguard of electromedical research.

Becker isn't the sort of person to give up easily and persisted in trying to help frogs regenerate limbs. He succeeded in causing some regrowth, but wasn't the first to do so. As a young anatomy professor at Smith College in the 1940's, Dr. S. Meryl Rose had achieved partial regeneration in frogs, the first time anybody had achieved that in an animal normally lacking in that capability. After the publication of Becker's research, he got a call from Dr. Rose and then a visit. Dr. Becker's wife, Lillian, remembered him; she'd studied at Smith and it turned out she'd helped treat the frogs he used in his experiment.

When Robert Becker began his reevaluation of the place of electricity in biology, he discovered an important ally in Albert Szent Gyorgy, the Nobel Laureate who discovered Vitamin C. Szent Gyorgy pointed out that when experimenters broke living things down into their constituent parts, somewhere along the line, life slipped through their fingers and they found themselves working with dead matter. "It looks as if some basic fact of life were still missing," and for that missing part, Szent Gyorgy proposed electricity. He pointed out that the molecular structure of many parts of the cell was regular enough to support superconduction. That manner of movement of electrons, fundamental to computers and solid-state electronics, occurs only in materials having an orderly molecular structure, such as crystals. Semiconductors can carry only small currents, but can carry them over long distances. Becker notes in *Body Electric* that when the discoverer of Vitamin C proposed this concept in *Introduction to Submolecular Biology* in 1960, it was seen as "evidence of his advancing age".

With Szent Gyorgy's suggestion in mind, Becker writes, "I put together a working hypothesis. I postulated a primitive... information system closely related to the nerves but not necessarily located in the nerve fibers themselves. I theorized that this system used semiconducting direct currents and that, either alone or in concert with the nerve impulse system, it regulated growth, healing, and perhaps other basic processes."

In research, it pays to know the right question to ask. Having figured out the question, it took Becker a few years, but he did prove the existence in all living animals of a direct current system that operates in the perineural cells along the nerve cells. The perineural cells constitute more than one half the bulk of the brain and accompany even the smallest nerve fibers. Therefore, this system, with its semiconducting ability to transport small amounts of current, permeates the entire body - The Body Electric.

Becker found that this system controls growth and healing and, in the salamanders, regeneration. The current of injury, then, is a local expression of this DC system.

His breakthrough in understanding the semiconducting properties of the body was a staggering discovery, of Nobel Prize magnitude.

Fundamental to electricity is the fact that where there is a flow of electrons, there is a magnetic field. Becker writes in *Cross Currents*, "In the early 1960's, I predicted that the flow of this DC current in the brain would produce a magnetic field that could be observed at a distance outside of the head if one had a magnetometer of sufficient sensitivity. When I made this statement at a scientific meeting, there was considerable laughter from the audience. I was told that such a device would never be made, and that even if such a magnetic field could be measured, its strength would be so small that it would be of no physiological consequence whatsoever." A few advances in solid-state physics and electronics eventually permitted the development of the device Becker predicted; the superconducting quantum interference detector, or SQUID. And the SQUID easily reads the brain's magnetic field as far as several feet from the head in what is called a magnetoencephalogram, or MEG.

In the 1960's, Dr. Becker also predicted that living organisms could be influenced by external electromagnetic fields as the fields interacted with the DC currents he had discovered to be flowing within the organisms. Conducting research in mental hospitals, Becker found that right after disturbances in the Earth's magnetic field caused by sunspots - magnetic storms on the sun - admissions rose and patients' behavior was more agitated.

In order to cause regeneration, Becker knew that he had to figure out how to induce a blastema, and to do that, he needed primitive or dedifferentiated cells. These are the cells in an embryo that eventually differentiate or specialize into skin or bones or eyes, etc. In conventional science, it was accepted as fact that once a cell has differentiated, it can never retrace its steps back to its embryonic stage and de-differentiate, with the exception of bone marrow cells. This is why regeneration in humans can happen in fracture healing, where bone marrow cells are available.

Becker was surprised to find when he studied fracture healing in frogs that it was not bone marrow cells which dedifferentiated, but red blood cells. This was a surprise, since such cells are a long way from bone marrow cells. It turned out that frog red blood cells have a nucleus which contains DNA, which can be reactivated to direct the cell to return to its primitive state. Human red blood cells, on the other hand, contain no nucleus and no DNA to re-program. Therefore, red blood cells could not serve humans as raw material to be dedifferentiated into primitive or "stem" cells to produce the blastema needed for regeneration. Since there would not be enough bone marrow cells to serve this purpose, Dr. Becker came to the reluctant conclusion that regeneration in humans - his El Dorado - probably was impossible.

However, Robert Becker did succeed in dedifferentiating frog red blood cells. This had never been done before and was considered impossible. He achieved this by exposing the cells to just one-half billionth of an ampere of current. After four hours of exposure to this current, all red blood cells in the experiment had reactivated their DNA and had become unspecified in form - they had dedifferentiated. What happened indicated the reactivation of the DNA, since the process continued even after the current was totally shut down. The process only worked with frogs' red blood cells, not with their white cells. The experiment was filmed on electron photomicrographs, pictures taken through an electron microscope. Charlie Beckman, a member of Becker's research team, had helped develop the electron microscope, and his presence contributed to Becker's credibility. Even so, when Becker presented the pictures at the NY Academy of Sciences, seeing wasn't believing. Many people stated that they didn't believe what they had seen, for everyone *knew* that cells can't be dedifferentiated.

After four years of such research, Dr. Becker turned his attention to seeing if the electric currents he had been observing could be used to accelerate human bone healing. He demonstrated that non-union fractures - bone fractures that won't heal - could be stimulated to do so with small DC currents, or with low-strength slowly-pulsing EM fields. In 1970, having deciphered the electrical control mechanisms governing fracture healing, Becker wrote a major article on the research and published it in *Clinical*

Orthopedics and Related Research. He found it the most satisfying of his publications, since this was his first work that led
directly to a technique that helped patients. Electrical stimulation
of bone healing was quickly accepted by clinical medicine and
was soon put to wide use.

Getting grants from the Veterans Administration proved
almost as difficult as doing the research. To look for other support, Becker submitted a proposal to the Department of the Army.
Suggesting that DC currents might stimulate wound healing, and
that the Army's business often produced a lot of wounds, he figured there might be interest. There was, but not what he expected. First, his grant proposal was quickly turned down. Then about
a month later, he got a call from a prominent orthopedic surgeon
who had served on the Army's committee that had turned him
down. The surgeon told Becker, "I have a grant from the Army to
study the possibility that direct currents might stimulate wound
healing, and I wonder if you might have any suggestions as to the
best approach to use." No-nonsense Bob Becker quickly told his
caller what to do with his grant.

There was another offer which Becker declined. With only
minor amounts of research funds, he was publishing more than all
his supervisors combined. One of them came to him one day with
"an offer you can't refuse" - all the VA funds he could ask for, so
long as the supervisor's name was added to all Becker's publications. Becker found out more about the politics in research than
he wanted to.

During his orthopedic research, Dr. Becker discovered something of conceivably great value to a lot of people, something that
has never been followed up. Becker explains in *Body Electric*,
that "bone is composed of collagen, the main structural material
of the entire body, and apatite, a crystalline material that's main-
ly calcium phosphate". Both materials turned out to be semiconductors. Becker and his assistants found something else in bone
they had not been aware of - copper. He found that the electrical
forces of copper hold the apatite crystals and the collagen together just as wooden pegs hold old chairs together. Writes Becker,

"Unfortunately for victims of osteoporosis, the copper peg discovery still hasn't been followed up, even though it was published in 1970. Regenerative growth was our primary target, so I reluctantly dropped osteoporosis."

Another of Dr. Becker's experiments would be of interest to anyone who recalls the unpleasant grogginess of coming out from under anesthesia. Studying the effects of magnetic fields on salamanders, Dr. Becker placed a salamander between the poles of an electromagnet and gradually increased the magnetic field. Delta brain waves (which characterize anesthesia) appeared at 2,000 gauss. At 3,000 gauss, the animal was motionless and completely unresponsive to stimuli. Then as he decreased the strength of the magnetic field, "normal EEG patterns returned suddenly and the salamander regained consciousness within seconds." Becker also tried anesthetizing the salamanders with direct current. It worked, but a half hour after the current was shut off, the animals remained groggy and unresponsive, just as after chemical anesthesia. Electromagnetic anesthesia seemed to Becker as "the best possible...allowing prompt recovery with no side effects". Becker tried to follow this up but got no takers at the VA. Proposing "to get a bigger electromagnet to try the method on larger animals and eventually humans, we never even got a reply."

In the Lazarus Heart chapter of *Body Electric*, Robert Becker describes one of his most incredible experiments. Studying red blood cells from salamanders, the animals were so small that the only practical way to extract blood was to cut the hearts in two and throw away the carcasses. One day his assistant, Sharon Chapin, asked "What would happen if I sewed these three up?" Becker assured her that they would be dead within minutes, since it was known that no animal's heart could repair major wounds. A few days later, Sharon brought the three salamanders back, looking perfectly healthy. Astounded, Becker anesthetized the miraculous creatures and dissected them. Their hearts showed no signs of having been damaged and were perfectly normal. Becker found that the salamanders' hearts regrew to normal in four hours after being mutilated, showing no sign of injury. Red blood cells formed a blastema within one-half hour of the injury, occupying the entire space where the missing part of the heart had been. After 2-3 hours, most of the blastema cells redifferentiated into heart muscle. After 4 hours, the heart was normal in appearance and was pumping blood. Becker wrote a report on this for *Nature* magazine but "even toned down", he writes in *Body Electric*, "it sounded like science fiction". "This is ideal healing", he summarized. "Spilled blood closes a wound at the body's center and replaces the missing part in a few hours. You can't get much more efficient than that."

After President Nixon went to China in 1970, interest in acupuncture surged. Dr. Becker secured a grant from the National Institutes of Health (NIH) to see if acupuncture worked electrically. He confirmed that thesis, finding less resistance and greater conductivity over the acupuncture points. Becker's research showed that the acupuncture meridians were conductors of direct current, the points being gateways to the body's electrical system. Just as he was going to start the next phase of his study, the NIH cancelled the grant.

Dr. Becker found that the shock of spinal cord injuries produced a prolonged positive charge. This seemed to be the main roadblock to spinal cord repair, since a negative charge is the current of regeneration. But, Becker speculates, it should be possible to cancel that positive polarity and replace it with a growth-stimulating negative charge by using a proper electric current. With sufficient funds, Becker believes he could achieve spinal cord regeneration. As far as he knows, no one has ever brought his work to the attention of America's most famous spinal cord injury victim, Christopher Reeve.

As his research progressed, Robert Becker became more and more aware that human beings, and indeed all living creatures in the plant and animal kingdoms, exist within an electromagnetic system and that we all are basically electromagnetic in nature - in effect, we all live in electric bodies. This keen awareness of the body's EM qualities and how little it took to affect them made him ever more concerned over the global smog of EM pollution that has come to exist world-wide.

In *Cross Currents*, Dr. Becker spells out some of the potential perils of certain frequencies. He describes a Swedish test of rats exposed to the EM frequencies from standard TV sets. The sets were placed about 12 inches above the animals for four hours a day. "Male rats were exposed for thirty-five to fifty days and then examined. Testicular weights were found to be significantly reduced." Prolonged exposure to unshielded TV electromagnetic frequencies is unique to the second half of the 20th century. One can only wonder if there is a connection between the Swedish study and the sharp drop in human male sperm count that has been observed in all parts of the world.

Here's another example of the sort of thing that concerns Becker. In the 1970's, a machine to monitor fetal heartbeats was developed which is not passive but invasive; it sends out an electromagnetic (EM) signal to the fetus. A study was done in 1989 which compared babies monitored by the device with those monitored the old-fashioned way, by ear. Over a period of 18 months, babies monitored by the EM device had a much higher rate of cerebral palsy than babies monitored by ear. This study is like an alarm signal going off.

Becker notes that 40% of children born in the 1990's are exposed to significant EM fields equal to what rats were exposed to in a study done by the NYS Department of Health; the rats later developed learning disabilities.

Current conventional concepts about cancer assume that cancer cells can never dedifferentiate and revert to normal cells. Such thinking holds that once a cancer cell, always a cancer cell, so therefore the only thing to do is to try to remove it with surgery or to kill it by radiation or chemotherapy. Becker's research, on the other hand, points to a different understanding; possibly a cancer cell is stuck in a state of incomplete dedifferentiation. It has already dedifferentiated back far enough to pick up the ability of the primitive cell to proliferate rapidly. It has not gone far enough to become a normal primitive cell, which by nature will specialize or differentiate into a cell of whatever organ it is part of.

Recent discoveries suggest that a cell may become cancerous because of a genetic alteration (the wrong genetic sequence being expressed) caused by - whatever. Dedifferentiation unravels the cell's malignant genetic program, permitting it to be reprogrammed as a normal cell. Becker believes that cancer cells would revert to normal if they could be fully dedifferentiated.

The possible link between regeneration and cancer occurred to a young researcher at the National Cancer Institute (NCI). One month after he submitted his proposal to his superiors with a request for funding, he was forced out of NCI.

In the 19th century, it was known that silver had antibacterial qualities; it is said that the early pioneers would put a silver dollar in a quart of milk to keep it from going sour while crossing the prairies. The knowledge of silver's value goes back even further. In the Middle Ages, doctors would advise putting a silver spoon in a child's mouth to protect against the plague. Since only the rich had silver spoons, this may have been the origin of the saying "born with a silver spoon in the mouth".

Dr. Becker rediscovered silver. By this time, he knew that he could turn on growth with negative current or turn it off with positive current. If he applied negative current, he could stimulate growth of a bone, but would it also stimulate growth of bacteria?

In preliminary lab tests, he had seen that silver electrodes, "when made electrically positive, would kill all types of bacteria, apparently because of positive silver ions driven into the culture by the applied voltage. This was an exciting discovery, because no single antibiotic worked against all types of bacteria." And this was accomplished with voltages harmless to human cells.

A big problem with his silver electrodes, however, was that their effects were too local, extending only 1 inch from the electrode. Needing something larger, like a screen made of silver, Dr. Becker stumbled onto a nylon cloth impregnated with silver ions. Since silver is highly conductive, direct current could be delivered all over the cloth.

Becker soon had a challenging case for trying the silver nylon cloth. His patient, John, had suffered a badly broken leg in a snowmobile accident. The bone had become infected - osteomyelitis, an even worse nightmare for an orthopedic surgeon than a non-union fracture, and that was present too. A cavity in John's leg was infected by five different kinds of bacteria. Becker explained to John his plan to use the silver nylon first with positive current to control the bacteria and later to use the negative current to try to heal the bone. Cleaning out the wound during the operation, Becker packed a large piece of silver nylon into the excavation, which ran almost from John's knee to his ankle. He then connected a battery to the silver nylon, which thus served as an electrode adapted to the shape of the wound. By the end of two weeks, all five kinds of bacteria had disappeared. The first problem was solved, and this represented the conquest of osteomyelitis. Taking an X-ray, Becker found that there had been some bone growth - all the pieces were stuck together. He kept using the positive electrodes and at the end of one month found that the non-union fracture was practically healed and by two months, the patient was walking on the leg. How could this be? The current used was positive and should have killed the bacteria but not have helped with the healing. The mystery was soon solved.

During one of his osteomyelitis treatments with silver nylon, while checking a culture of material from a patient's wound, Robert Becker found something completely unexpected and serendipitous. It could never have been predicted, and it reopened his old dream of human regeneration. Faced with the fact that he couldn't regenerate without cells that could be dedifferentiated, which were hard to come by in humans, Becker had sadly concluded that human regeneration was impossible. Now, inspecting the culture, he found dedifferentiated, primitive, human cells. Quickly jumping on this lead, he combined the electrically-generated silver ions he had used in the wound with fibroblasts, a common human cell type found throughout the body. Incredulously, he saw that he soon had a petri dish full of dedifferentiated cells. Until then, it was accepted that once cells differentiate, or specialize, that was the end of the line and there was no way back to square one. But Becker had found a way to dedifferentiate human cells, which even he had thought to be impossible. This could mean the elimination of the main obstacle to regeneration in humans, the lack of cells which could be dedifferentiated.

Furthermore, Becker realized that the silver electrode technique could be used to dedifferentiate large quantities of a patient's cells to primitive or stem cell state to be stored for use in an emergency when tissue healing is necessary, such as after an operation. It is for just such a purpose that companies have been set up to store stem (primitive) cells from the umbilical cords of newborn children.

On June 1, 2000, National Public Radio announced some interesting research on stem cells and pointed out that if only we knew how to produce stem cells in mass, it would revolutionize medicine. But we do know how to do this, for a dedifferentiated cell can do anything a stem cell can do. Dr. Bob Becker published the above research in the late 1970's, but nobody paid any attention. It's time somebody did, because the NPR announcer was right; it would indeed revolutionize medicine.

Dr. Becker patented his silver electrode technique, pointing out in the patent that silver is not toxic or harmful to tissues, is not cytotoxic, not carcinogenic, not mutagenic (doesn't change genes), but is a destroyer of bacteria and fungi, and is a dedifferentiating agent. In this process, Becker explains that the work is done by silver ions which bind right at the site being treated. They do not get into the bloodstream, and therefore cannot cause argyria, a graying of the skin which occasionally has happened to people taking a lot of colloidal silver.

He also found an application to cancer. When he used a positive charge delivered through silver electrodes to cancer cells in his lab, cell division (mitosis) stopped completely. While growing tissue is negatively charged, cancer is the most negative of all. This was not the result of the positive current but of the silver ions being released from the electrodes. If the electrodes used are made of any material other than silver, the electric voltage and current will cause cancer cells to increase their rate of mitosis, or growth.

Electricity in cancer has a long history. In 1880, the British medical journal *Lancet* published a letter from a doctor telling of a patient whose cancer of the chin gradually vanished over two weeks after he was struck by lightning. Also in the 1880's, Dr. Apostoli, a French surgeon, reported reversing tumors by passing between 100 and 250 milliamperes of positive polarity direct current through an electrode inserted into the tumor. Learning of Apostoli's work, Dr. Frederick Martin, who later founded the American College of Surgeons, published several papers confirming Apostoli's work. In a more recent application of this method, Swedish Dr. Björn Nordenström (who invented needle biopsies) has reversed tumors with 10 volts of positive DC delivered through stainless steel electrodes placed directly into tumors.

Dr Becker has observed that anything over 1.1 volts creates electrolysis in the body, *i.e.*, the splitting of water into hydrogen and oxygen. In *Cross Currents*, Becker states, "In biological tissues, this produces gases such as hydrogen, that are extremely toxic to the cells. Hydrogen immediately turns into hydrochloric acid, which dissolves cells. Since Nordenström used 10 times the current that causes electrolysis, Becker assumes that Nordenström's results, as well as those of Apostoli and Martin, have come from electrolysis, and not from any biologically significant electrical current or polarity.

Since Becker has seen both negative and positive currents stimulate tumor growth, he is concerned that this method could result in the stimulation of other tumors in the area. This phenomenon did occur in some of Nordenström's cases, Becker observes. However, Becker points out, the targeted tumors were destroyed, so even if the method achieved cell destruction by hydrochloric acid created by electrolysis, it works and is useful.

Before his lab closed, Dr. Becker demonstrated the dedifferentiation of one type of cancer cells by placing them in a petri dish with silver electrodes delivering positive direct current and releasing silver ions. Such a method goes right to the heart of what a cancer cell is, a once normal cell that went astray. It reverses the cancer cell back to a primitive cell, which then red-ifferentiates as a normal cell of whatever organ it is part of. Becker later used the method to reverse two skin cancers. Becker states in *Cross Currents*, "While we do not have firm evidence at this time, what probably happens is that the silver ion is shaped so as to connect with some receptor site on the surface of the cancer cell membrane".

What a lead to leave hanging! But that is just what happened, because this research occurred just before the Veterans Administration cut off his funding on January 1, 1980.

The cause was politics at its worst. His research having shown the sensitivity of human cells to the most miniscule amounts of current, Dr. Becker began to realize that human health may be affected by the incredible electromagnetic smog of the second half of the 20th century. He was asked to serve on a special environmental committee to advise the U.S. Navy on Project Sanguine. This was a plan conceived by the Department of Defense at the height of the Cold War to permit communications with nuclear submarines submerged to a depth of 120 feet. The system involved creating signals of 45-70 hertz from an enormous antenna to be buried under a large part of northern Wisconsin. Meeting in Washington, the committee learned of research where 9 out of 10 human volunteers exposed for just one day to the magnetic field component of the Sanguine signals showed a significant increase in serum triglycerides. A rise in triglycerides is part of the body's response to stress. The system was shelved, but the Navy never released the impact statement.

Returning to New York State, Dr. Becker learned of a plan to construct ten ultra-high frequency (765 KV) transmission lines across the state. The potentially harmful Sanguine frequencies were similar to those of the proposed power lines. He wrote to the NYS Public Service Commission (PSC) and informed them that the Navy had substantial evidence of possible harm to the population in the vicinity of the proposed lines, and told them the name of the person to call. A few weeks later, a man from the PSC called Becker to say that the Naval officer whose name Becker had given him had said that there was no such thing as Project Sanguine, that there was no such committee, and that he'd never heard of Becker, who had not been there. "That's funny", Becker replied. "I just got the minutes of the Project Sanguine committee meeting from the Office of Naval Research in this morning's mail". When Becker assured the PSC man that he could see the minutes, since they were not classified, the man said "I'll be over tomorrow". After reading the minutes of the meeting that never happened of the Navy committee that wasn't supposed to exist, the PSC set up public hearings on the proposed lines. Becker and others testified. When information on Project Sanguine came out, Wisconsin's Senator Gaylord Nelson was furious with the Navy over its proposed experiment on his constituents. After the hearings, the PSC adopted Becker's recommendations for a 5-year moratorium on the proposed lines, and for a 5-year, $5,000,000 study of possible hazards, with costs assessed to the utilities proposing the lines. As final fallout, the PSC required a wider right-of-way for the lines.

On the national level, no one paid much attention to Dr. Becker's warnings about possible dangers to human cells from frequencies carried by high tension lines, except behind the scenes. Meanwhile, other voices were raised. *New Yorker* staff writer Paul Brodeur wrote *The Zapping of America* in 1977. In *Electromagnetic Man* (1989), British researcher Cyril Smith, PhD, described how, after a major power line was constructed right over the main street of Fishpond, a tiny hamlet in Dorset, England, most of the villagers became ill in one way or another. There were numerous cases of cancer and also mental disturbances. Having moved to Fishpond, Smith also became sick, which precipitated his research into EM frequencies and his book.

On December 14, 1990, the *Atlanta Journal* reported that when the Environmental Protection Agency (EPA) did a study that linked EM fields to leukemia and brain cancer in children, White House aides in the Bush Administration delayed release of the report, concerned that the public "might misinterpret the report's conclusions". An earlier version of the EPA study had proposed to classify EM fields as "Class B" carcinogens (meaning probable sources of human cancer). This proposal was removed upon "revision".

In July 1997, the *New England Journal of Medicine* published a study done by the National Cancer Institute (NCI) claiming that there was no evidence that powerline EM fields increased the risks of childhood leukemia. However, an article in the Oct-Nov 1997 issue of *Nexus* magazine pointed out that the researchers dismissed as a "statistical fluke" a 24% increase in leukemia risk for children exposed to especially high magnetic fields. The NCI researchers dismissed this fact by setting a 2 milligauss level as a cut-off point for their calculations. *Nexus* asked Dr. Ross Adey, one of the most respected bioelectromagnetics researchers in the U.S., to comment. Dr. Adey pointed out that if the NCI had taken a 3 milligauss level as their cut-off, the conclusions would have been exactly the opposite, *i.e.*, that there is a significant risk of childhood leukemia.

Finally, in early 1999, a committee set up within the National Institutes of Health (NIH) issued a report acknowledging that, yes, there is a statistically significant relationship between children with leukemia and exposure to EM fields. Becker again was vindicated.

Becker points out that, "We've filled the electromagnetic spectrum with all manner of frequencies which have never before existed on the planet, frequencies with which humans and other species have never before coexisted."

After his PSC testimony, Becker noticed increasing resistance to renewing the VA grants which were funding his research. Finally, all grants ceased and his lab closed on January 1, 1980. It was the only one in the world doing any research in regeneration.

Ruth Harvey was right; had Dr.Becker's funding continued, he probably would have shown how to regenerate limbs. With all the significance this could hold for so many U.S. veterans, it was ironic that it was the Veterans Administration that cut off his funds. And he probably would have demonstrated practical ways to cause cancer cells to "dedifferentiate" and revert to normal. As noted earlier, in retirement, Becker refused to "shut up" and wrote *Body Electric*. In it, he writes, "I wanted the public to know that science isn't run the way they read about it in the newspaper... As research is presently funded and evaluated, we're learning more and more about less and less, and science is becoming our enemy instead of our friend".

During the twelve years his lab was operating, Dr. Robert Becker and his staff discovered:

1) the secrets of how the salamander regenerates its limbs;

2) a DC control system existing in all animals, travelling in semiconducting currents through the perineural cells along the nerves, controlling growth and healing;

3) techniques for electrical stimulation of bone healing including healing non-union fractures;

4) the effects of low frequency electromagnetic (EM) fields on human cells;

5) how to dedifferentiate frogs' red blood cells - something known to be impossible;

6) how to dedifferentiate human fibroblast cells- something known to be impossible;

7) how to dedifferentiate some cancer cells - something known to be impossible;

8) aspects of the electrical nature of the acupuncture system;

9) the quantity of voltage which causes electrolysis in the body;

10) how to cure osteomyelitis - infected bone;

11) electromagnetic anesthesia;

12) a clue to the cause of osteoporosis, thus to a cure.

All these discoveries were published in medical journals, and many are Nobel Prize material. Why Dr. Becker has not been awarded the Nobel Prize is as great a mystery as was the way the salamander regenerates his limbs - until Becker figured it out.

One more sad story, the reader might think, but after so many stories of what might have been or should have been, this one proceeds on a happier note.

Over the years, Ruth Harvey has often said, "I pray that someone will fund Dr. Becker, so that he can continue with his brilliant work".

Ruth has demonstrated the power of prayer in this case. When she and her husband put their Montana home up for sale, Bruce Kania came to take a look. A partial amputee, he had devised a plastic pad to place between stump and prosthesis, which he was marketing and selling like hotcakes. In gratitude for his new-found success, he told Ruth, he had a deep desire to help someone's research. Meanwhile, he was looking for some material to place on the pad to prevent infections. Ruth immediately thought of Becker's silver nylon, loaned him her copy of *Body Electric*, and put him in touch with Dr. Becker. As an amputee, Bruce had to be interested in someone who was researching regeneration. He went to visit Becker and made arrangements, within his means, to fund the continuation of Becker's research, which had just about ground to a halt by that time. So this story isn't over yet. Once more the prospect is alive that this should-be Nobel Laureate will have the opportunity to show the world the science of human regeneration.

Dr. Robert Becker inaugurated the scientific discipline now called Bioelectromagnetics. Its basic tenets, the electrical properties of all living things, were denied as quackery when he first came along. However, the wonders of electromedicine were greeted with about the same enthusiasm as Official Medicine greeted Rife in the earlier part of the century. But there was a younger generation coming on, and younger generations are often not too impressed by orthodoxy.

As a young woman, Ruth Harvey once had a dream that

someday she would be working with electrical machines used in healing. And so it was that when I first met her in 1982, she was demonstrating and distributing a remarkable device called the Alpha-Stim 2000. This was the brainchild of Dr. Daniel L. Kirsch, PhD in neurobiology, and produced by Electromedical Products International Inc. (EPII), a company he founded in 1981. Kirsch started studying acupuncture at age 13, and later studied other health disciplines such as chiropractic and naturopathy. He acquired quite a bit of clinical experience, too, serving as Director of the Center for Pain and Stress-Related Disorders at Columbia Presbyterian Medical Center in New York. He also studied electronics and took a great interest in Eastern European work in electromedicine, particularly something then called "electrosleep". Examining the existing devices, he decided he could do a better job and founded EPII. Moving to the Los Angeles area, he found time to serve as Clinical Director of the Electro-Acutherapy Medical Group in Laguna Beach, California, the Sports Medicine Group in Santa Monica. and wrote the curriculum for a graduate degree program in electromedicine at City University, Los Angeles.

Dr. Kirsch's Alpha-Stim 2000 was loosely classified as TENS (transcutaneous electrical nerve stimulation) but had its own unique twist. While TENS units suppress pain by overriding body electricity with stronger currents, Kirsch's device used microcurrents similar to the body's own electricity, the ones Becker found to be normal to the body. Acupuncture holds that illness results from alterations or blockages in the body's flow of energy. The Alpha-Stim 2000 was able to measure the body's normal current, determine to what extent it was altered at the site of a problem, and supply the appropriate microcurrent wave form to restore the normal flow of bioelectricity, thus healing the underlying cause of the problem. An ordinary TENS unit is designed to provide current strong enough to override a pain signal. While connected, such a unit will relieve pain, but the pain often returns when the unit is turned off. Kirsch's version usually resolved pain permanently by eliminating electrical blockage, or by restoring the normal flow of current to the problem area. The Alpha-Stim also had a way to administer its microcurrents through earclips in a variable square wave form designed by Dr. Daniel Kirsch so that it would not "entrain" brain waves; if the wave were repetitious instead of variable, the brain would get used to it and ignore it. His variable wave form thus would interrupt the chaotic brain waves which characterize stress, inducing or permitting them to return to a normal, harmonious pattern. This use of earclip electrodes is known as cranial electrotherapy stimulation, or CES, not invented or discovered by Kirsch, but improved on by him. Several other manufacturers were producing devices of this sort, all stimulated by the electrosleep research of Eastern Europe, where electromedicine is considered more "mainstream".

Learning of this interesting device, my late mother and I decided to acquire one around 1982. By then she was in an advanced state of arteriosclerosis and all too often exhausted by anxiety. When Bob Kirsch, Dan's father, drove to my mother's home in northern New York State to deliver the machine, she was in bed in just such a state. Observing her, Bob Kirsch said to himself, "This is going to be a challenge". After confirming that a doctor had prescribed the device (in conformance with FDA regulations), he unpacked the device and placed the earclips on my mother. As she dozed off, he sat down in the kitchen to talk with Ordetta Sharpe, her housekeeper. About 45 minutes later, my mother awoke and came out to the kitchen, refreshed, relaxed, even effervescent, as she was when at her best. Bob Kirsch could not believe how much better she was, nor could she herself. The Alpha-Stim's microcurrents had done their magic, melting away her stress and revitalizing her.

In the winter 1985 issue of the *American Journal of Electromedicine*, the organ of the National Institute of Electromedical Information, Ruth Harvey published an article on remarkable results she had observed while working with the Alpha-Stim 2000:

Sister Louise Hentzen had been a nun for fifty years. For

*thirty-five of those years, she suffered excruciating pain
as a result of the amputation of her right leg. She could
not tolerate analgesics because of severe allergies, yet she
remained stoic... When I met Sister Louise, she was sitting
on an examining table in one of the best pain clinics in the
midwest. Her doctor, a prominent neurosurgeon, had
asked me to see if I could ease her pain. In less than five
minutes, her pain was gone! Only once before had she
known this kind of relief. A week before, her doctor had
treated her with acupuncture, leaving the needles in for
twenty minutes. The present treatment, however, took only
five minutes and no needles were used. This is typical of
the results we see with electromedicine.*

When Ruth Harvey demonstrated the Alpha-Stim at a convention in Madison, Wisconsin, she wrote in her article that "a
lady wondered if the instrument could help her hearing. Although
the Alpha-Stim 2000 had FDA clearance only for the relief of
pain, I treated her on a point where acupuncture had been known
to help. The following day, the lady excitedly informed us that her
hearing had returned to normal."

In *Body Electric*, Dr. Robert Becker wrote; "There's reason to
believe that gifted healers generate supportive electromagnetic
effects which they convey to their patients." When he wrote that,
he was not aware that Ruth Harvey had measured just such a
capability with a close friend, the late English healer Rose
Gladden. Before Rose started to perform a healing, Ruth took a
microcurrent measurement with the Alpha-Stim on a place on the
patient's body. Then Rose placed her hands on that area of the
patient. After she had finished her healing, Ruth took another
measurement on the same spot. The original reading had
increased by 75%.

Blanche Hanks, a therapist using the Alpha-Stim 2000 while
working under Lyle Brooks, MD, a family practice physician in
Edmond, Oklahoma, told Ruth of a remarkable case, which Ruth
included in her article:

Elbert Jones...first came to our office as a stroke patient... He had no use of his left side...couldn't move his arm at all and could only barely drag his left leg. He couldn't walk unassisted. When I first saw Mr. Jones, I placed two electrodes at the base of his brain and two at the sacral area of his spine... His improvement was phenomenal. With each treatment, we watched him gain more and more use of his limbs. With two treatments a week, his activity increased to mild exercises and swimming, and in three months, he was playing racketball at the 'Y' with much younger men. Then in late February, 1983, he suffered another stroke affecting the same side and leaving him just as disabled as before. When he was able to leave the hospital, we started treating him again and had the same phenomenal results. He can now walk two miles a day, but no longer plays racketball - doctor's orders!

William Bauer, MD, MS, while an assistant professor at Case Western University School of Medicine and Chief of Otolaryngology at the VA Medical Center in Cleveland, Ohio, acquired an Alpha-Stim 2000 and found electromedical treatments effective in relieving tinnitus and even multiple sclerosis. Bauer wrote a paper entitled "Neuroelectric Medicine" which was published in the *Journal of Bioelectricity* in 1983. He described the biological mechanisms involved...not only for pain relief but the mechanisms by which the body is healed when stimulated with the appropriate electric currents. Bauer presented this paper at the First Symposium of the International Society for Bioelectricity in Boston on October 1, 1983, at which both Dr. Robert Becker and Dr. Björn Nordenström were present.

Explaining to Ruth Harvey his theories as to why Alpha-Stim works, Dr. Bauer said "There is evidence that there is a balancing process going on. Cells that are performing at sub-optimal levels are stimulated to 'turn on' and produce what they're supposed to produce, probably through DNA, which is stimulated through the cell membrane. I believe that normal cells simply resonate with the electrical impulses we send in because they're already doing their job. But diseased cells will take up this energy and literally be turned on. The thing that's nice is that you can't damage anything where you're treating since you're only bringing things back into balance, up to the optimal level, which is normal."

However effective, Dan Kirsch's Alpha-Stim 2000 cost $5,850 and was not selling all that well. To keep his company alive, he needed something that could be marketed in larger volumes. Going back to the drawing board, he designed a miniaturized Alpha-Stim. Getting it into production was another matter. Being brilliant in electromedicine wasn't enough; he needed to be a good entrepreneur as well. His adventures with venture capitalists were incredible and sometimes traumatic. At one point, he felt certain he could write a best seller on his experiences; then the profits from that might permit him to afford to return to electromedicine. There was a bad period when he was at a complete standstill and almost went through the floorboards. But he persisted, obtained the capital he needed, and launched a miniature Alpha-Stim in 1989. It sold well, and a few years later, he came up with his present version, the handsomely-designed "Alpha-Stim 100". By this time, his work had been noticed by Michael Hutchinson, who wrote a chapter on it in *Mega Brain*. He was written up twice in the *Los Angeles Times*, in Kathy Keaton's *Omni* magazine, in *USA Today*, the *Denver Post*, the *Seattle Post-Intelligencer*, *Saturday Evening Post*, *Houston Chronicle*, and *Rolling Stone Magazine* as well as in publications in South America, Australia, Japan, and Europe.

No larger than a cellular telephone, the Alpha-Stim 100 delivers microcurrents of the type and strength compatible with normal bioelectricity either through earclips or two electrodes, which can be self-adhesive or in the form of hand-held probes. Thus microcurrents can be steadily delivered to a sprain or strain. One of Dan Kirsch's most treasured pieces of promotion is a TV clip of the Dallas Cowboys' famed running back Emmitt Smith wearing an Alpha-Stim 100 at half-time. Since then, many if not most major professional sports teams use Alpha-Stim technology.

Just like its predecessor, the Alpha-Stim 100 cuts through stress like a hot knife cuts through butter, and I would not leave home without it.

Dr. Robert Becker has long been concerned that in the excitement over electromedicine, people might use currents that are too strong, which might do harm. He remembers hearing Dr. Dan Kirsch state at a conference in the 1970's that "some people think that if a certain current is good, more is better, and that's not true!" When I brought up Dan Kirsch's name, Becker said "He's the only one that's doing it right; the rest are using too much juice".

As Kirsch's cranial electrotherapy stimulation (CES) device gained momentum, there was the ever-present FDA, not paying a lot of attention at first, but always there. FDA could not conceive that medicine could be other than a pharmaceutical; for pain, you'd take a drug; for stress, you'd take another drug; what did microcurrents have to do with it? The FDA understood drugs, and a great many FDA higher-ups (some estimates say as many as 65% of FDA employees) upon finishing their FDA careers, go off to high-paying jobs in the pharmaceutical industry - if they have not made waves while at FDA. By the early 1990's, FDA regulation of medical devices had become more and more complex, approaching that for drugs. It was not intended to be that way.

The late Dr. Andrew Bassett, an early pioneer with Dr. Becker in using microcurrents for bone healing, served on a committee to plan the law (passed in 1976) governing regulation of medical devices. Bassett felt the law was good, but the problem was in getting the FDA to obey it. The law's intent was quite clear; medical devices should not be regulated like drugs. And devices which were "substantially equivalent" to devices on the market before the law was passed should be "grandfathered" and allowed on the market with no undue fuss. Electrosleep had inspired Dan Kirsch's original work. While he clearly had designed a better technology, there had been several such devices on the market. Thus getting grandfathered with the FDA as substantially equivalent to one of those devices should not have been a problem. The law requires that the FDA should grant such "510(K)" approvals in 90 days; for Kirsch's Alpha-Stim, it took 22 months. When approval was granted, FDA declared he could not market it for anxiety, depression, and insomnia - which were its main purposes. Kirsch hired a lawyer, something he was to do a great deal of in the years ahead. The lawyer wrote FDA pointing out that it was out of step with its own law, and that his client intended to go ahead and market his product if he didn't hear from the FDA. The FDA made no comment, so Kirsch proceeded to market.

In 1978, FDA set up a panel of experts to study CES. They recommended that CES be accepted for treatment of anxiety and addictions. The reference to addiction brings up one of the most interesting of electromedical products, a device invented by Dr. Margaret "Meg" Patterson of the United Kingdom. Her device was successful in enabling several famous British rock stars, such as Pete Townshend of The Who, to escape from heroin addiction. In October, 1999, Dr. Patterson opened a charity clinic in Tijuana, free if one cannot pay the $750 fee. Cocaine, heroin, alcohol, or smoking addictions are generally reversed in ONE WEEK. CBS carried a segment on the Patterson clinic on February 13, 2001. Why does such a breakthrough as this have to go outside the U.S.? Dr. Meg died in July 2002, but the technology survives.

As Kirsch was trying to survive the FDA, serious researchers were beginning to take notice, and he was happy to lend his CES devices for a large variety of studies. An early one looked at the effect of CES microcurrents on learning abilities. College students with no typing experience had Alpha-Stims hooked up to their earlobes. Some were turned on and some were not. Microcurrents in the CES device were set so low that they could not be felt, so students did not know whether they were receiving microcurrents or not. When the results were in, it was clear that those whose devices had been activated had learned significantly more quickly than those whose devices were not on. Also, a group of stenography students who had failed their test as much as four times passed on the fifth attempt when using Alpha-Stims.

Stress could be considered as a condition in which normal,

harmonious, coherent brain waves become incoherent and chaotic, reflecting the distressed state of an anxious person. Dr. Michael Heffernan conducted a study that graphically illustrated the above; two pictures of brain waves, one of a distressed person before an Alpha-Stim treatment and one after, with the previously spiked waves smoothing out (see page 300).

In 1992, tumultuous riots and fires in Los Angeles kept Dan Kirsch and his wife Tracey from getting to their office. For a few days, they didn't even know if they still had an office. Reluctantly deciding to leave the West Coast, the small city of Mineral Wells, Texas, came to their attention at an industrial relocation exposition. Once a booming resort, Mineral Wells might as well have changed its name after 1947, when the FDA appeared and shut down their wells, their main business, on a labeling pretext. The 14-story, 400-room Baker Hotel still stands, closed, in downtown Mineral Wells as an elegant reminder of the pre-FDA era. It is with considerable frustration that the people of Mineral Wells realize that in Europe, doctors prescribe and government health insurance pays for "taking the waters". Before 1947, people used to take the waters in Mineral Wells, coming from all over the U.S. by the trainloads.

The Kirsches decided that Mineral Wells met their criteria and moved Electromedical Products there in 1994. Happily and comfortably resettled, Dan and Tracey Kirsch, now the company president, would have liked nothing better than to concentrate on building their business in a pleasant small city near the Dallas-Fort Worth Metroplex. Tracey even became the chairperson of the local chamber of commerce. However, how long could they stay there? Increasing pressure from the FDA made them seriously consider relocating to Europe. On one of several scouting trips, a European industrial development official welcomed them with open arms and told them, "We love the FDA. They send us some of your most technologically-advanced companies, which can't stand their excessive regulation". Kirsch learned from the Medical Device Manufacturers Association (MDMA) that 24% of the American medical device industry had relocated to Europe.

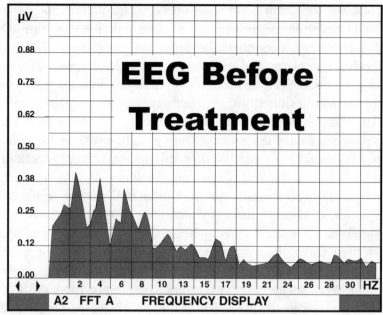

This first chart shows a typical pain patient's brainwaves averaged over two minutes. This is an abnormal frequency pattern.

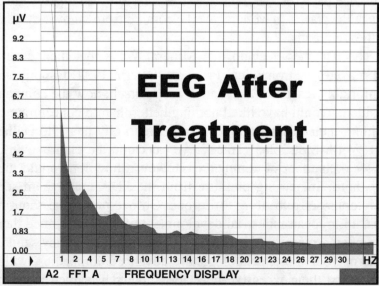

This second chart was taken from the same patient after 10 minutes of Alpha-Stim use. It shows beneficial smoothing of the brainwaves to a normal pattern.   (NOTE: EEG = Electroencephalogram)

These were companies like Kirsch's EPII, on the cutting edge of the technological breakthroughs in which the U.S. excels, the high-tech companies which epitomize and symbolize the U.S. competitive advantage in the world.

During the 1980's and early 1990's, Dr. Kirsch was one of six or seven FDA-registered manufacturers in the CES field. This was to change in a very dramatic way.

One day in August, 1995, Dan Kirsch called me and said "the FDA is trying to put me out of business". Aware of the earlier pressures that had led him to contemplate moving to Europe, I asked, "what have they done now?" While the FDA was directed by law not to try to regulate devices like drugs, they were proceeding to do just that. Part of the drug regulatory process requires the preparation of a Pre-Marketing Approval or PMA before a new product is placed on the market. Preparing a PMA is a monstrous process, requiring the history of all scientific research on all similar products, a history of the marketing of the product, and all other relevant information. PMA's are not that common; the FDA only gets about 40 per year, *i.e.*, 40 new products. However, there are 12,000 or more "510(K)" applications for product updates; the comparison indicates how FDA requirements for exhaustive paperwork stifle the introduction of anything new. What the FDA had done, Dan Kirsch explained, was to publish a proposed regulation requiring all manufacturers of CES devices to prepare a PMA within 90 days or go off the market. In his case, this would be a pre-marketing approval not for a new product to go on the market, like a new drug, but so that a product which had already been on the market for 16 years could stay on the market. Consulting several experts, Kirsch learned that to hire someone to prepare the PMA would cost about $250,000 and take probably one to two years or more, at least four times longer than the period allowed. Not having the time or money to hire anyone, he set out to do the job himself.

Apparently assuming that nobody could possibly prepare a PMA in 90 days, the FDA entered in their computer that Electromedical Products International Inc., was "out of business". EPII products were manufactured in Asia, so this meant that when they arrived at Customs in Los Angeles, it would take Tracey Kirsch two to four weeks to clear a shipment. On one occasion, she threatened to call their congressman, who had already given public support to EPII against the FDA. FDA released the shipment the same day.

Having noticed an increasing volume of static from FDA over the previous couple of years, the Kirsches had had the good sense to seek the help of their congressman, Charles Stenholm (D-TX), who took a keen interest in their situation, as did Congressman Joe Barton (R-TX), chair of the committee which oversees the FDA. So when real trouble came, the Kirsches had some friends in Washington.

On Halloween Day, 1995, Dan Kirsch was literally working around the clock in a desperate attempt to finish the PMA and thus stay in business, the business he'd spent most of his life building. On that day, the FDA decided to stage an inspection, which lasted three days. In came two inspectors from the FDA Dallas office, led by an agent of the Texas Department of Health (TDH), who was acting jointly as an FDA inspector (the two agencies work closely together). It was a memorable inspection.

Very much on their guard, the Kirsches had arranged for Jonathan Emord, their Washington attorney, very experienced in FDA matters, to participate by telephone in any FDA visit. Dennis Rudder, the FDA/TDH chief inspector, strenuously objected but finally agreed to the attorney's participation. On several occasions, Emord had to point out that Rudder's questioning was outside of his authority, such as, "where are your bank accounts?" Emord reminded Rudder that EPII's finances were not the business of the FDA. There was a reason for the FDA's question. When the FDA decides to target a firm, they have a disturbing pattern of seizing and freezing its bank accounts, leaving such a firm unable to fight back.

All these matters were on Tracey Kirsch's mind as she tried to find out what the FDA group really wanted. They said they were there to investigate a complaint, but refused to provide the nature of the complaint, which they are required to do. She had earlier informed the *Mineral Wells Daily Index* of the FDA visit, and the newspaper had sent reporter Charles McClure to see if there was a story. There was, and he was soon to become a big part of it. Seeing himself being photographed, Rudder demanded to know "Who is THAT?" Informed that it was the press, there to cover the public business of a government agency doing its regulating, Rudder and his agents stormed out of the office, refusing to talk in the presence of the press. He returned sometime later, saying that his superior, whom he refused to identify to Attorney Emord, had said it was all right for the press to be there. However, on his way back in, Rudder told reporter McClure, "Don't you photograph ME!" and lunged at him, pushing the reporter back into some file cabinets. Meanwhile, McClure snapped a picture of Rudder and his thumb coming at the camera. The picture appeared on the front page of the *Index* the next day, November 1, 1995. The entire proceedings were videotaped by EPII, much to the distress of the FDA agents. Attorney Emord had to tell them sharply that EPII was entirely within its rights to videotape and audiotape the inspection. When the dust finally settled, the FDA inspectors asked a few minor questions which were quickly answered. The "complaint", a legally defined term indicating that someone had been injured, turned out to be nothing more than a competitor complaining that EPII was marketing devices for CES applications - not exactly a secret.

The Freedom of Information Act, passed in the wake of an earlier time of government excesses, enables any citizen to demand any government documents that are not classified. Hiring a firm specialized in this area, Dan Kirsch asked for every document on EPII in the FDA files. When the file finally arrived after the FDA had stonewalled for two years, the Kirsches saw how close they had come to a raid. After the inspection, the Dallas FDA office had recommended stern measures against EPII and had drafted a severe warning letter to be sent, threatening seizures, injunctions and civil penalties. However, FDA headquarters in Washington, aware that Congressmen Barton and

Stenholm took an interest in EPII, overruled the Dallas FDA office. In a raid, inventory, files, even computers, might be taken.

Dealing with the FDA, Dan and Tracey Kirsch found, was not for the faint-hearted.

As the rumpus of the inspection was going on, Dan Kirsch was in his back office feverishly working to finish the PMA, which he did with five days to spare. The FDA wanted the PMA in six copies, which he had his attorneys hand deliver. Each copy weighed 18 pounds and six ounces.

The next move for the FDA upon receiving a PMA would be to "file" it for review. The Office of Device Evaluation (ODE) in the FDA's Center for Devices and Radiological Health (CDRH) informed Dr. Kirsch that it would not "file" the document he had spent 85 days and nights preparing. It outright refused to review his work, meaning that he would be out of business after all; if they didn't accept it, he was done.

The only preliminary review given the PMA at ODE was by a mechanical engineer, a woman who repeatedly demonstrated that she knew nothing of electromedicine, of electricity, of medicine, of behavioral sciences or of stress and anxiety. At their first meeting, she asked questions making it very evident that she had not read the document at all. Given FDA hostility, Dr. Kirsch informed those attending the FDA meeting that his company would almost certainly have to move to Europe. That being the case, Kirsch told the mechanical engineer, "please hold onto those six copies of my PMA, since I can probably use part of the documents in Europe." A few weeks later, the engineer called Tracey Kirsch, asking for six more copies, since the previous ones had been destroyed. Since FDA was supposed to retain them on microfiche, Mrs. Kirsch told her to get them from that.

Given the FDA's attitude, Attorney Emord agreed to do whatever the Kirsches wanted, but he was not optimistic. EPII then hired a different lawyer, Larry Pilot, a former FDA counsel, and an expert on the FDA devices law. When Pilot saw how arbitrary and capricious FDA's treatment of EPII and its PMA was becoming, he filed suit against the FDA. He demanded that the FDA obey its own laws and that a review of Kirsch's PMA be carried out by independent persons qualified to do so, as the law requires. FDA produced an electrical engineer to pronounce on the relationship between anxiety and depression; EPII and Pilot maintained that electrical engineers, while important, are not qualified to render medical or psychiatric opinions. FDA even had a government dentist say that although CES research shows that CES will help anxiety in dentistry, she could not see any need for that. Dan Kirsch wondered if she had ever been to a dentist herself.

Finally, FDA agreed to "file" the PMA, but sent EPII a "major deficiency" letter. In a manner designed to create a problem rather than settle one, the letter asked questions, but said that if the questions were answered, FDA would restart the clock of review of the PMA upon receipt of the answers. This was calculated to mean that EPII would thus have missed the 90-day deadline for submitting the PMA. Then it would have to stop marketing, and thus be out of business in the U.S. - just as FDA had entered into its computers months earlier. FDA suggested that EPII devote itself to full-time research, but gave no suggestions as to how to pay for the research if the company had no cash flow.

The legal battle had its ups and downs; Pilot won some stages for EPII and lost some. At one point, it seemed the cause was lost. But then came a surprise.

On January 28, 1997, the FDA announced that it would completely withdraw its proposed regulation of August 1995 requiring CES manufacturers to file a PMA. Dan Kirsch had won; he had beaten City Hall. But as Tracey Kirsch commented, "The FDA is a lot bigger than City Hall".

Commercially, all the commotion had produced an unexpected effect; EPII was the last man standing. All the other CES manufacturers had folded when faced with FDA's demand for the PMA.

In March 1999, Dr. Dan Kirsch attended the 10th International Congress on Stress in Montreux, Switzerland, to give a paper entitled "Cranial Electrical Stimulation: An overview of its application for the treatment of pain, anxiety, insomnia, depression, and other stress-related disorders". A senior FDA official was there, also to give a talk, and he knew who Dan Kirsch was. He told Kirsch, "It was really unnecessary that you were put through all that, for after all, the treatment is harmless." He added that, "The FDA should not bother companies with a 20-year marketing history." The FDA man was absolutely right, for the bottom line is; if something is harmless, why do we need the FDA protecting us from it?

In the late 1990's, ABC's *20/20* literally accused the FDA of being responsible for killing people with excessive red tape, and for giving the impression of being more interested in paperwork than scientific fact. In a show devoted to the over-regulation of medical devices, ABC told of FDA's refusal to approve "Breastpad", a very simple lubricated pad with an established 20-year history intended to aid women in self-examination for breast tumors. The manufacturers won quick approval in Japan, Europe, and Canada. But after 1,200 pages of documentation and $2,000,000 spent over nine years on attempting to obtain approval, FDA classified this simple pad as "high risk", like pacemakers. In another case, *20/20* told how the FDA had gone after defibrillators, a device the American Heart Association calls "the most important treatment for cardiac arrest". FDA forced some defibrillator manufacturers to shut down because of insufficient paperwork; ABC estimated that this may have cost 1,000 lives. Originally introduced at the end of the 18th century, defibrillators were denounced by religious leaders at the time, since they considered that reviving people from the dead had to be the work of the devil. It took a lawsuit to get the FDA off of defibrillators. ABC also told how FDA barred the use of heart pumps, standard equipment on ambulances in Europe and Japan, since the patient had not given informed consent for their use. The FDA did not volunteer how a patient with no heartbeat could give informed consent. ABC estimated that this resulted in another 20 lives lost each day because of FDA regulations.

From the first, the Alpha-Stim has been considered a Class III device, meaning significant risk, and thus requiring a doctor's prescription. For years, the FDA also considered acupuncture needles as Class III devices, "significantly risky, dangerous devices". Finally, at an August 1996 meeting, the head of FDA's Office of Device Evaluation openly granted that there was no safety issue with EPII's CES device. Since the PMA flap, EPII has applied to FDA for reclassification of CES to Class II or Class I (harmless). It would seem that Dr. Kirsch put the safety issue to rest once and for all in 1997 by completing the rigorous examination to secure registration of the Alpha-Stim 100 CES device by the Underwriters Laboratories (UL), a good way to handle safety questions for any electromedical device. The Alpha-Stim also passed the strict safety requirements to market in Europe having earned their CE Mark of Approval.

Part of the PMA asked about the efficacy of CES devices. In answer, Dr. Kirsch pointed to seventeen independent scientific studies maintaining that Alpha-Stim technology is effective in reducing anxiety and related symptoms. Kirsch further notes that his PMA application contained 155 CES studies, 28 of them double-blinded, and 20 experimental animal studies. He also notes that in 1995, the Harvard School of Public Health published a thorough statistical review of selected CES research in the *Journal of Nervous and Mental Diseases* confirming the modality as an effective treatment for anxiety. Kirsch published a summary of all the CES studies listed in his PMA in 1999 in a book entitled *The Science Behind Cranial Electrotherapy Stimulation.*

Despite the dubiousness of the FDA, cranial electrotherapy stimulation (CES) is regarded as an important anti-stress treatment in most of the world. Following the Gulf War, Kuwait, which knows something about stress, invited Dr. Kirsch to come teach their doctors, and treat Kuwaiti veterans suffering from stress and anxiety. The VA never offered such help to U.S. veterans.

Kirsch notes that it has been estimated that stress is the cause, or at least a contributing cause, in 75% to 80% of all diseases. "If that is indeed the case", says Kirsch, "then I believe that CES and the Alpha-Stim can make a big contribution to preventing such things as cardiovascular disease and stroke, thus reducing health-care costs."

Studies by Official Medicine often tend to confuse the issue. The National Institute of Drug Abuse, part of the NIH, carried out a study to see if use of CES devices could help people cut down on smoking, or stop completely. The Institute pronounced that they were ineffective. However, the study was set up to fail; it used far too little current to treat addicted persons, only 10% of the current necessary to achieve results. In the next two chapters, similar tests that were set up to fail will be described, carried out by another branch of the NIH, the National Cancer Institute, only those cost lives. In a way, cheating by Official Medicine is the greatest of compliments, showing that a therapy is being taken seriously.

The sky seems the limit for what electromedicine can accomplish. Consider one of the most dreaded calamities that can befall anyone - a stroke. Ruth Harvey reported on someone whose paralysis was reversed twice with electromedicine. Dan Kirsch heard of another such case, not an old man but a young girl, only 25. As a medical student, she had had a stroke at age 20 and hadn't walked or been able to move one arm in five years. She got hold of an Alpha-Stim, used the earclips, but other than resting her, it didn't help her main problem; she couldn't walk. Then someone told her that when the clips are placed on the earlobes, microcurrents are sent through the lower part of the brain, which controls the emotions and automatic functions of the heart and lungs. But if the clips are placed on the top of the ear, they send microcurrents to the cerebral cortex. Three days later, she reported that she had just gone for a slow one-mile walk and could rotate her arm at the elbow after using the earclips on the top of her ears.

Apologists for Official Medicine would aerily dismiss such stories as mere anecdotes. To be sure, two cases do not make a double blind study, but what anecdotes! Strokes are still among the costliest illnesses in the U.S., and among the most numerous. Surely these anecdotes are a signpost, an incredible lead, pointing to a solution for a dreaded problem.

The stroke reversals point a tantalizing finger to the vastness of the electromedical potential, whose limits we do not yet know. Chinese acupuncture charts show numerous points on the scalp; our medicine has no notion that anything can be accomplished through electrical stimulation of such points. Many years ago, Ruth Harvey was using the Alpha-Stim 2000 on a woman who had had a disc operation on her back. A nerve was cut that should not have been, and the woman dragged her right leg. Knowing that the left side of the brain governs the right side of the body, and studying a scalp acupuncture chart in a book Dan Kirsch wrote in 1978, she looked for the area of the brain governing the leg. The Alpha-Stim 2000 could measure bioelectricity, and when she found the point, it registered dead - no electricity at all. She treated the point until the machine indicated that normal electric flow had been restored. Within a half hour, feeling returned to the woman's leg. Two other therapists, using an Alpha-Stim on the scalp of Parkinsons patients, saw tremors come to an abrupt halt.

These are indications of a dramatic therapy, something that works quickly, the sort of things Americans like. Dr. Bill Bauer saw improvement in MS patients after treatments on the tops of the ears and on the scalp. Conventional medicine has nothing for these conditions - strokes, Parkinsons, MS. Does the list stop there? Could CES treatments help epileptics? Or Alzheimers? Nobody knows. Dr. Kirsch and other manufacturers should be free to tell the truth about what electromedicine can do, based on facts, and doctors should be free to use such harmless therapies (there has never been any report of any harm coming from a CES device). Until then, the poor unfortunates suffering from such diseases will continue in their adversity and be told "there's no drug for this".

Were we as a society organized to greet medical breakthroughs as eagerly as we do computer breakthroughs, our health costs would plummet.

With Dan Kirsch having enough trouble with the FDA just over claims for effectiveness in stress and anxiety, the last thing he wants is to do is to open Pandora's box and talk about these other CES capabilities. For the FDA, that would be making claims, even though he would simply be telling the truth and announcing interesting scientific events that happened. Dr. Kirsch has had to put a great deal of resources and attention just into surviving. Someday, as a neurobiologist also trained in acupuncture, homeopathy, chiropractic, and naturopathy, perhaps he will have the freedom and resources to organize research in other CES capabilities. Such research will have to be done abroad, far from the FDA - unless things change.

Already well situated in Europe, Kirsch's next focus is China, where a young doctor, who also earned a PhD in electrophysiology from the University of Arizona, is interested in Kirsch's work. Together, they plan to open an electromedical treatment center based on Alpha-Stim therapy. There, Chinese stroke victims, or Parkinson's patients, will be able to receive Alpha-Stim treatments. Meanwhile, news of the very existence of such treatments is censored from American stroke victims by the FDA.

For continuing CES research, it would be nice to have the capabilities of the earlier Alpha-Stim 2000, which is out of production. When it measured low electricity at certain points, you treated until the reading came to normal. Kirsch would love to produce a modernized version of the old 2000, but there is just one problem; money. He's still paying the legal bills he ran up to sue the FDA to stay in business. He feels that it would cost about $5,000,000 to reengineer the 2000 and bring it up to the latest in computerization. While good, his business does not generate that kind of cash. Ruth Harvey has declared a new prayer objective; funds to produce a new 2000. With her demonstrated track record, it may happen.

After a lecture, someone asked Dr. Kirsch to present a "best case". Kirsch referred to one written up in the October 1998 *American Journal of Pain Management* about a U.S. government official named Wilson Hulley who has global reflex sympathetic dystrophy (RSD), one of the very worst pain-related illnesses. Usually this is just in one limb, Kirsch explained, but Hulley had it throughout his entire body. He was in such extraordinary pain that he felt tempted to commit suicide. Using nothing more than the Alpha-Stim's earclips applied to his earlobes, Hulley's pain was reduced significantly during his very first treatment. After 18 months of Alpha-Stim, his pain was further reduced sufficiently to allow him to continue his activities as an executive for President Clinton's Committee on Employment of People with Disabilities. He again can work 30-40 hours a week, is completely off morphine, and has reduced his need for other drugs.

On a perfect summer day in June 1999, at a restaurant in Alexandria Bay, NY, overlooking Boldt Castle and the Thousand Islands, Robert Becker and Daniel Kirsch and their wives finally met. They had paid their dues as pioneers, blazing hard trails, and immediately became friends. Kirsch gave Becker an Alpha-Stim and they laid plans for close collaboration.

After some months of experience with his patients, Becker commented, "In the majority of cases when you're dealing with a pain syndrome where you can't locate the source, what we call neurogenic pain, the Alpha-Stim does a pretty decent job, although not in every case. In pain, as a substitute for pharmaceuticals, it has considerable value."

CES is a field that would not have happened without the pioneering efforts of Dr. Robert O. Becker and Dr. Daniel L. Kirsch. Looking at the unfulfilled potential of electromedicine is kind of like a walk on the wild side - It can stop pain, dissolve stress, accelerate learning, raise I.Q.'s, reverse stroke damage of long standing, stop Parkinsons tremors, regrow bones, regenerate flesh, even dedifferentiate cancer cells. Future Science, we could call it, except that it already exists. Dealing with the basic forces of life, the secrets of the body's currents, frequencies and resonances, electromedicine is surely the medicine of the new millennium. We will hear much more of it, for it will save many lives, much suffering, and fortunes in healthcare costs - if the government will just get out of the way.

Hydrazine Sulfate

In May 1998, an article on the front page of the *New York Times* described a potential breakthrough in cancer achieved by Dr. Judah Folkman of Harvard Medical School. Folkman reported that he had developed two compounds to stop angiogenesis, the formation of new blood vessels which supply tumors with nutrients. Folkman's compounds stopped angiogenesis in cancerous mice, after which tumors shrank and even vanished. The prospect of such a simple way to deal with cancer won well-deserved praise for Dr. Folkman. Then cancer researchers warned that his compounds would be hard to produce in volume, that it would be a long time before they would be available, and that people should calm down. Stopping angiogenesis is how shark cartilage works.

Cancer orthodoxy holds that the best way to deal with cancer cells is to cut them out with surgery, destroy them with radiation, or kill them with poisonous chemicals (many of which evolved from the mustard gas used in World War I). The idea is for the poison to kill cancer cells faster, hopefully, than it kills normal cells (and perhaps the patient). Sometimes it works, but it is profoundly damaging to bone marrow, which produces vital immune cells. Many cancer patients die from chemotherapy rather than from cancer. Thus starving a cancer by cutting off its blood supply is an attractive alternative to flooding a patient with poison.

Stopping angiogenesis is an excellent idea but so is stopping gluconeogenesis, another path to the same goal of preventing the body from feeding a tumor. Was there selective myopia in mentioning one and not the other?

Gluconeogenesis refers to how the liver processes lactic acid and other small molecules into glucose (sugar). In 1968, Dr.

Joseph Gold of the Syracuse Cancer Research Institute in Syracuse, NY, published a paper suggesting that if a way could be found to stop gluconeogenesis, it might stop cachexia (caKEKsia). This is the wasting process that kills about 70% of cancer victims; the other 30% die when a tumor's invasion of a vital organ brings life to an end. (Cachexia kills AIDS patients as well, but AIDS was not known in 1968.) Gold stated that cancer cells draw on the body's glucose for energy and produce lactic acid as waste. The liver then reprocesses the lactic acid back into glucose, thereby supplying the cancer with more energy. In the meantime, protein (muscle) is breaking down into its constituent amino acids and the liver is reprocessing these, too, via gluconeogenesis, into glucose. The process repeats over and over in a vicious cycle, with the cancer getting stronger and the patient getting weaker, wasting away (cachexia) as the cancer robs the body of glucose and energy. Preventing cancer's process of wasting a person's energy by stopping gluconeogenesis in the liver or kidney would be very important, just as important as stopping angiogenesis.

The next year, Gold heard biochemist Paul Ray give a paper showing that the chemical hydrazine sulfate would deactivate the enzyme in the liver needed to produce glucose from lactic acid. Hydrazine sulfate (HS) is a common, cheap chemical, a derivative of which is sometimes used in rocket fuel. As a product, HS is unpatentable.

Setting up experiments in mice, Gold confirmed his theory. After cancerous mice were given hydrazine sulfate, not only did they stop wasting away from cachexia but their tumors shrank and some vanished. Gold published his initial animal experiments with HS in *Oncology*, an international cancer journal, in 1969 and 1970, and thence from 1971 through 1975.

If hydrazine sulfate were indeed useful in cancer, Gold realized that it had a big advantage by being extremely inexpensive, in welcome contrast to costly chemotherapies. One session of chemotherapy would buy a ten year supply of hydrazine sulfate.

As a chemical, HS could itself be considered chemotherapy,

but unlike conventional chemo, it is virtually non-toxic.

Applying to the National Cancer Institute (NCI) for a grant to do research with hydrazine sulfate on cachexia in rats and mice, Gold was funded by NCI from 1973 to 1976. However, once HS began to catch on as being effective in humans, NCI refused him further grants.

Introducing a new cancer therapy, Gold knew, would not be easy. However, Dr. Joseph Gold had in-depth experience with difficult projects. As a U.S. Air Force medical research doctor, he was a member of the elite USAF team which selected the Mercury Astronauts (including John Glenn), who made the first U.S. manned space flight. Gold was awarded a Presidential Citation by President Eisenhower for his work on the Mercury Project.

Dr. Gold presented his ideas to the New York Academy of Sciences in 1973. After his talk, a doctor came up to him and said, "I have a patient with terminal Hodgkins disease who will certainly die in three or four days. I'd like to try hydrazine sulfate."

Gold suggested a dosage. The doctor later reported to Gold that his patient experienced an extraordinary turnaround and was "up and about" in a few weeks. This was told by Gold to veteran researcher Wayne Martin in 1977, and quoted in Ralph Moss' *The Cancer Industry*. In his book, Moss reports that, "by August 1973, there were about 20-30 patients taking HS in various parts of the country. By the middle of September, 200-300, and by October, over 1,000."

Closely following Gold's progress was his friend and fellow scientist, Dr. Dean Burk, who spent forty years as head of cell chemistry at the NCI. Writing in the *New England Natural Food Association Bulletin* in 1974, Burk called hydrazine sulfate "the most remarkable anticancer agent I have come across in my 45 years experience in cancer…this material is so cheap because it is made by the trainload for industrial purposes".

Ralph Moss writes in *Cancer Industry* what Burk told officials at Sloan Kettering in New York when he met with them in August, 1973:

Let me tell you this perfectly true story. There is nothing mystical or poetic about it - and I could give you many (such stories). A woman with Hodgkin's disease who had been flat on her back for seven weeks, who had no appetite and who had lost all her weight - a 'paper-thin' patient - took hydrazine sulfate. One week later, she was shopping in the grocery store with her own bag; five days later she was spending most of the day in her garden. I don't give you that as any miraculous story - it is simply the plain truth.

In September 1973, Sloan Kettering proposed to Dr. Gold that a joint study on the use of hydrazine sulfate in terminal patients be carried out between them and Gold's Syracuse Cancer Research Institute. Because it was a chemical, HS was assigned to the Sloan Kettering chemotherapists to evaluate. It was agreed that the dosage would start at 60 milligrams (mg) a day for three days, then 60 mg twice a day for three days, and then 60 mg three times a day from then on. Dr. Gold soon learned that Dr. Manuel Ochoa, the supervising physician, had lowered the dose to 1 mg a day the first day, 2 mg a day the second day, then increasing 1 mg a day until reaching 20 or 30 mg a day, far less than the agreed dosage. When Gold protested, Ochoa agreed to return to the correct protocol. Deciding to pay a surprise visit, Dr. Gold found the stubborn Ochoa continuing to change the dosage. As patients started to improve, Ochoa gave them a single dose of 120 to 190 mg, which had the effect of short-circuiting their recovery. The brother of one of the patients called Gold to report that Ochoa had told him he had "no enthusiasm or interest" in hydrazine sulfate, and that the drug was "worthless" in cancer. (Moss, *Cancer Industry*) When Ochoa later reported that HS had caused some nerve damage, Gold reprimanded him at the March 1974 meeting in Houston of the American Association for Cancer Research, "You should know by virtue of your training that in critically ill patients, it is quite easy to produce serious toxicities with any cancer drug by overdosing". Gold also pointed out that only the patients who were overdosed had experienced nerve damage, which was temporary and ceased when the medication was stopped. Dr. Gold believes that any treatment with HS of less than one month is inadequate to produce results. Of the Sloan Kettering patients, 4 received HS for less than 2 weeks and 12 for 14-28 days. Only 13 patients received HS for more than 28 days; these included some who were underdosed and some who were overdosed.

By breaking the protocol not just once, which could have been a mistake, but persistently, Dr. Ochoa and his team of chemotherapists broke Sloan Kettering's agreement and Ochoa broke his own word to Dr. Gold. That made the trials worthless. Was it Dr. Ochoa's purpose from the beginning to mess up the trials and thus discredit hydrazine sulfate? Even though the test had been mishandled, Ochoa moved ahead to publish.

In 1975, a Sloan Kettering researcher leaked to Dr. Gold an advance copy of the statement Sloan Kettering was preparing to release. It stated that "negative results were obtained despite strict adherence to Dr. Gold's protocol" (Moss). Through his lawyers, Gold demanded that all reference to following his protocol be removed. Sloan Kettering withdrew the offending remarks, but in mid-year, it announced that it was no longer treating patients with HS. Sloan Kettering claimed that it had "adequately" treated 29 patients, with none of the patients responding positively and some showing nerve damage (Moss).

Dr. Gold then experienced the phenomenon of whoever has the loudest microphone wins the debate. He strongly protested that no one was "adequately" treated with HS at Sloan Kettering, but Sloan Kettering's decibel level was much higher than his. Sloan Kettering never disciplined Dr. Ochoa for not being able to follow a very simple protocol, which any intern could have done. Apparently Sloan Kettering wasn't embarrassed at all. Perhaps Ochoa was not acting on his own initiative in making so many mistakes.

Dr. Gold told a friend, "I've heard of cancer politics, but I've never seen anything like this... I wouldn't believe it if I hadn't seen it with my own eyes." (Moss)

In 1975, Gold published in *Oncology* a study carried out under the auspices of Calbiochem, a California pharmaceutical company. The study showed that 70% of 84 advanced cancer patients, when treated with the correct HS protocol, had subjective improvements such as weight gain and decrease in pain; "17% showed objective improvements including tumor regression...or more than a year-long stabilization of their condition". Dr. Gold reported that in seven of the improved cases where there had been previous therapy, improvement occurred only after HS was added to the protocol. He also pointed out that of the "objectively" improved cases, 50% were on HS alone. Gold noted that about 2% of the patients, after several months of three 60 mg tablets a day, experienced pain or weakness in their limbs (the nerve damage reported at Sloan Kettering); however, this condition was easily corrected by lowering dosage or giving Vitamin B-6 (Moss).

Dr. Gold advises anyone interested in hydrazine sulfate that certain substances are completely incompatible with it. Among these is Vitamin B-6, which counteracts the drug. Other incompatibles (some of which can do harm if taken with HS) are alcohol, tranquilizers, and barbiturates. Also to be avoided are any foods containing large amounts of the amino acid tyramine, which blocks the action of HS. Such foods include raisins, nuts, and fermented foods such as yogurt and certain cheeses.

In his *Oncology* article, Gold called HS a "new type of chemotherapy" and "the first of a class of new agents designed to interrupt host participation in cancer" (*i.e.*, the body feeding the cancer). Gold stated that "hydrazine sulfate is apparently not a tumor-specific agent, since virtually all types of cancer... appear susceptible to its actions... Reports which have reached this laboratory indicate that the spectrum of disease beneficially affected by hydrazine sulfate extends to cancers arising from all organ systems and/or tissues in the body."

Attracted by the low cost of hydrazine sulfate, Dr. Mikhail Gershanovich, Dr. Vladimir Filov, and other Russian researchers at the Petrov Institute in what was then Leningrad, later renamed St. Petersburg, took note of Dr. Gold's work in 1972. In 1975, the Russians published two studies, both showing HS effective in controlling cachexia, Dr. Gold's main point. The Russians reported 54% of patients deriving the "subjective" benefits described earlier (Moss). The Russians did not give HS as the initial cancer treatment, but rather to late-stage, terminal patients who were not getting useful results from radiation or chemotherapy. Six weeks after completing radiation or chemo, the Russians then gave HS by itself. While American chemotherapists insist that cancer drugs must kill cancer cells (*i.e.*, be cytotoxic), the Russians had no such hang-ups over using the non-toxic HS.

Ralph Moss summed up the Russians' findings as follows:

HS reverses cachexia.
HS stops the growth of animal tumors.
HS works by stopping gluconeogenesis.
HS is relatively non-toxic.
HS controls cancerous growths in humans.
HS causes a remarkable improvement in patients' mood, sometimes to the point of euphoria.

The American Cancer Society (ACS) apparently could not find anyone who could read Russian. In March 1976, the ACS magazine, *CA*, stated, "After careful study of the literature and other available information, the American Cancer Society does not have evidence that hydrazine sulfate is of any objective benefit in the treatment of cancer in human beings". This language placed HS on the ACS "unproven" list, a kind of blacklist which also includes Dr. Koch's glyoxylide, the Hoxsey treatment, and Krebiozen. In thus blacklisting HS, the ACS failed to mention a conflict of interest, its ownership of 50% of the rights to a competing chemotherapy, the extremely toxic "5-FU" (Rorvik, 1977). Skipping around in the medical literature, the ACS quoted the flawed Sloan Kettering tests, ignored the Calbiochem tests and Gold's other published work, and chose to overlook or misconstrue the Russian testing of hydrazine sulfate.

The ACS wasn't the only part of Official Medicine that couldn't or wouldn't read Russian. In 1976, Representative Jim Hanley, congressman from Syracuse, wrote to the NCI requesting a status report on HS. NCI wrote back, "Hydrazine sulfate has been tested in the Soviet Union at the Petrov Institute... No evidence of meaningful anticancer activity was reported". One week later, Hanley received a copy of the actual Petrov study, which stated exactly the opposite. The taxpayer-funded NCI had lied to a member of Congress. Senator Paul Douglas would not have been surprised (Chapter 8).

By 1978, Gold estimated that about 5,000 cancer patients in the U.S. were being treated with HS by hundreds of physicians (Moss). One of these was Dr. R. O. Bicks, professor of medicine at the University of Tennessee in Memphis. Bicks told the *Medical Tribune* in 1978 of several patients with inoperable pancreatic cancer who, when put on HS, survived twice as long as he would have expected. He would have kept using it but the FDA got in touch with him and claimed that HS causes bone marrow toxicity.(Moss) Gold has never seen any such results in the thousands of cases he has monitored, quite unlike conventional chemotherapy, which does not just damage bone marrow, but destroys it. This was about the time when the FDA was putting out the word that DMSO might cause cataracts, an assertion contradicted by DMSO research.

In September 1978, the NCI announced that it was interested in research in cachexia. Apparently they were only interested if the drug used was not hydrazine sulfate. When Dr. Gold applied for a grant, he was turned down flat.

During the time of the Soviet Union, everything was a state secret. That even included the Petrov Institute's HS results, which did not get out of the USSR easily even though they had been published in a Russian medical journal. The late industrial magnate Armand Hammer maintained contacts in the USSR right to the top; his private jet was always allowed to land at Moscow airport at any time. On one visit, he pried loose the Petrov results and forwarded them to Gold and the NCI.

In the 1970's, regular meetings between Russian and American cancer doctors were scheduled on an annual basis. Since such a gathering was approaching, Gold urged that the NCI invite Dr. Mikhail Gershanovich, the chief HS researcher. The NCI refused to issue the invitation, and Gold called Armand Hammer. Hammer called Joseph Califano, Secretary of Health, and Stuart Eisenstadt, adviser to President Jimmy Carter. Both called the NCI, which finally issued the invitation, stating that opportunities would be arranged for the Russian data to be presented.

Upon Gershanovich's arrival, a seminar where he would present his research was set up at the NCI. However, determined bureaucrats have many ways to achieve their ends; NCI simply did not publicize the meeting, so very few people knew about it. Instead of the expected 500-600, only 16 showed up.

The old boy network wasn't through yet in showing what it could do when pushed. It had also been proposed that Dr. Gershanovich should speak at the American Association for Cancer Research (AACR) at New Orleans in May 1979, where he would be introduced by Dr. Gold. At the last minute, AACR chairman Dr. Bayard Clarkson, a chemotherapist from Sloan Kettering, abruptly canceled Gershanovich's appearance. It was too late, however, for Clarkson to stop the abstract of Gershanovich's paper from being published in the AACR conference Proceedings. The abstract stated, "Initial studies indicate hydrazine sulfate to be clinically effective in reversing cachexia and producing disease stabilization in late-stage cancer patients".

A reporter spoke to Dr. Clarkson and commented on the Russians having carried out the first wide-scale trials of hydrazine sulfate, reporting good results. He asked Clarkson, "Shouldn't the paper be presented?" Clarkson replied, "Our decision is final. The Gershanovich paper is not going to be presented, and that's it." (*Medical Tribune*, May 16, 1979)

In *Cancer Industry*, Ralph Moss noted that just before the AACR conference, according to the Sloan Kettering house journal, Dr. Clarkson and a colleague received grants totaling

$123,000 from the American Cancer Society - which had HS on its "unproven" list. If this influenced Clarkson's treatment of Gershanovich, the wind was soon to shift. Later that year, the ACS took HS off its "unproven" list. The change may have been influenced by Dr. Frank Rauscher, former director of the NCI, who had not long before gone to the ACS to direct its research.

In 1980, Dr. Vincent DeVita became director of the NCI, where he would stay until 1988. Having pioneered a frequently successful chemotherapy protocol for Hodgkin's lymphoma, Dr. DeVita had a right to be proud of his achievement. However, he seemed to be biased against anything other than toxic chemotherapy. "We throw away better drugs than hydrazine sulfate", he told Geraldo Rivera on ABC's *20/20* in 1981.

Until 1980, the Petrov Institute was receiving grants from the NCI. Shortly after Dr. DeVita took over, Petrov's funding was canceled. This was after they had released their favorable studies on HS. It happened to be the year the Soviet Union invaded Afghanistan, when a chill began to pervade Soviet-American relations. Thinking the Afghan invasion was the cause for the canceling of the NCI grant, Dr. Bulaev, Petrov's international liaison officer, wrote her friends at the NCI asking "Isn't cancer more important than politics?" She received no answer. (Kamen, *Penthouse*)

Ironically, Dr. Gershanovich and his colleagues at the Petrov Institute found that in cases of non-Hodgkin's lymphoma where the DeVita chemo protocol failed, they got favorable results by then giving patients hydrazine sulfate. This is the type of cancer which killed Jacqueline Onassis, who may have received the DeVita treatment (and probably did not receive HS). At the beginning of the 21st century, HS is the treatment of choice in Russia for this type of cancer (after failure of chemotherapy).

The Russian research was published as an interim paper in 1981 in *Nutrition and Cancer*, a medical journal founded by Dr. Gio Gori, who had left the NCI because of its disinterest in nutrition. (*Penthouse*)

In 1981, Dr. Rowan T. Chlebowski and his team at UCLA's

Harbor Hospital in Torrance, California, started what became ten years of research with hydrazine sulfate. Applying to the ACS for a grant to replicate the Russian work, Chlebowski was turned down by one branch of ACS, but Dr. Rauscher reversed that decision and funded the project. Noting that not everyone responds favorably to HS, Chlebowski presented overall positive results to an April, 1982, meeting in St. Louis of the American Society for Clinical Oncology. He told Ralph Moss, "We have confirmed the rationale which Gold originally proposed for hydrazine sulfate". (Moss)

In 1983, Dr. Chlebowski presented another paper confirming HS's effectiveness at the American Society of Clinical Oncology. After the presentation, Dr. DeVita came across Dr. Gold. Poking him in the chest, DeVita warned, "I'm going to take off my gloves on hydrazine sulfate". (Moss)

Two years later, Dr. DeVita published a massive cancer textbook entitled *Cancer: Principles and Practice of Oncology*. He asked his NCI Deputy Director, Dr. Jane Henney, to write a chapter on "Unproven Methods of Cancer Treatment". On page 2340 she wrote: "hydrazine sulfate has been subjected to clinical testing and found ineffective". She thus blew off the Russians' published studies, all of Dr. Chlebowski's published clinical studies, Dr. Gold's work, and the Calbiochem tests. In dismissing Dr. Gershanovich's work in St. Petersburg, Dr. Henney wrote, "objective measures of antitumor activity were observed in only 3 patients of more than 225 evaluated". Dr. Gold explains that, in the language oncologists speak, the word "objective" very specifically means over 50% reduction in tumors. However, in the abstract of his study, Gershanovich reported quite a different story: "initial studies indicate hydrazine sulfate to be effective in reversing cachexia and producing disease stabilization in late-stage cancer patients". In other words, the wasting away which is what finally kills most cancer patients was reversed, so people went on living. Disease stabilization means that their tumors stopped growing, which is what happens when HS stops the liver from reprocessing lactic acid and amino acids into glucose, at great cost to the body.

When HS stops this process, tumors stop growing. Dr. Ralph Moss' summation of the Russian work reported that HS reversed cachexia, stopped the growth of tumors in animals and humans, and caused an improvement in patients' mood. It may be suspected that the Russian patients were satisfied with the results; they went on living even though some still had tumors (which were no longer growing) and they were feeling better.

By selectively focusing on just tumor reduction, which is not HS' strong point, and ignoring what HS really can accomplish, Dr. Henney misled all the cancer professionals who read Dr. DeVita's book, which is considered a very important text in the field. Dr. Henney's embarrassingly inaccurate evaluation of HS was dropped in the next edition of DeVita's book, and her chapter disappeared entirely from later editions. Thus the damage she may have caused was curtailed. Still, had she written objectively, many doctors might have used HS, and lives might have been saved. Dr. Henney had access to all previous clinical trials on hydrazine sulfate. Was her misleading inaccuracy on HS part of Dr. DeVita's "taking off the gloves"? Or was she simply an inept researcher? Dr. Henney's report on HS is reminiscent of the NCI committee which pronounced Krebiozen ineffective 35 years earlier. All the committee members were found to have received NCI grants, and their distortion led Senator Paul Douglas to pronounce his distrust of the NCI (Chapter 5).

Dr. Jane Henney became Commissioner of the FDA in 1998. The position became vacant when her predecessor, Dr. David Kessler, was forced to resign after being caught fudging on his travel vouchers. He then became Dean of Yale Medical School. Official Medicine takes care of its own.

In 1985, Joe Gold's ship almost came in. He received a letter from Dr. Maxwell Gordon, then senior vice-president of the Science and Technology Group of Bristol-Myers. At that time, Gold held a patent (which expired in 1995) on the use of hydrazine sulfate against cachexia. Convinced that HS could save a lot of lives, Gordon proposed a world-wide licensing agreement. Bristol-Myers would test the drug in all kinds of cancer, market the drug throughout the world, and would provide a big pay-off for the Syracuse Cancer Research Institute and the pioneering Dr. Gold. It didn't happen. Gordon's bosses called off the deal when one of the Bristol-Myers top brass, a former member of the NCI establishment, threatened to quit if the firm took on hydrazine sulfate (Moss).

In February 1987, Dr. Rowan Chlebowski published additional favorable double-blind results using HS on cachexia in cancer patients in *Cancer*, the journal of the American Cancer Society. In August of the same year, Dr. Chlebowski published a study of HS's ability to prevent protein breakdown in cancer patients in *The Lancet*, the prestigious British medical journal. With his research thus internationally recognized, he then applied to the NCI for a grant for "Phase III" trials of hydrazine sulfate. "Phase III" is an FDA term for double-blinded, randomized, and placebo-controlled tests to determine how a drug will perform. Such tests, then, would show how effective HS really was. It would seem that people would want to know such information at this stage of the research, but the system didn't work that way. The NCI, still directed by Dr. Vincent DeVita (who'd told Gold he would "take off the gloves") turned down Dr. Chlebowski.

In the summer of 1987 in Sarasota, Florida, Erna Kamen was sent home to die within a few days from metastasized lung cancer, shrinking daily from cachexia. The three "accepted" cancer therapies, surgery, radiation, and chemotherapy, had failed to help. Her cancer doctor had read about hydrazine sulfate and offered it as a long shot. Her son Jeff called the NCI's hotline (800-4-CANCER) and was told that HS had no value. His mother took one pill and the next morning asked Jeff to join her for breakfast. Her recovery was rapid. Jeff Kamen, an Independent Network News TV journalist, contacted Dr. Gold and became very interested in HS. He prepared seven TV news stories which were carried on more than 100 stations all across the U.S. His mother appeared on one of them, enthusiastically explaining how hydrazine sulfate had brought her back to life.

Jeff Kamen's TV journalism got results. Dr. Frank Rauscher called for nationwide testing of HS. Several months later, Jeff got a call from Dr. Henry Masur, chair of the experimental AIDS drug screening committee at the National Institutes of Health (NIH). Dr. Masur told Kamen that the NCI had stopped saying HS was worthless on its Cancer Information Line. Instead, they were referring people to Dr. Chlebowski's Harbor/UCLA studies.

Four months after starting hydrazine sulfate, Erna Kamen, a one-time athlete, had gained back 23 pounds. Then her oncologist suggested changing horses in the middle of the stream, stopping something that was working - that was "proven" at least in her case - and trying a new experimental chemotherapy. Dr. Gold strenuously advised against the change. He was overruled. Erna Kamen took the chemotherapy and was dead in five days.

In 1988, Dr. Alexander Fleming at the FDA announced that he was looking for a pharmaceutical company to carry out Phase III trials of HS with a view to wide-scale marketing of the drug. Before Bristol-Myers had a chance to change its mind, a "sponsor" stepped forward. However, it was not a pharmaceutical company, but the NCI. Yet on May 17, 1988, NCI director Dr. Vincent DeVita told the *Washington Post* that he considered hydrazine sulfate a "ho hum" idea. The NCI, which had lied about hydrazine sulfate to Congressman Hanley, which had spent most of the previous ten years claiming that HS was of no value, which had just turned down Dr. Chlebowski's request for a grant to do Phase III trials, did a surprising about-face and offered to sponsor the tests itself. These would be preparatory to FDA approval of hydrazine sulfate as a treatment for cancer. There had been a lot of pressure on the NCI to sponsor such tests, just as there was twenty years before to test Krebiozen. But there's an old saying, "beware of what you pray for - you might get it".

It seemed a moment of triumph for Dr. Joseph Gold, after twenty years of persistent plugging. It would have been hard to predict at that time what a sandbagging hydrazine sulfate would receive in the 1990's from Official Medicine.

The January 1990 issue of the *Journal of Clinical Oncology* carried Dr. Chlebowski's latest Harbor/UCLA study, with "Phase-III"-type controls; this showed that HS increased the survival time of 65 end-stage lung cancer patients. However, the journal also carried an editorial on HS written by Dr. Steven Piantadosi of the Johns Hopkins Oncology Center, who was on the FDA's oncology advisory panel. Piantadosi panned Chlebowski's study for being "too small" to be relevant. Twelve other studies in the same issue had far fewer patients than Chlebowski's, but escaped Piantadosi's selective criticism. Both Gold and Chlebowski were concerned that the editorial would scare off researchers, and they were right. It did.

Dr. Chlebowski received a grant to study the effects of hydrazine sulfate on cachexia in AIDS. Shortly after the grant had been approved and funded, Chlebowski learned that the FDA planned regulations that would result in it taking months just to obtain HS, which he had been using for ten years. His boss at Harbor/UCLA, Dr. Jerry Block, had "high hopes that HS would be effective against AIDS cachexia. Cachexia isn't a trivial problem. It isn't only cancer, it isn't only AIDS... It is a part of advanced aging as well". (Kamen. *Omni*, September 1993) Dr. Block told Kamen that no other drug had ever been subjected to the "gauntlet of scientific criticism" that HS had been forced to run. He probably was not aware of the similar problems of DMSO.

Stung by the editorial, disgusted by the FDA obstructionism, Dr. Rowan Chlebowski turned down the AIDS grant and stepped back from hydrazine sulfate research. After ten years of excellent work, he remained convinced that HS could help millions. Soon after giving up HS research, Dr. Chlebowski was invited to become a member of the executive board of the American Society for Clinical Oncology, which publishes the journal that had criticized him.

The fact that a pioneer often gets little recognition was forcefully brought home to Dr. Gold in the July 1990 issue of *Cancer Research*. The journal contained two articles on cachexia, which people hardly knew how to pronounce until Gold came along.

Neither mentioned Gold's work, and one stated that there is no effective treatment for cachexia.

Cachexia is the same condition whether in cancer or AIDS. If it sounds a bit like anorexia nervosa, at least one doctor has reported the quick disappearance of this serious and sometimes fatal eating disorder after his patient was given hydrazine sulfate.

From the earliest days of the research, Dr. Gold had warned about the products that are incompatible with hydrazine sulfate. Gold's advice on incompatibles was rigorously followed in the Calbiochem, Harbor/UCLA, and Russian studies. Even the FDA, in the numerous individual compassionate use exemptions it approved for the use of hydrazine sulfate on a case-by-case basis, warned in no uncertain terms that no tranquilizers, barbiturates, or alcohol were to be taken while a patient was on HS.

Before the NCI's Phase III trials started, Dr. Gold supplied NCI with animal studies which underlined the problem. These tests showed that "when tumor-bearing rats were given hydrazine sulfate together with widely used tranquilizers known as benzo-diazepines, 100% of the rats went into coma and 50% to 60% of them subsequently died. Rats receiving either the HS or the tran-quilizers alone had neither of these frightening outcomes." (Jeff Kamen, *Penthouse*, November 1994). Based on these studies, Dr. Gold was concerned that similar results might occur in humans. He wrote the NCI on the importance of excluding the incompati-bles.

Dr. Maxwell Gordon heard about the NCI trials similar to the ones he had planned at Bristol Myers before he left that company to become head of the Ajinomoto Co.'s American operations. Learning that Dr. Michael Kosty of the Scripps Clinic in San Diego would direct the first of three NCI trials, Gordon called Kosty. Dr. Gordon told Jeff Kamen (*Penthouse*, April 1993): "I emphasized the importance of the exclusions (of the incompati-bles)... Kosty answered 'You're right' and said that he would fol-low my advice." Jeff Kamen states: "Gordon even sent Kosty a letter dated September 19, 1989, emphasizing in writing the importance of the exclusions". Dr. Kosty told Kamen, "We talked with many individuals prior to finalizing the study and made no commitments to include or exclude specific medications". "Not only did Kosty fail to exclude the incompatibles", wrote Kamen, "but he said in an interview…'we just think this is a non-issue'".

It wasn't a non-issue for the rats in Gold's study. If you want to test a new high octane gas knowing that it won't work if you put sugar in the tank, what would you think of a test of the gas where sugar was indeed put into the tank?

Not surprisingly, when the final results of Dr. Kosty's study were in, they were negative. Curiously, some months before, Kosty told a different story to veteran reporter Naomi Pfeiffer of *Oncology Times*. Kosty told her in April 1991, she reported, that he and his staff had just reviewed preliminary results of the HS study. These showed that "those patients who received hydrazine sulfate had 'far superior' survival than patients in studies where HS was not used". (Kamen, *ibid.*) Pfeiffer asked Dr. Kosty in her telephone interview "Are the definitive data (at the end of the study) likely to be different?" Kosty replied "No, they (the data) can only get better". (Kamen, *ibid.*)

Kosty insisted to Kamen that he had been misquoted. But Pfeiffer told Kamen, "I did not misquote him. I remember what he said". Kosty claimed to Jeff Kamen that he could not have known the results Pfeiffer reported, since he was "blinded" to the results until the end of the (double blind) test. In that case, asks Kamen, "Why did he and his group meet to discuss and then report on preliminary results in April 1991?"

Similar changes to protocols happened in the other two NCI studies at the Mayo Clinic. The Mayo protocol read, "Patients [admitted] to the study would have to be previously untreated with chemotherapy". Mayo changed that. In a letter to Dr. Gold, Mayo test director Dr. Loprinzi wrote, "We have written into the protocol that (the hydrazine sulfate) should not be started for several days until the first (vomiting) from the first cycle of chemotherapy has cleared". While it had been agreed in the protocol that, for a change, early-stage patients would be treated with HS, patients actually put into the tests were mostly late stage, some with only a few weeks to live. A physician involved with the North Central Tests, as the Mayo tests were called by the NCI, "is reported to have remarked", Jeff Kamen wrote in the November 1994 *Penthouse*, that some of the patients in the study "'were so far gone, they had one foot in the grave, the other on a banana peel'". In the Kosty study (which also was to include early-stage patients) about 60% were late-stage, in violation of the protocol. So Dr. Kosty and the Mayo Clinic, like Sloan Kettering before them, could not or would not follow a simple protocol.

Like Sloan Kettering in 1975 and like Kosty, Mayo changed the protocol and, like Sloan Kettering and Kosty, Mayo announced negative results.

Something certainly was radically different about the NCI tests carried out at the Mayo Clinic and at the Scripps Clinic by Dr. Kosty. In Gold's early work, in the Calbiochem trials, in the four Harbor/UCLA trials, people improved and got well. In the Russian tests of 1,000 people, about 50% improved, with 40% showing a halt or regression of tumors. Many got well and are alive in the Year 2000. If the three NCI tests, totaling 600 patients, had followed the previously well-established pattern, about 200-300 should have improved, and some would have recovered completely. But out of the NCI's 600 patients, nobody improved; in fact, there were no survivors at all. Something was different.

Through a hard-hitting series of articles in *Penthouse* and *Omni* magazines, Jeff Kamen became a player in the hydrazine story as well as a reporter of it. At a rally in the Shoreham Hotel in Washington on election night, 1992, he noticed the name tag of a young doctor attending an AIDS conference going on in the same hotel. "Do you work in cachexia?" Jeff inquired. "Yes", the doctor answered, "why did you ask?" That was Jeff's opening to talk about hydrazine sulfate, "the only substance that has demonstrated its ability to arrest and then reverse the terrible wasting away of body and spirit that is cachexia". The AIDS doctor was amazed and asked "Why don't I know about this?"

Kamen told the above as part of the whole story of hydrazine sulfate in "Hope, Heartbreak, and Horror" in the September 1993 issue of *Omni* magazine. He concluded the article with a summation by Dr. Joseph Gold, "Each year 500,000 Americans die from cancer, and there are over a million new cases annually in this country alone. The UCLA data indicate that over half of these afflicted patients would be helped by hydrazine sulfate, some achieving significant extensions in survival. The Soviet data, consistent with the UCLA results, indicate that of every million late-stage cancer patients, 500,000 would receive significant symptomatic improvement, 400,000 would show a halt or regression in tumor growth, and some would go on to long-term survival." Commenting on the seemingly intentionally flawed NCI tests, Gold added, "That the NCI should be a part of an effort to snuff out hydrazine sulfate constitutes what is truly one of the most shameful, scandalous medical undertakings in this country's history, depriving vast numbers of people of their health, happiness, and lives."

While hydrazine sulfate is a common, cheap and non-toxic chemical, it is not approved by the FDA for use as a drug. Until 1993, under its "compassionate use" program, FDA routinely approved doctors' requests to use HS on a case by case basis. Seizing NCI's announcement of negative results in the three trials as an excuse, FDA stopped giving "compassionate use" exemptions. That meant that formal, FDA-approved research with hydrazine sulfate stopped in 1993, although some doctors continued to use it quietly.

Jeff Kamen flew to St. Petersburg in 1994 to interview Drs. Gershanovich, Filov, and the other Russian researchers. He wrote of their success with hydrazine sulfate in "From Russia with Love - Stonewalled in the U.S.", which appeared in the July 1994 *Penthouse*. Kamen found that the Russians had raised some venture capital and put HS into production. In their clinical work, they had scrupulously followed Dr. Gold's recommendations on avoiding the "incompatibles". When Kamen told the Russians that NCI not only had failed to do so but had actually even given

patients the incompatibles, they were shocked at what they took
to be incompetence. Incredulously, one of them asked him, "Are
Communists now running the NCI?"

Bob Guccione, publisher of *Penthouse* (circulation over
1,000,000) and *Omni*, started running articles on hydrazine sulfate in the 1980's. He and his wife, Kathy Keeton, gave Jeff
Kamen strong support and set up a section at *Penthouse* to distribute materials on HS. While doctors could no longer prescribe
it, hydrazine sulfate remained a cheap legal chemical, so those
needing it could still pop three 60-mg pills a day in the privacy of
their homes.

In 1994, Bob Guccione joined Joe Gold on a Washington
radio talk show hosted by Jeff Kamen to discuss hydrazine sulfate and the NCI scandal. (After Kosty's tests, Kamen had predicted in *Penthouse* that the remaining two would similarly be
flawed.) The three demanded that Congress force the FDA to
reverse its cancellation of compassionate use permits for HS.
They also demanded that Congress direct its investigational arm,
the General Accounting Office (GAO), to investigate the NCI and
its handling of the Phase III tests on HS. They urged the public to
call Congress, and gave out the phone and FAX numbers of
Representative Edolphus Towns (D-NY), then chair of the House
Intergovernmental Relations Subcommittee. This was the committee with authority to investigate the NCI. In a very short time,
Towns' office called, urgently asking Kamen to stop giving out
their phone numbers, since they were being swamped with phone
calls "making it impossible for us to get our jobs done". A year
earlier, Kamen had left a lot of material on HS and the NCI for
Congressman Towns and had gotten no response. He kept on giving out the numbers. The next call came from the Congressman's
administrative assistant, who promised to get Towns to read
Kamen's material.

Jeff Kamen writes in the September 1997 *Penthouse*, "Within
a week, the chairman ordered the GAO to conduct an investigation into the matters raised by *Penthouse*. When GAO investigators called on senior officials of the NCI, they ran into anger and

resentment. At one point, informed sources say, there was considerable shouting and screaming, and a sense of gloom over the possible outcome of the congressional investigation." Having stirred up the GAO, Bob Guccione and Jeff Kamen were looking forward to seeing NCI officials forced to testify under oath before a Congressional investigation.

Guccione and Kamen loaded down the GAO investigators with documentation collected over the previous six years. At first, NCI officials told GAO investigator Barry Tice that they knew nothing about a protocol prohibiting the "incompatibles". Then Tice called Dr. Gold and told him "I think we have a 'smoking gun'". He'd located an internal NCI memo discussing the protocol in detail, revealing that NCI knew very well what patients should not take while on hydrazine sulfate.

The Congressional investigation never happened. Barry Tice prepared a "Final Draft Report" which told exactly what NCI had done wrong. When sent to the NCI on June 5, 1995, for comments, the roof fell in. After a tense meeting two days later between NCI and the GAO, GAO backed off. In late 1995, the GAO issued its official report to Congress entitled, "Contrary to Allegations, NCI Hydrazine Sulfate Studies Were Not Flawed". "It upheld the NCI's testing methods...making the GAO probe...a veritable whitewash."(*ibid.*) Jeff Kamen writes "The NCI brass shouldn't have lost much sleep... The GAO slapped the wrists of the NCI for sloppy, inaccurate record-keeping on drugs other than hydrazine sulfate used in the trials" (the incompatibles).

As part of NCI's penance, the leaders of its HS trials wrote a letter which was published in the June 1995 *Journal of Clinical Oncology* (the one that had panned Chlebowski). The letter admitted "what they hadn't bothered to disclose in their original report to the medical community - that 94% of the patients had received one or more tranquilizers". (*ibid.*) The letter did not state that the tranquilizers were incompatible with hydrazine sulfate and could do mortal harm to the patients (Gold's study). If a reader of the NCI letter did not already know that, then their "mea culpa" letter seemed just to confess to "not having fully reported other drugs consumed by patients in the study". (*ibid.*)

Penthouse hired Richard Wilkins, a medical statistics consultant and former statistician for a large pharmaceutical company, to evaluate the NCI's analyses of its HS trials. Wilkins' report came back to Jeff Kamen with a note saying "You are to be congratulated for bringing the important, indeed truly scandalous hydrazine sulfate story to the attention of the American people. The enclosed should provide more ammunition for it". His analysis demolished NCI's statements.

The patients in the NCI trials all signed "informed consent" statements agreeing to let the government experiment on them by taking hydrazine sulfate. They hoped HS would help them, as it had in numerous cases in previous studies (some of the patients were aware of the Harbor/UCLA studies). By supplying NCI with his animal studies, Dr. Gold had showed the urgency of avoiding the incompatibles. Not one patient, on the consent forms, was informed of the incompatibles or that he or she could be imperiling life itself by taking one of them along with HS. The NCI admitted that patients in one test were not advised of the incompatibles, and that 50% of the 94% who received them were given them on a long-term basis. Jeff Kamen wrote that Dr. Michael Kosty had told him "face-to-face that 'Lorazepam', a benzodiazepine, was the 'major tranquilizer' used by the patients" ("The Cancer Empire Strikes Back", *Penthouse*, November 1994). Benzodiazepine was the type of tranquilizer Dr. Gold had used in his animal tests which, when given with HS, threw 100% of the rats into coma, with 50% dying. To repeat, nobody survived the NCI tests. In the Russian tests of 1,000 patients, 50% actually improved.

Kathy Keeton, Bob Guccione's second in command as well as his wife, was originally from South Africa. Once a Royal Ballet School dancer in London, she founded *Longevity* magazine as part of the Guccione General Media family of publications. In 1995, Bob and Kathy went to the Cannes film festival and Kathy came down with what seemed to be food poisoning. When it persisted, they flew home and she checked into Mt. Sinai hospital in New York. Having just passed a thorough physical exam six weeks earlier, she presumed that the problem could not be serious, but it was. After a series of tests, she was told that she had widely metastasized "galloping breast cancer", which had developed so rapidly it had not shown up on the mammogram done as part of her recent physical. She had perhaps six weeks to live, the doctors told her. Thus there was no time to lose in getting started with aggressive chemotherapy, which, they admitted, had at the most a 20% success rate in cases like hers. Having advised thousands about hydrazine sulfate over the previous ten years, she and Bob called Joe Gold. He felt it was worth a shot, so she refused chemo and started on HS, to the disapproval of the doctors. Because she was in a great deal of pain, a skin patch was applied which provided a powerful narcotic. One week after starting HS, Kathy no longer needed the patch. In 2 ½ weeks, she was functioning normally. After 2 ½ months on hydrazine sulfate, a CAT scan showed that many abdominal tumors had either diminished or cleared, as well as those occluding major blood vessels. However, one tumor around the common bile duct had increased, causing some jaundice, so a stent was installed. To improve the situation, it was decided to use radiation to diminish the tumor. Dr. Gold advised that HS would enhance radiation, so a smaller than usual dose should be given. Kathy explained this to the radiotherapist, who nevertheless gave the maximum dose; this burned Kathy's liver and later caused scar tissue. Still, she sailed past the six weeks she was supposed to live. Six months later, the tumor had not just diminished slightly from the radiation, but had disappeared. A year later, her metastasized galloping breast cancer was in remission.

Kathy Keeton became a living, breathing, very high profile testimonial for hydrazine sulfate, telling her story on national TV or wherever she found an opportunity. The September 1997 issue of *Penthouse* featured Kathy's successful battle against cancer in an article entitled "The $200 Billion Scam" by Jeff Kamen. Kamen stated in his article that the money spent "has produced so little bang for the buck that it makes the Pentagon's $600 toilet seats (an earlier scandal) look like bargains for every American home". $200 billion is a rough estimate of the amount spent by the NCI and other professional cancer researchers in the 25 years since President Richard Nixon and Congress declared "War on Cancer". The figure may be low. It was estimated that cancer research, cancer treatment, cancer care, and cancer administration was costing $160 billion a year by the end of 1996.

In the 1970's, Dr. Gold started writing about the useful qualities of little-known Vitamin K-2 and about how it hits cancer tumors directly. He pointed out that it acts somewhat like a chemotherapy called Adriamycin, having a very similar molecular structure, but, unlike the chemo, is non-toxic. He also noted that K-2 greatly enhances the action of hydrazine sulfate. The Hoffman LaRoche pharmaceutical firm manufactured Vitamin K-2 from around 1952 until 1992. Then the FDA asked it to cease production of the vitamin. Hoffman LaRoche complied with the request of the agency which regulates it. Bob Guccione told this story when he appeared on the Art Bell radio talk show in August 1997. He told of his world-wide search for the vitamin when Kathy got sick. There was a supplier in Japan, but its product contained something incompatible with hydrazine sulfate. Finally, he found K-2 in Italy. It was used with HS to help Kathy Keeton recover from cancer.

Convinced that the NCI's unethical handling of its Phase III hydrazine sulfate trials had caused deaths, perhaps 600 of them, Bob Guccione announced in the September 1997 *Penthouse* that he was considering a class action suit against the NCI for genocide. A very curious federal law prohibits the NCI from revealing the names of people who have died in NCI-sponsored tests. So in order to find out who the 600 or so victims were, Guccione was forced to advertise, inviting relatives of patients who had died in the NCI trials of 1989 to 1993 to contact him and Kathy about joining the lawsuit.

As minority counsel to the Permanent Subcommittee on Investigations of the Senate Committee on Governmental Affairs,

Jeff Robbins was monitoring the GAO/NCI situation. In a letter of October 15, 1997, to the GAO, Robbins wrote, "Clearly, the NCI did not respond to inquiries about its testing in a way that inspired confidence. It is apparently undisputed that the NCI first denied that tranquilizers were used in any of its hydrazine sulfate studies. It was only after its studies were scrutinized that it admitted that its prior statement was false and that, in fact, 94% of the patients in the principal NCI study had tranquilizers administered to them concurrently with hydrazine sulfate."

The bottom line is that either the NCI administered tranquilizers on purpose, or it didn't. If it did so on purpose, endangering patients' lives by flying in the face of Dr. Gold's animal studies (which were replicated by the Russians) showing the perils of giving "incompatibles" with HS, then justice needs to take its course. If it did not administer incompatibles on purpose, then NCI's having done so is a matter of sheer incompetence. This is in an institution which spent around $2.5 billion dollars in 1998, whose findings have major influence all over the world. Why are the people who did this still in their jobs and not in jail?

The Canadians, for one, decided to part company with the NCI on hydrazine sulfate. The Canadian Breast Cancer Research Initiative (CBCRI) is a partnership made up of the Canadian Cancer Society, Health Canada, the Medical Research Council of Canada, and the National Cancer Institute of Canada. While the GAO found the NCI studies "not flawed", the CBCRI found the exact opposite in a report entitled "Hydrazine Sulfate", published in December 1996. The report stated, "Unfortunately, all three (NCI) clinical trials had significant methodological flaws and the results are therefore inconclusive".

In October 1997, the tragic news went out that Kathy Keeton had died. Knowing of her struggle with cancer, many assumed that she had finally lost the battle. However, this extraordinarily talented and beautiful woman died, unbelievably, of complications following surgery in a major New York City hospital.

The September 1998 issue of *Penthouse* contained another feature story by Jeff Kamen entitled "Intent to Kill", and subtitled

"The Government's Conspiracy to Destroy Hydrazine Sulfate". Kamen tells in graphic detail the story of the GAO caving in to NCI pressure and withdrawing its Final Draft Report, which actually told the truth about what had happened. In the increasingly incriminating story of the use of the incompatibles in the NCI tests, FDA medical officer Dr. Eileen Parish expressed surprise at the Mayo Clinic having changed the protocol, as noted earlier. Dr. Parish told GAO's Barry Tice that "NCI knew from the (medical) literature that there is an incompatibility of hydrazine sulfate with alcohol, barbiturates, and tranquilizers". She added that she "found it bizarre that the Mayo Clinic would include such a statement (in their protocol allowing tranquilizers) since the reason for conducting the Mayo-directed trials was to exclude the use of substances that are alleged to be incompatible with hydrazine sulfate". (*ibid.*)

Jeff Kamen also reported that on April 23, 1998, the FDA raided Great Lakes Metabolics in Rochester, Minnesota, a distributor of hydrazine sulfate, looking to seize whatever was on hand. Donna Schuster, owner of the company, is the former daughter-in-law of a retired CEO of the Mayo Clinic. She also was a friend of the late Dr. Dean Burk (head of cell chemistry at NCI for 40 years). In 1974, Burk asked Mrs. Schuster to get into the distribution of hydrazine sulfate, since "someone reputable should be doing it". The FDA previously raided her in 1989 although hydrazine sulfate is a legal chemical. In 2000, FDA raided and indicted her supplier, so she closed her business and retired, having lost her source.

Looking back at the clinical trials that were done properly, it is curious to note that hydrazine sulfate has virtually never been tested alone in the early stages of cancer (when any drug has a better chance of working). The NCI was supposed to give HS to early stage patients, but didn't. The Russian protocol is to give HS when conventional chemo and radiation have failed; at that point, the patient's immune system has very likely been gravely weakened by the chemo. Even with all that, the Russians still get better results than any chemotherapists can claim in the U.S.

There was no Internet in the 1970's and 1980's, but there is in the 21st century and there's a lot of information on it about hydrazine sulfate. Here are some testimonials from one Internet site:

► In less than two weeks on HS, two tumors are gone and two others have reduced in size by 50%.

► Began HS on January 21, 1997. On February 20, 1997, reports no pain medication taken for two weeks; colon/incontinence improved by 90%. Calls it a miracle drug.

► Thirty days on HS and tumor almost disappeared from neck.

► Seven weeks on Hydrazine Sulfate. Brain and lung lesions disappeared.

► Patient doing great. Back to work. Attending physicians do not understand how cancer can reverse in such a short time.

► Oncologist report in today. No cancer anywhere, after 2 ½ months on HS and vitamins/minerals and supplements. They have no idea where cancer went.

► I'm doing so well on HS. I feel like a million dollars. My husband says he can't hold me down since I'm on that rocket fuel.

► Started HS on February 1, 1997. Gained 14 pounds in two months. Feeling great. Praise the Lord.

► I purchased some HS for my sister a few weeks ago. Too early to tell, but she went from near death at the hospital on chemo to a campground some place, with a fishing pole.

► Glioblastoma multiforme (brain cancer). Four months on HS. Recent MRI indicates 40% shrinkage of tumor.

► Fourth week on HS therapy. Spots on lung are gone. One of the lumps in lymph has disappeared and the other one has shrunk by 60%.

► Started HS in July 1997. Tumor markers reduced
from 339 to 13. Three months on HS. CT scans show
nothing. Lesions in the liver are gone.

That's enough to provide a good sample. Orthodox oncologists would dismiss these as "anecdotal", the ultimate put-down.
Because of the NCI/FDA debacle, formal research with
hydrazine sulfate in the U.S. is on hold, so we have few ongoing
ways to learn about HS other than anecdotes. The FDA, it has
been reported, is studying what it can do about "misinformation"
on the Internet. Unless the FDA finds a way to censor the
Internet, perhaps certain websites could gather research on cases
where only HS is given right at the very first sign of cancer, since
most cancer cases are not terminal when first discovered. With
some careful guidance on the Internet, after a year or so, we
might find out the following: where HS and nothing else is taken
at the first diagnosis of cancer, what is the success rate? What is
the percentage of regression? What is the speed of regression,
when it occurs?

Nothing works all the time, but the principle behind
hydrazine sulfate therapy, stopping gluconeogenesis, should
work all the time if not interfered with by "incompatibles". How
many people for whom HS did not work took some nuts or raisins
for quick energy, or had some bread pudding with raisins or some
nice healthy raisin bread served to them in the hospital? If staff in
the NCI trials disregarded the incompatibles, one can bet the
dietitians never heard of them. Nuts and raisins contain tyramine.

Any food containing tyramine is a no-no with HS, because
tyramine is an amino acid which blocks HS. How many people
for whom HS did not appear to work were taking a good multivitamin pill? Any multivitamin pill contains Vitamin B-6 (pyridox-
ine). B-6 stops the action of HS. Can the Internet get this sort of
information to cancer victims? It's a better bet than the NCI.

The Internet would be a good place to spread information on
Vitamin K-2 and its apparent ability to enhance the effectiveness
of hydrazine sulfate. The combination worked for Kathy Keeton.

The vitamin is not illegal in the U.S.; it just isn't available. The Internet could create a market for the vitamin, which could be imported.

From 1989 to 1994, the long hoped-for NCI trials turned into a nightmare and the FDA stopped giving permission to doctors to use hydrazine sulfate in individual cases. Within a few short years, Dr. Joseph Gold's hydrazine sulfate went from being the fair-haired subject of prestigious NCI-sponsored trials to being almost outlawed. Somebody - various somebodies - evidently did take off the gloves. If Senator Paul Douglas were still alive, he would understand perfectly. On December 6, 1963, he stood on the Senate floor and denounced in specific details the deceptions of the NCI and the FDA concerning Krebiozen. He then uttered historic words, prophetic words, "It is a terrible thing that we cannot really trust the NCI or the FDA".

During a period in 1996 when there had been a lot of publicity about hydrazine sulfate, Dr. Joe Gold recalls getting twenty calls in one day from Sloan Kettering doctors wondering how to get HS for patients with cancer. About 2/3 of these patients were members of the doctors' own families. Six of these doctors were known to have refused HS to other Sloan Kettering patients, who had then called Dr. Gold to ask him to intervene.

As we enter the 21st Century, hydrazine sulfate is a legal drug in Canada and the treatment of choice for several types of cancer in Russia and in the Eastern European countries. In the U.S., Official Medicine has stalled HS and is trying to do worse.

Having tried obfuscation about hydrazine sulfate in her chapter in Dr. DeVita's book, FDA Commissioner Dr. Jane Henney is now trying Prohibition. Her FDA has proposed to remove hydrazine sulfate from the list of chemicals which compounding pharmacies can sell. As things stand, they cannot sell HS as a treatment for cancer, but they can sell it. "De-listing" HS would make it an illegal drug, and those selling it could find themselves in jail. This means that Donna Schuster and others like her would be out of business. Dr. Joseph Gold has protested vigorously in an exchange of letters with Commissioner Henney and her assistant,

Dr. Janet Woodcock. A number of Congressmen are fighting the proposal.

To make such a "de-listing", the FDA is obliged to go through a process of appointing a committee to hear testimony. Dr. Gold pointed out that the committee invited several known enemies of HS, and not one proponent such as himself, Dr. Chlebowski, or Dr. Gershanovich. Dr. Charles Loprinzi was invited, who had been director of the NCI trials of HS at the Mayo Clinic. While the Mayo protocol had stipulated that patients in the study were to be previously untreated with chemotherapy, as noted earlier, Dr. Loprinzi changed the protocol. Then there was the all-important matter, discussed earlier, of giving things incompatible with HS. These were given to 94% of the patients in the trials, presumably including those at the Mayo Clinic. As trial director, Dr. Loprinzi could hardly have been unaware of this, unless he was inept. There were no survivors of Dr. Loprinzi's trials of HS at the Mayo Clinic.

In a letter of January 18, 2000, to Dr. Gold, the FDA's Dr. Janet Woodcock stated that "we invited Dr. Loprinzi (because he was) associated with the largest, best controlled studies of hydrazine sulfate to date, the two studies conducted by the North Central Cancer Research Group.... sponsored by the NCI (this included the Mayo Clinic study). These studies have been exhaustively reviewed and have been found to be well-conducted, valid studies." That's not what the first report from the GAO said, and that's not what the Canadian analysis of the NCI studies of HS said. This is an old Official Medicine trick; cheat on a test and then quote it as proof that the medicine tested was no good. The best word to describe this ploy is "chutzpah", from the Hebrew, meaning unmitigated gall.

Unlike Krebiozen, hydrazine sulfate is sold in commerce as a legal chemical (if not a legal drug) and cannot be stamped out, although "de-listing" could drive it underground. Will Congress get tough enough to head off the FDA? It would be ironic - and tragic - if people in need of HS were forced to obtain it through the same channels used by people buying cocaine or heroin.

In the unlikely case of a thorough Congressional investigation, the fight will be bitter. Boston attorney Jeff Robbins, former counsel to the Senate sub-committee which monitored the GAO report, recalls what one government official told Jeff Kamen (incensed over Kamen's reporting), "When you get your tumor, go have it treated in Russia!"

The Fiercest Battle

The first impression on meeting Dr. Stanislaw Burzynski of Houston, Texas, is strength, cheerfulness, and calm. He's needed them in double measure. Official Medicine greeted this Polish immigrant researcher-physician with the longest and most intense of any of the persecutions seen in this book - the fiercest battle of all. In 1983, the FDA began a harassment of Dr. Burzynski that included the summoning of four grand juries, an indictment, and a trial which the FDA lost.

Growing up in post-World War II Communist Poland, Stanislaw Burzynski seemed headed for an academic career. Studying at the University of Lublin, Burzynski prepared his PhD thesis on a series of blood analyses. Most were readily explained, but certain patterns that appeared in all blood tests were puzzling.

Not to worry, said his professor; no one has ever figured out what those mean. In Poland, as in many European countries, candidates for a PhD degree defend their theses in public; the events are announced and many people attend. There was always a chance that someone might ask about those unknown patterns and young "Stash" Burzynski did not want to be publicly embarrassed. Putting his nose to the grindstone, he found that the blood fractions not previously identified were a series of peptides, which are clusters of amino acids, the building blocks of protein.

He breezed through the exam and won his PhD.

As a matter of fact, Stanislaw Burzynski earned both his MD and his PhD by age 24, the youngest person in Poland to gain both degrees in the 20th century. Seen as a rising star, he soon came under strong pressure to join the Communist party. When he refused to do so, his position in the country became uncertain. Managing to obtain a passport, he came to the United States in

1970 at age 25 with $20 in his pocket - and his analyses of the blood peptides.

Shortly after Dr. Burzynski's arrival in the U.S., he landed a job as assistant professor at the Baylor College of Medicine in Houston, working under Dr. George Ungar in the Anesthesiology Department. Ungar was interested in the use of peptides for the purpose of enhancing memory. Had Burzynski been given a job in the cancer section, his research would have been to do what he was told to do; under Dr. Ungar, however, he was free to follow his own inclinations. In 1974, he won a grant from the National Cancer Institute (NCI); this enabled him to purchase equipment that did not exist in Poland, and thus to carry his peptide research much further.

In Poland, Burzynski had found 39 peptides; in Houston, he was able to break these down into 119 peptides of 10-15 amino acids each. Until Dr. Burzynski came along, peptides had been largely ignored on the presumption that they were waste products, or artifacts, a term scientists sometimes use to pass over what they don't understand. In the eyes of many researchers, Burzynski said, "they were some type of chemical UFO's which some people were seeing and some people were not seeing" (*The Cancer Industry*, by Ralph Moss, PhD). He had suspected while in Poland that his peptides had anti-cancer activity after noticing that one of them was almost totally lacking in the blood of a prostate cancer patient. In Houston, he carried out a series of experiments to test for the peptides' biological significance. In 1974, he and Dr. Ungar published an article reporting that they had found the peptides to cause up to 97% inhibition of DNA synthesis and cell division in cancer cells in tissue cultures. In other words, if the DNA were inactivated and the cells did not divide, cancer cells could not spread. He called the peptides Antineoplastons, a term meaning anti-cancer.

If the human body did not have multiple back-up systems for stopping cancer, deaths from the disease would be even worse. Dr. William Koch (Chapter 3) spotted one such system and a way to enhance it. Dr. Andrew Ivy postulated the existence of such systems in an article that brought Dr. Stefan Durovic and Krebiozen to his attention (Chapter 5). Dr. Burzynski discovered yet another such mechanism, naturally occurring peptides.

Dr. Burzynski had first studied peptides in blood. Since obtaining blood was sometimes difficult, in 1970, he switched to another source - urine, in which a fellow Pole had found peptides in 1897. (The drugs urokinase and Premarin are derived from urine.) Before making the switch, Burzynski was finding that it was not easy to get a lot of blood for his research. He told the 1990 World Research Foundation Congress in Los Angeles, "Basically, I was getting blood from my friends, but then the friends began avoiding me and I finally decided to try something else" (Moss, *op. cit.*).

Burzynski's mentor in Poland was Dr. Marian Mazur, an expert on cybernetics, the theory of messages. Mazur's work led Burzynski to develop a theory that antineoplastons were, in fact, transferring messages to the cells. Where they existed in abundance, there was no cancer. Cancer patients almost invariably had smaller quantities of peptides than healthy persons. Rather than thinking of peptides just as substances, Burzynski says "I looked on them as words, pieces of information" (Lang, 1987). Cancer, then, would be "a disease of information processing", *i.e.*, a virus in a body's computer. Peptides would be the program which, when in abundance, would keep cells from becoming abnormal. Or, if in short supply, when supplied, they would tell errant cells to return to normal. As Dr. Burzynski puts it, "Cancer is really a disease of cells that are not programmed correctly. Antineoplastons simply reprogram them so that they behave normally again." (*Burzynski Breakthrough*, Tom Elias)

During the Baylor years, Burzynski married a fellow Polish doctor, Barbara Szopa, MD, who also had taken her degree from the University of Lublin. Passing an exam to permit him to practice medicine in the U.S. in 1973, he opened a private practice. Continuing peptide research in animals, Dr. Burzynski found that antineoplastons were so nontoxic that it was almost impossible to find an "LD-50" value, a technical term for the dose at which half of the tested animals die. He did find, however, that his peptides were "species specific" - *i.e.*, each species makes its own. Human antineoplastons, then, would not work in mice, nor would animal antineoplastons work in humans.

Conducting numerous lab tests on cancer cells, Dr. Burzynski published studies in the 1970's showing that he had found anti-neoplastons "active against every type of human neoplasm we tested, including myeloblastic leukemia, osteosarcoma, fibrosar-coma, chrondrosarcoma, cancer of the uterine cervix, colon can-cer, breast cancer, lung cancer, and lymphoma. All antineoplas-tons inhibited up to 100% of the growth of neoplastic cells with less inhibitory effect on normal cells" (Moss, *op. cit.*). In addi-tion, Burzynski reported, effectiveness of the peptides was dose-related; the more given, the better the results, *i.e.*, the opposite of toxic chemotherapy.

In 1976, Dr. Burzynski presented a paper in Anaheim, California at a convention of the Federation of American Societies for Experimental Biology (FASEB). In *The Cancer Industry*, Dr. Moss reports, "Out of 3,700 papers, Burzynski's became the lead *Associated Press* (AP) story from the confer-ence:

> *A chemical with the power to change cancer cells back to normal cells has been extracted from human urine... It apparently detects cells that are getting out of line and feeds them new information that returns them to normal.*

> *If the naturally occurring substance can be made artifi-cially, Dr. S. R. Burzynski of Houston said Wednesday, it would be valuable in cancer therapy (Houston Chronicle, April 15, 1976).*

After the *Houston Chronicle* story, the Baylor Cancer Research Center invited Burzynski to become a member of the Center - on condition that he give up his growing private practice. The invitation signified recognition, but he had seen how institu-tions smother initiative in Communist Poland. In addition, his private practice was flourishing and making him financially independent.

The *Chronicle* article had precipitated an attractive offer, but it did not bring a pharmaceutical company to help develop his discoveries. Antineoplastons were increasingly his focus and after he had determined nontoxicity, he was determined to test them in humans. Because of their being species specific, his peptides had only indifferent results in animals. However, under FDA rules, before testing in humans he would have to show efficacy in animals, and this he knew he could not do. If he wanted to test in humans, he would just have to start doing so, knowing that sooner or later this could bring the FDA and the state medical board down on him.

After Dr. Ungar, his Baylor superior, was forced out of Baylor in 1976, Ungar's successor was not sympathetic to Burzynski's research. Not anxious to leave the protected world of academia but feeling boxed in, Burzynski was laboring over how to proceed when his old mentor from Poland, Dr. Mazur, came to Houston to lecture at Rice University. When Mazur heard Burzynski's dilemma, he resolved it with a simple observation, "If you're right about these peptides, everyone will eventually have to acknowledge it" (Moss).

In 1977, Stanislaw Burzynski decided to leave Baylor and dedicate himself completely to his private practice and research. As he was receiving a certificate for meritorious service from the Baylor College of Medicine, his department chairman, Dr. Lawrence Schuhmacher, prophetically warned, "Just wait, Burzynski. They're going to kick your ass" (Moss).

Since his plan was to research the use of antineoplastons in cancer, his next step was to check where he stood legally. At that time, it was not illegal to make and use within the State of Texas drugs not approved by the FDA. Since the FDA governed interstate commerce, he could not ship antineoplastons out of Texas. Through a lawyer, the FDA confirmed orally that as long as he restricted his antineoplastons to Texas, he was within his legal rights. The Texas Attorney General gave a letter with a similar favorable opinion.

The next challenge was to find a place to test the antineoplastons. Burzynski found a kindred spirit in Dr. William Mask, chief of the Jack County Hospital in Jacksboro, Texas. Mask and Burzynski conducted a clinical trial, which was successful. Dr. Mask later testified in 1985 (during one of Burzynski's legal problems), "There's no doubt in my mind. I'm convinced that in my 40 years of experience in seeing cancer, this (treatment) is the best" (*Houston Post*, October 11, 1985). Ralph Moss writes (*op. cit.*), "He also cited the case of a Wichita Falls man cured of bladder cancer... Mask told the judge that he would recommend antineoplaston treatments in place of traditional chemotherapy and radiation which 'kill the good cells as well as the bad cells' (*Houston Chronicle*, October 11, 1985)."

The Jacksboro results enabled Burzynski to convince the institutional review board of Houston's Twelve Oaks Hospital to let him try the peptides there. As soon as Burzynski published a paper (1977) stating that antineoplastons showed "profound anti-tumor activity without any significant toxicity in 21 patients" (Moss), the Twelve Oaks Hospital cancelled permission to let him do any further testing.

The next year, the Harris County Medical Society's Board of Ethics investigated Burzynski on the basis of his making his own non-FDA approved medicine. This was somewhat off-base, since it is traditionally within a doctor's prerogatives to prepare his/her own medicines. The Board asked Dr. Burzynski not to talk to the press. He refrained from doing so for awhile but in 1979 Gary Null wrote about him in an article in *Penthouse*.

In 1980, Dr. Burzynski, an eternal researcher, learned how to synthesize antineoplastons. This became possible after the development of mass spectrometry technology. This, in combination with high performance liquid thermatography, enabled him to identify every single molecule. Once that was done, he could make antineoplastons from standard amino acids, a huge breakthrough. Until then, he had had to make arrangements with public places to collect urine, which was then purified and processed into a white powder. His brother, Tad, was in charge of manufacturing. "Thank God for mass spectrometry", Burzynski told writer Tom Elias (*Burzynski Breakthrough*, 1997). "Without it, we'd still be depending on urine."

It is unfortunate that the technologies Dr. Burzynski used were not available when Krebiozen was around, so that, too, could have been identified. The spectrographic analysis the FDA fraudulently used to try to discredit Krebiozen is not in the same ballpark with mass spectrometry, which could have told us the identity of the molecules that comprised Krebiozen.

ABC's *20/20* put the national spotlight on Burzynski on October 22, 1981. Its commentator, Geraldo Rivera, said (Moss, *op. cit.*):

> *The deeper we looked into the story, the more we realized that Stanislaw Burzynski is really not a maverick at all. His work is very much in the scientific mainstream, that burgeoning field of cancer research that's pinpointing the body's own natural materials, its own proteins, to control irregular cell growth... Burzynski has simply decided to do things his way.*

In effect, Stanislaw Burzynski had become an entrepreneur in the best American fashion, like so many immigrants before him.

The *20/20* show brought a huge flow of cancer patients and attention from other quarters. The NCI asked Burzynski for samples of his compounds to use in their standard "P388" mouse leukemia test. Burzynski warned that his "A-10" antineoplastons were "species specific" and unlikely to prove effective in mice, but sent along the samples so as not to appear uncooperative. As he'd predicted, antineoplastons were not effective in mouse leukemia.

Because of production complexities, antineoplastons were an expensive therapy and cost patients $342 per day (still low, however, compared to chemotherapy). The price would fall to ¼ of this, Dr. Burzynski calculates, after the product is approved by the FDA; then it could be put into mass production. Although sometimes given orally, the treatment usually is administered intravenously through an implanted shunt or catheter. It needs to be given continuously, and may go on for 6-12 months or even longer. Although costly, it showed effectiveness, especially in brain tumors.

In January 1983, the American Cancer Society (ACS) attacked Dr. Burzynski in their magazine *Ca*. In their usual language, the ACS stated that it "does not have evidence that treatment with antineoplastons results in objective benefit". Yet, Ralph Moss pointed out in *Cancer Industry*, "ACS included in its article data which undercut its own conclusions. For instance, it reported that in Burzynski's 1977 study, 'twenty-one far-advanced cancer patients were treated with Antineoplaston A' and 'some degree of clinical improvement was noted in 18 of the 21 (86%)'.   It also stated that there were 'minimal or no side effects' and presented without criticism a chart showing complete remission in four cases, or 19%, and partial remission in another four."

Moss quotes Robert Houston: "'In contrast', wrote Robert Houston, 'a study on Interleukin-2 in 25 patients with advanced cancer by Dr. Steven Rosenberg (1985) at the NCI produced an avalanche of attention because one out of 25 patients had a complete remission' (Houston, 1987). But Rosenberg was President Reagan's surgeon and a powerhouse at NCI, which may have accounted for his technique's ready acceptance."

In terms of complete remission, 4% for Interleukin-2 gained acceptance while 19% for antineoplastons - nearly five times as much - gained a "no evidence" from the ACS.

Now the prediction "they'll kick your ass" began to come true. During Easter Week, 1983, (the same time of year the FDA attacked Dr. William Koch in 1942) the FDA sued Dr. Burzynski in civil court without warning. It asked the court to "force permanent cessation of all... scientific and medical work on the development, manufacture, and administration of antineoplastons" (Lang, 1986). By chance, Dr. Burzynski's lawyer was in the courtroom on another matter, heard what the FDA was requesting, and told the judge that such an order would cause people's deaths. The next month, Judge Gabrielle McDonald refused the FDA's request. However, she granted an injunction against interstate shipments until Dr. Burzynski filed for and obtained FDA approval of an Investigational New Drug (IND) application. The judge specifically allowed Dr. Burzynski's work to continue within the State of Texas. Robert Spiller, lead FDA attorney, did not accept Judge McDonald's ruling with grace. He told the judge that if she would not shut down Dr. Burzynski, the FDA would be forced to use other methods such as seizures and criminal prosecution, in effect outlining its game plan for the next 14 years.

Burzynski applied for an IND the same month, but before the end of May, 1983, the FDA turned him down. The FDA knew full well that antineoplastons would not be effective in the P388 mouse test, as is the case with some other useful drugs. However, the FDA used that as its grounds for not moving forward and constantly demanded more and more data.

Side effects of antineoplastons were minor. "About half the patients reported...transient rashes, headaches, flushing or dizziness, but generally of only one or two days duration during treatment that lasted from 42 to 872 days" (Moss, *op. cit.*). No hair fell out, the immune system wasn't destroyed, and the patient was not in danger of dying later from the effects of the treatment. The side effects were small compared to those from treatments already approved by the FDA.

Ron Wolin was diagnosed with lymphocytic lymphoma in September, 1983. A one-time antiwar organizer, by July, 1984 he was at Stage IV, nearing the end. Dr. Michael Schachter of Suffern, NY, suggested Dr. Burzynski, who began Wolin's treatment in August. In 1988, most of his tumors were gone. "I'm doing sixty sit-ups a day", he wrote that year, "and my overall health is better than at any time in the past five years. I owe it all to Dr. Burzynski and his antineoplastons."

On July 17, 1985, Ron Wolin was taking antineoplastons at Dr. Burzynski's when the FDA raided the office. Waving search and seizure warrants, FDA agents, accompanied by a U.S. marshall, loaded up eleven four-drawer file cabinets and carted them off to the FDA office. Some of the files were urgently needed for treating current cases. Under order of Judge McDonald, Dr. Burzynski was allowed to install a xerox in the FDA office and to send staff to make copies when needed. Ron Wolin and his companion, Avis Lang, quickly organized a Patients Rights Legal Action Fund which sued the FDA for the return of the files, but the case was lost in lower court. Then a three-judge panel in the U.S. court of Appeals took the side of the FDA, in effect giving it the right to seize doctors' confidential patient records. The court said, "This court... must not allow sympathy for the plight of persons suffering from cancer to cause us to interfere hastily with the mission of the FDA". The Supreme Court refused to hear the case. As we enter the 21st century, the FDA still has not returned Dr. Burzynski's files. Doctor-patient files are considered confidential and privileged. There was a huge press flap when the Nixon Administration's "plumbers" lifted patients' files from a doctor's office in the 1970's. The press paid little attention to Dr. Burzynski's case.

With every blow, Dr. Burzynski just dug in his heels a little deeper. Back in 1979, he had told Gary Null, "I'm going to fight no matter what they do because I believe I'm doing the right thing. I believe this is our obligation to people. If you find something that's valuable, you must continue; I believe that we've found something that may be able to save lives." (Moss)

During hearings following the raid, several of Dr. Burzynski's patients testified that when their insurance ran out, Dr. Burzynski continued to treat them. One of the patients, William Cody, had been treated gratis for years. "Why do you continue to treat Mr. Cody?" an FDA lawyer asked. "Because we care about his life", Dr. Burzynski replied (Lang, 1986). Shortly after the raid, the FDA began sending misleading information to Dr. Burzynski's patients, whose addresses it had obtained from the raid. Letters were also sent to insurance companies, many of which had been paying for antineoplaston therapy. On October 24, 1985, Judge McDonald directed the FDA to stop releasing false information about Dr Burzynski.

Following the raid, the FDA got the U.S. attorney's office to set up a grand jury to investigate Burzynski. The FDA has authority over interstate commerce, but not intrastate commerce such as within the state of Texas. From 1985 on, the FDA was fully aware that patients were coming to Houston from other states, starting treatment with Dr. Burzynski, and taking antineoplastons home with them. FDA took no exception to this procedure, so long as the doctor did not ship the medicine across state lines. FDA could find no evidence that he had done this, so the grand jury disbanded without returning an indictment.

In 1985, by request of the FDA, the Texas Legislature amended the Texas Health and Safety Law to make it illegal to distribute in Texas any drug not approved by the FDA. However, Judge McDonald's order of 1983 permitting Dr. Burzynski to treat patients in Texas protected him from attack under this change.

In Japan, Kurume University was interested in testing antineoplastons (which were also being tested in Poland). On April 17, 1986, the FDA denied Kurume University's request to obtain the therapy from Dr. Burzynski.

In 1986, the United States Postal Service got into the act. It sent letters to Burzynski patients informing them that "an investigation is being conducted into the activities of Dr. S. R. Burzynski and particularly regarding alleged improper insurance billing practices" (Moss, op. cit.) Ralph Moss added, "Despite such harassment, Burzynski was not about to fold his clinic and leave the country." He maintained a serene confidence that his work on antineoplastons would eventually be vindicated, and that the American establishment would wake up to the facts.

On January 13, 1988, the FDA wrote Dr. Burzynski stating that it now believed antineoplastons had shown anticancer activity, thus acknowledging what had been known for ten years. However, it again denied his request for an IND, demanding more data. During 1988, while the FDA was asking for more data, another 400,000 Americans died of cancer.

On March, 1988, New York City talk show hostess Sally

Jessy Raphael had Dr. Burzynski on her program. She was so besieged with calls that she scheduled a second program, on which the doctor was to be joined by three recovered patients. She received such strong protests from the National Cancer Institute (NCI) that her sponsor cancelled the second show.

The effects of antineoplastons continued to be impressive. In an article in the June, 1988 *Advances in Experimental and Clinical Chemotherapy*, Dr. Burzynski reported the case of a woman with astrocytoma, a rapidly growing and generally lethal brain tumor. "On January 8, 1986, she began treatment with AS2-1 (one of the antineoplastons). After five months, she no longer had any signs or symptoms of her disease by physical examination. Two years later, she still did not have any symptoms, felt well, and was living a normal life. She continued to take a maintenance dose of antineoplaston capsules." (Moss)

On September 23, 1988, the Texas Board of Medical Examiners, whose officials had so mercilessly hounded Harry Hoxsey thirty years earlier and any doctor who worked with him (Chapter 2), opened a hearing on whether or not to revoke Dr. Burzynski's medical license. No patients had complained; the Board itself brought the charges. The organizing skills of Ron Wolin and Avis Lang caused the Board to be inundated with letters, copies being sent to the governor of Texas and its congressmen and senators. Here is what one letter said:

> *I am 13 years old and I have a 7-year old brother. We love our father very much. Thanks to Dr. Burzynski's treatment, my father's tumor has stopped growing. All of the doctors in my home state of Missouri said there was no cure for my father's disease. Dr. Burzynski gave him a chance for life again. Please don't take that away from us (Moss).*

On a split vote, the Board postponed taking a decision.

In 1989, the NCI began distributing incorrect and false data about antineoplastons based on its ineffectiveness in the P388 mouse test, which by this time the NCI itself had abandoned. Le

Trombetta, Dr. Burzynski's spokesperson, wrote the NCI a strong protest.

Elsewhere in 1989, the Polish equivalent of the FDA award-ed Dr. Burzynski a special medal for his achievements in the field of cancer chemotherapy. Antineoplastons were indeed chemo-therapy, but nontoxic chemotherapy.

While one branch of FDA investigated him, Dr. Burzynski persisted with his IND application at another part of the agency, which also did not make things easy for him. No matter what he submitted on the IND, a request would come back asking for more data. He would painstakingly comply, only to receive another request. The IND application was in the name of the Burzynski Research Institute (BRI), since no pharmaceutical company, large or small, had yet shown interest. If antineoplas-tons were to be developed, either Burzynski would do it, or the job wouldn't get done. In 1982, Dr. Richard J. Crout, then Director of the FDA's Bureau of Drugs, minced no words when he stated, "I never have and never will approve a new drug to an individual, but only to a large pharmaceutical company with unlimited finances" (*Spotlight*, January 18, 1982). It was a year after his statement that the FDA sued to halt Burzynski's produc-tion of antineoplastons. Dr. Crout was the FDA official who caused big problems for DMSO some years earlier (Chapter 6).

In most fields, innovation is done by individuals or small teams, often working in modest circumstances. The personal computer did not come out of IBM but from two teenagers, Steve Jobs and Steve Wozniak, working in a garage. Some of Dr. Burzynski's early Houston research was done in his garage labo-ratory. The FDA left little doubt that it did not welcome such innovation in the health field.

However, on March 16, 1989, the FDA unexpectedly approved Dr. Burzynski's IND application for one of his antineo-plastons, but for study only in breast cancer. The documents in his IND application made a stack six feet tall by the time approval finally came, six years after filing. IND applications from phar-maceutical companies are generally approved by the FDA in 30 days. From 1983, when Burzynski's IND application was filed, to 1989, when it was approved, between 2,500,000 and 3,000,000 Americans died of cancer.

After his IND approval, Dr. Burzynski optimistically made a comment to Dr. Ralph Moss that was both prophetic and premature, "We are at the end of the war", he said, "but at the end of the war comes the fiercest battle". In *Cancer Industry*, Moss entitled his Burzynski chapter, "The Fiercest Battle", from which the title for this chapter has been borrowed with Dr. Moss' permission. The fiercest episodes of all lay well ahead, after Moss completed the 1989 edition of his book.

In 1990, Le Trombetta put out a circular to Dr. Burzynski's supporters alerting them that for the first time, all the forces against the doctor were preparing to attack at the same time. Shortly thereafter, as if to say, "Why won't you just go away?", the FDA convened a second grand jury. Again, thousands of documents were subpoenaed as well as most of Dr. Burzynski's employees. Again, the grand jurors could find no reason to indict Dr. Burzynski.

There was some good news in 1990. The July-August issue of *Oncology News* put on its front page an article about a "completely new type of anti-tumor agent that is non-toxic and seems to make malignant cells revert to normal". The report came from the 9th International Symposium on Future Trends in Chemotherapy, which was held March 26-28, 1990, in Geneva, Switzerland. Mutual Benefit Life's Winter 1991 issue of *Discoveries in Medicine* told its readers:

> *The new agents are called antineoplastons, naturally occurring peptides and amino acid derivatives which were first isolated in human blood and then in urine. They are currently being synthesized by a biotechnology research facility in Texas. Research indicates that there is a marked deficiency of these peptides in cancer patients. Research also indicates that antineoplastons are components of a biochemical defense system. Unlike the immune*

system which protects us by destroying invading agents or defective cells, the biochemical defense system protects us by reprogramming or normalizing defective cells.

A special session was devoted to antineoplastons, where seven papers were presented, including preclinical and clinical results by researchers from Japan, Poland, China, and the U.S.

Some of the most exciting preclinical research was reported by Dvorit Samid, PhD, from the Uniformed Services University of Health Sciences in Bethesda, Maryland. She reported that 'Antineoplaston AS2-1 profoundly inhibits oncogene expression and the proliferation of malignant cells without exhibiting any toxicity toward normal cells'. Dr. Samid explained that AS2-1 does not kill cancer cells, rather it reprograms them to behave like normal cells.

The Geneva session was the culmination of 23 years of research by Dr. Stanislaw R. Burzynski, MD, PhD, who first identified these peptides in 1967.

Dr. Dvorit Samid had sought out Dr. Burzynski in late 1988, showing great interest in his work. He provided her with antineoplastons and a small grant to do some research for him, about which she reported at the Geneva conference.

After the momentum provided by the Geneva conference, Dr. Burzynski was contacted by a number of pharmaceutical companies, proposing collaboration. One, Elan Pharmaceutical, based in Ireland, signed a letter of intent with Dr. Burzynski on June 20, 1990. The agreement, when finalized, would give Elan the right to license and distribute antineoplastons. Elan was to sponsor FDA Phase II trials in brain tumors, prostate cancer, and non-Hodgkins lymphoma, and to secure FDA approval in those areas. It seemed like a major breakthrough; at last a significant pharmaceutical company had taken note of Dr. Burzynski's work. The letter of intent provided for a 90-day period during which Elan would have almost unlimited access to Dr. Burzynski's "know-how". Dr. Burzynski introduced Elan to Dvorit Samid, since her research was supportive of his work.

After discovering in 1980 the chemical identities of his anti-neoplastons, Dr. Burzynski patented a number of them. One of the antineoplastons, his "AS5", turned out to be the chemical phenylacetate. He had not used it since 1981, noting that it stayed in the body much less time than other antineoplastons and as a result was much less effective. He saw no point to use it when other antineoplastons were much more effective, so he did not patent it.

At the end of the 3-month period, Elan announced that it would not sign a contract with Dr. Burzynski, citing as an excuse his lack of patent protection for the use of phenylacetate in cancer.

Shortly after cancelling its agreement with Dr. Burzynski, Elan gave a grant to Dvorit Samid to research phenylacetate. Neither she nor Elan would answer author Tom Elias' questions as to the size of the grant, but Elan executive Dr. David Tierney told Elias, "We got involved through Dr. Samid" (in phenylac-etate) (Elias, *Burzynski Breakthrough*). Sometime during 1991 Dvorit Samid went to work for NCI's Clinical Pharmacology Branch.

On October 4, 1991, Dr. Burzynski received a visit from six NCI scientists, who spent a day reviewing the records of seven terminal brain tumor patients treated with antineoplastons. After returning to Washington, they began making favorable noises. In an internal memo, Dr. Michael Friedman, then associate director of NCI's Cancer Therapy Evaluation Program (CTEP), wrote the director of NCI's Division of Cancer Treatment that "Antineoplastons deserve a closer look. It turns out that the agents are well-defined, pure chemical entities...The human brain tumor responses are real. We will keep you informed."

In December, Dr. Burzynski made a presentation at the NCI at their invitation. On January 6, 1992, NCI announced that it had indeed found anti-tumor responses in antineoplastons during its October site visit. NCI also stated that it would sponsor them through the FDA approval process, with clinical trials to start as early as March. After the disappointment with Elan the year before, this was a major boost. (But, of course, the NCI undertook to test hydrazine sulfate, too.)

Three weeks after the NCI announcement, the Texas Department of Health filed suit against Dr. Burzynski and his lab, seeking a permanent injunction against the selling and distribution of antineoplastons in Texas. It also asked the court to order that all antineoplastons be destroyed. The Health Department's suit was based on the 1985 change (requested by the FDA) in the Texas Health Law which prohibited the distribution in Texas of any drug not approved by the FDA.

Perhaps the most curious aspect of the Health Department's case was: where had it been before? Why just now, after the NCI had found anti-cancer effect in Dr, Burzynski's antineoplastons, was the Department of Health finding him and his therapy a threat to the health of the people of Texas? If the Department were to prove successful, then what would happen to the 200 or so patients who were then on the antineoplaston treatment? What, Le Trombetta asked in her announcement of the suit, would happen to Ryan and Paul, two children with brain tumors who had exhausted conventional treatment? The NCI had confirmed that Ryan's tumor had gone into complete remission and that Paul's tumor was reduced by 40%-50%. The Health Department stated that "our action will not prevent the NCI from conducting independent clinical trials". But NCI officials called Dr. Burzynski's office wondering how they could conduct trials if all the antineoplastons were destroyed. Dr. Burzynski's lawyers once again went to work to defend him.

The NCI had said trials would start in March, 1992, but the month came and went with nothing from the NCI but excuses - somebody critical to the program having suddenly taken a 6-month leave of absence, things like that.

On June 3, 1992, another blow fell. The JAMA published an

article on antineoplastons by Dr. Saul Green. It could be compared to the JAMA's "Status Report on Krebiozen" of October 27, 1951, which put the kebosh of Official Medicine on Krebiozen (Chapter 5). As in the Krebiozen report, there was no mention whatsoever of the many cases where antineoplastons worked, such as the successes reported at the Geneva conference in 1990, as well as the NCI findings announced earlier in 1992. Green suggested that Dr. Burzynski did not really have a Ph.D, and never bothered to place one phone call to ask about Dr. Burzynski's Polish degree. Green stated that "the FDA would not confirm that it had stated in writing that Burzynski's plant was in conformance with Good Manufacturing Practices". Another phone call would have revealed that Dr. Burzynski had such a letter from the FDA dated October 30, 1985. Green referred to a 1990 NCI test indicating ineffectiveness of antineoplastons, but omitted to note that the test was conducted at 10,000 times less than the recommended dose. Green also omitted to report that in 1992, NCI repeated the tests at the recommended dosage, which then demonstrated anti-cancer effect.

Green also reported that Dr. Tsuda at Kurume University in Japan had told him that he saw no evidence of any biological effect of antineoplastons. Dr. Burzynski wrote Dr. Tsuda in some amazement, since he had received favorable reports from the Kurume doctor. Dr. Tsuda's response was quite revealing. What he had written to Green, Tsuda told Burzynski, was that since Green was not an MD, he "will not pick up any biological effect of antineoplastons even though there is evidence there". He added, "Since we are not native English speakers, he took the meaning different way".

Furious, Dr. Burzynski wrote the JAMA a detailed rebuttal, including a sworn statement from the president of the Medical Academy of Lublin confirming Burzynski's PhD in biochemistry and his MD with honors. Going over Green's statements point by point, Burzynski charged that "Green seriously misrepresented over 20 years of research by selective omission". Dr. Burzynski wondered how such an article could ever have passed "peer review", a system which, when used properly by professional journals, prevents the publication of erroneous material. This was the same question Dr. Andrew Ivy had asked in 1951 about the JAMA "Status Report" on Krebiozen. The JAMA refused to print Dr. Burzynski's rebuttal. In 1951, it refused to print Dr. Ivy's rebuttal; he was then one of the most respected scientists in America. Forty one years later, the JAMA had not become any more even-handed.

By the fall of 1992, Dr. Burzynski had still heard nothing from the NCI. Unbeknownst to him until later, some reconsideration was going on within the organization. An internal memo to Dr. Michael Friedman revealed that antineoplastons had been discussed at a September 14 meeting. The memo stated, "There is reason to believe from preclinical data provided by Dr. Samid of the Clinical Pharmacology Branch that the active component of the antineoplastons is phenylacetic acid (PAA) (phenylacetate), the final breakdown product of the antineoplaston preparations. It would be preferable to study PAA (since it is easier to produce and obtain, and since a pharmaceutical company has been identified that is more likely to reliably provide drug supplies) rather than the more complex mixtures of antineoplastons."

The first Dr. Burzynski knew of all this was when the NCI journal announced in the fall of 1992 that NCI had contracted Elan Pharmaceutical to do a series of clinical trials with phenylacetate. Phenylacetate was Burzynski's one-time "AS5", which he had not patented. He had not used it since 1981 since it was far less effective than his other compounds - "the more complex mixtures", as the NCI called them.

There was another indication that all was not well at NCI. Dr. Nicholas Patronas, NCI's Chief of Neuroradiology, was part of the NCI team which verified Dr. Burzynski's brain tumor results in 1991. On May 24, 1993, Dr. Patronas testified in Austin at a hearing on the Board of Medical Examiners' move to suspend Dr. Burzynski's license and place him on probation. Dr. Patronas testified that "antineoplastons are the most effective treatment for brain tumors I have ever seen". When asked what would happen to patients deprived of the drug, Dr. Patronas testified, "I believe these patients will die".

When Dr. Patronas returned to Washington, he was severely reprimanded for having supported Dr. Burzynski. Under pressure, on May 28, he withdrew a paper on antineoplastons he was scheduled to give at a cancer conference in Sweden. If the NCI were serious about moving antineoplastons through the FDA, who, then, would have wanted to reprimand Dr. Patronas over his appearance in Austin? Was the NCI speaking with forked tongue?

On another front in 1992, Chryssie Schiff, age 4½, developed a malignant brain tumor. Her parents, Ric and Paula, took her to the University of California at San Francisco (UC/SF) hospital. Dr. Michael Prados, UC/SF head of oncology, assured them that he knew of no alternatives to the chemotherapy and radiation he urged be administered. Believing him, they gave the go-ahead and Chryssie went through six months of hell. During that time, Ric, a San Francisco police sergeant, heard of Dr. Burzynski, but Dr. Prados told him that antineoplastons did not work. Ric and his wife took Chryssie to Dr. Burzynski anyway. Dr. Burzynski showed them letters from the same Dr. Prados reporting on California businessman Jeff Keller's recovery from a brain tumor following antineoplaston therapy. From 1989 to 1993, Dr. Prados had sent Dr. Burzynski no less than fourteen two-page letters documenting Keller's condition. On September 6, 1991, with Keller in complete remission, Prados wrote, "Mr. Keller...seems to be having an excellent response to antineoplaston therapy" (Dr. Julian Whitaker's *Health and Healing*, February 1996). A few weeks after writing that letter, Prados told Ric and Paula Schiff that he knew of no alternatives to chemo and radiation.

Dr. Prados and his UC/SF staff had earlier seen another success from antineoplastons, patient Pamela Winningham. Diagnosed with a Grade 3 astrocytoma in her brain stem in July, 1987, she received surgery and radiation, but neither stopped the tumor. One of Dr. Prados' staff urged her to "eat, drink, and be merry", for she had only a few months to live. Instead, she went to Dr. Burzynski and the tumor disappeared. Since UC/SF had assumed she was dead, they thought they were talking to a ghost when Pamela called to report her good health.

The Schiffs stopped antineoplastons after eighteen months, thinking Chryssie's tumor was in remission, but it came back aggressively. Dr. Prados opposed her taking any more antineo-plastons and proposed a new type of chemotherapy. Instead, the Schiffs put Chryssie back on antineoplastons and in six weeks, MRI scans showed that the tumor was gone again. Chryssie Schiff's story did not end as well as Jeff Keller and Pamela Winningham. Deeply injured by the chemotherapy and radiation she had undergone, she weakened and died of pneumonia. An autopsy showed no cancer. (*Health and Healing*, February, 1996)

Because Prados and staff had told him and Paula they knew of no other treatment, Ric Schiff was bitter. He had accepted what they told him; that aggressive treatment would buy time and little else. "They told us the treatment would likely kill her. They even-tually were proven correct about that one point... They only gave her so much radiation and chemotherapy because they thought she would die anyway". (Chryssie's total radiation and chemo-therapy bill was $800,000.) "They knew if you give a little girl 6,000 rads of radiation to the brain and 4,000 to the spine, she won't live long. She will lose her gag reflex and won't respond when things are swallowed the wrong way and go into the lungs." (Elias, *Burzynski Breakthrough*). The pneumonia Cryssie died from may have been brought about in just that way, but Ric and Paula did not know that until much later.

Had Chryssie never been treated with chemo and radiation, and only with antineoplastons, her story might have ended differ-ently. Dr. Prados and staff knew of the success of antineoplastons in Jeff Keller and Pam Winningham, but told Ric and Paula Schiff that they knew of no alternatives to chemo and radiation. Chryssie died.

In mid-1993, the NCI began moving on clinical trials. Tom Elias describes what happened (*op. cit.*), "A three-site trial of antineoplastons was authorized, with patients to be accepted at the National Institutes of Health (NIH, of which the NCI is part), the Mayo Clinic, and Memorial Sloan Kettering. No patients, however, were signed up until early 1994. In a letter signed by Dr. Michael Friedman, the NCI agreed that the trials would take in patients with anaplastic astrocytomas and glioblastoma multiforme, two of the fastest-growing and deadliest brain cancers. Thirty-five patients would be treated; none would have tumors that exceeded five centimeters in diameter and none would have multiple tumors or cancer that had spread elsewhere in the body."

The second patient accepted at NIH, in early 1994, was Ingrid Schultz, who had had two surgeries for a glioblastoma brain tumor but had refused radiation. The NCI trials required that patients should have undergone every form of conventional treatment and failed. Since Ingrid had not had radiation, she was initially rejected but obtained an exemption. She was treated for six weeks under the supervision of Dr. Alain Thibault, a close associate of Dr. Dvorit Samid, and an "investigator" for NCI in the antineoplaston trials. Curiously, he had also been appointed a "principal investigator" for NCI's competing phenylacetate trials.

Ingrid's roommate at the NIH hospital in Bethesda, Maryland, was a woman named Didi, the first patient accepted in the trials. Lon Schultz, Ingrid's husband, remembers that Ingrid suspected early on that something was off base. Ingrid called Lon one day and told him that Dr. Thibault had come into their room "amazingly ecstatic" - Lon remembers these were the words Ingrid used - over Didi's failure to respond to antineoplastons. This meant she would die, Thibault told Didi. Telling of his interview with Lon Schultz about his wife's case, Tom Elias writes (*op. cit.*), "When her treatment at NIH ended, Ingrid Schultz was convinced that most NIH doctors wanted the antineoplastons to fail. 'After several weeks, it was determined that the treatment was not working on her', Lon Schultz says. 'Ingrid felt Dr. Thibault was tremendously excited and pleased that it was not working. And after they pulled her off the drug, Ingrid met with four or six other doctors there who said she needed to go home and die. They emphasized that she needed to die, that it was the proper thing to do.'" But Ingrid would not pass away on schedule. She contacted

Burzynski, who agreed to treat her at no charge after he learned of her travails at NIH. His treatment had an effect on her tumor, which slowed and then stopped growing after three months. However, Lon Schultz reports, she died about six months later from another condition, not from the tumor.

While at the Burzynski clinic, Lon and Ingrid met a woman who had been in Dr. Thibault's phenylacetate trials. Deriving no benefit there, she came to Dr. Burzynski. Ingrid told her the strange incident of Dr. Thibault seeming so pleased that antineoplastons had not worked for her or Didi. The woman responded, "But he wasn't at all like that with me. When Dr. Thibault told me that phenylacetate wasn't working on me, he was very sad!"

During their stay in Houston, Lon and Ingrid heard rumors that the antineoplastons used in the NCI antineoplaston trials were diluted. Lon wondered "why, if she was in fact getting full strength antineoplastons at NIH, she didn't respond there, when she did respond at Burzynski's clinic." (Elias, *op. cit.*) If Ingrid received a diluted dose of antineoplastons for six weeks, Lon Schultz wonders if she would still be alive had the NCI given her full strength antineoplastons, to which she responded at Dr. Burzynski's. Effectiveness of the medicine is dose-related; more is more effective; diluted is less effective.

While the NCI trials were going on, Dean Mouscher, a consultant to Dr. Burzynski, was told by a doctor at the Mayo Clinic that they were diluting the antineoplastons four to one. When Mouscher expressed astonishment, the doctor then insisted that he really didn't know much about it, apparently realizing he might have said the wrong thing.

With only a handful of patients besides Ingrid Schultz admitted to the antineoplaston trials, Dr. Mario Sznol of NCI's Cancer Therapy Evaluation Program (CTEP) wrote Dr. Burzynski on March 24, 1994, stating that NCI proposed major changes in the protocol. The idea was to treat larger tumors, and patients with metastases - but with no change in the dosage. Dr. Burzynski realized that "treating larger and more widespread tumors without increasing dosage would bias the trial against antineoplastons and guarantee they would appear useless or at least no more effective than plain phenylacetate... Burzynski said, 'I told Sznol in the beginning that if he wanted to treat more advanced tumors, he would need more antineoplastons. Instead of giving them one gram of A-10 per kilogram of body weight, they might need five grams per kilogram'. This, Dr. Burzynski notes, is consistent with the finding of the NCI 1991 site visit, which reported that 'no significant (anti-tumor) activity was seen in tissue cultures when low concentrations were used.'" (Elias, *op. cit.*)

In answer to Sznol's letter Burzynski proposed that patients with tumors larger than the original proposal be placed in a separate trial and be given a different dosage. Drs. Michael Friedman and Sznol ignored his request and wrote Burzynski that the suggested amendments to the trial had been approved (without Dr. Burzynski's agreement) at the request of the investigators, *i.e.*, Dr. Jan Buckner of the Mayo Clinic and Dr. Mark Malkin of Memorial Sloan Kettering. However, Dr. Malkin wrote a letter to the chair of his hospital's Institutional Review board stating that "amendments have been made (to the antineoplaston trials) at the request of the NCI", directly contradicting Drs. Friedman and Sznol.

In 1994, the Texas Board of Medical Examiners moved in court to put Dr. Burzynski on indefinite probation. The Board had accepted testimony that many patients would die if Dr. Burzynski's practice were closed. However, the Board had stated, "the efficacy of antineoplastons in the treatment of human cancer is not of issue in these proceedings". Judge Paul Davis threw the case out and denounced the Board for being "arbitrary and capricious", and for "abuses of discretion". The Board appealed.

In 1994, Robert Spiller, the FDA lawyer assigned to the Burzynski case from 1983, convened a third grand jury to investigate Dr. Burzynski. Again, thousands of documents were subpoenaed. Again, no indictment was voted by the jurors.

It became clear that NCI had no intention of keeping Dr. Burzynski informed of what was going on in the trials. In May 1995, a CTEP official wrote a memo stating that the clinical trials monitoring service had been instructed not to send any clinical trial data to Dr. Burzynski.

In the summer of 1995, the NCI announced that it was canceling its trials of antineoplastons because "A consensus could not be reached with Dr. Burzynski on the proposed changes in the protocol" (Elias). Dr. Michael Friedman seemed to be the point man for scuttling the NCI trials, since his signature appeared on most of the relevant documents. So ended NCI's only trials with antineoplastons.

Having shot down the antineoplaston trials, NCI proceeded apace with its trials of phenylacetate, in which Dr. Michael Prados joined Dr. Alain Thibault as a principal investigator. However, Drs. Buckner and Malkin, also principal investigators, wrote a paper "conceding", Tom Elias states (*op. cit.*), "the major biochemical point Burzynski had been making for more than a decade. Burzynski maintains that phenylacetylglutamine, one of the two major components of antineoplastons, causes the activity of phenylacetate to intensify and be sustained over a longer period of time. Similarly, Buckner and Malkin conceded...that studies of blood drawn from their patients showed that those who received antineoplastons had a higher blood content of phenylacetylglutamine than those who received plain phenylacetate... Patients on antineoplastons did not excrete phenylacetylglutamine in their urine as quickly as patients who got plain phenylacetate - precisely the reason Burzynski gave up using plain phenylacetate more than a decade earlier." (it left the body too fast.)

"Prados gave the first formal report on the phenylacetate brain tumor trial at the 1995 meeting of the American Society for Clinical Oncology. Of the first 19 patients who could be evaluated, he reported tumor reduction in 5. One saw tumor shrinkage of 66%, one was reduced by 48%, and three others were in the 20-30% range." (Elias, *op. cit.*) Reacting to these results, the ever optimistic Burzynski said, "If they get good results using plain phenylacetate when our medicine is so much better, that has to help us" (Elias, *op. cit.*).

NCI's tilt in favor of phenylacetate confirmed Dr. Burzynski's conclusion that his version of antineoplastons are superior. The Prados report showed brain tumor reduction in 5 out of 19, a response rate of 29%, but with no complete remissions. In contrast, an analysis of 36 brain tumor patients treated with Dr. Burzynski's antineoplastons shows 28 responding (8 not) with tumor reduction for a response rate of 77%. Of the 36, 9 went into complete remission. So the track record is a response rate of 77% for antineoplastons vs. 29% for phenylacetate and a remission rate of 25% for antineoplastons vs. 0% for phenylacetate.

As a footnote to the NCI trials, the February 1999 *Proceedings of the Mayo Clinic* published a review of the nine patients who were treated with NCI's version of Dr. Burzynski's therapy before the trials were cancelled. The article reported the levels of antineoplastons in patients' blood after treatment. This data unwittingly provided solid evidence that the antineoplastons used in the NCI trials were indeed diluted, just as Dean Mouscher had been told. The concentrations in the blood reported by Mayo were 53 times less than the concentrations Dr. Burzynski routinely observes in his patients. The point of the NCI trials was to replicate Dr. Burzynski's treatment. Since NCI used very diluted concentrations of antineoplastons, obviously they did not replicate his treatment and thus could not duplicate his results. The patients were not told that they were not receiving the real thing, and should have been, since this was not a "double blind" test.

NCI knew from their 1991 visit to the Burzynski clinic that "no significant anti-tumor activity was seen in tissue cultures when low concentrations (of antineoplastons) were used". (Elias, *op. cit.*) By using a highly diluted dosage, the NCI might have contributed to the deaths of Ingrid Schultz and Didi and others in the NCI antineoplaston trials. It is all sadly reminiscent of the 1989-1993 NCI trials of hydrazine sulfate, where patients were given other drugs known to be incompatible with hydrazine sulfate and known to cancel its effectiveness. All 600 patients in the NCI's hydrazine sulfate trials died.

Randy Goss, a Burzynski patient from western New York State, was told by Roswell Park Cancer Institute that he was terminal with renal cell carcinoma and that chemotherapy and radiation would not help him. A few days later, Roswell Park officials arranged for him to receive free treatment with interleukin-2 at the NIH in Bethesda, Maryland. However, NIH told him that he would have about a 15% chance of surviving the interleukin-2 itself, which he declined. Instead, he went to see Dr.Burzynski in May 1994, began treatment with antineoplastons, and was cancer-free in six months. Back in the Buffalo area, he began making speeches about his recovery, noting that death was not in the air at the Burzynski Clinic. After one appearance, a Roswell Park official sitting in the back got up, confirmed that Goss indeed had had renal cell carcinoma and had gone to Houston. "But", said the official, "can we say that the medicine cured him? No. We have seen a lot of spontaneous remissions in renal cell carcinoma." (Elias, *op. cit.*) The American Cancer Society publishes figures on spontaneous remissions: about 1 in 100,000, and indicates they have almost no such cases in renal cell carcinoma.

On March 23, 1995, FDA agents made an unscheduled visit to Burzynski brain tumor patient Domenick Pugliese on Long Island. They had no search warrant but aggressively insisted on searching the house, telling the Puglieses that they had been trying to "get" Burzynski for years. The agents insisted that antineoplastons were ineffective and that Pugliese should seek other treatment. (*Health and Healing,* op. cit.)

The next morning, Dr. Burzynski was on the CBS morning show with three patients in remission. Hours later, the FDA raided his clinic again, once more confiscating boxloads of records and confidential patients' medical records.

In April, FDA prosecutor Robert Spiller convened yet a fourth grand jury, each month subpoenaing more documents and more employees.

In May 1995, former FDA Chief Counsel Peter Barton Hutt gave a credible explanation for what was behind the FDA's moves in an article in *Reason* magazine:

If you beat the FDA in court, you have an angry FDA that

is willing to slit your throat. When the FDA loses a case,
it has a mind like an elephant. It's just something you'd
got to understand about the FDA. Once the agency makes
a collective decision, trying to make it let go is almost
impossible. These are FDA crusades - in a real sense, they
are vendettas.

The Grand Jury went on through November. Even author
Ralph Moss was called, but the subpoena was withdrawn when
Moss pointed out that it violated six federal laws.

On November 15, Congressman Joe Barton held a hearing on
what the FDA was doing with Dr. Burzynski. FDA Commissioner David Kessler was questioned harshly over having convened
four grand juries to investigate a nontoxic therapy without being
able to find anything wrong. Barton put pressure on Kessler and
secured commitments that current Burzynski patients would continue to receive antineoplastons. Patients who stated that they
were being kept alive by another nontoxic therapy, LK-200, also
attended. There were fewer of them and their case was not so
famous. Since Kessler made no commitment to keep LK-200
available, it vanished from the market. A year later, two of the
LK-200 patients who had testified at the hearings were dead.

One week after the Barton hearings, David Kessler's FDA
secured an indictment against Dr. Burzynski on 75 criminal
charges, which would put him in jail for 229 years if convicted.

What was different this time from the previous grand juries?
From the beginning in 1977, Dr. Burzynski knew that he was
dealing with a product not approved by the FDA, which had jurisdiction over interstate commerce. Therefore, he had never
shipped across state lines. The FDA was looking for proof that he
had done so in its multiple raids, subpoenas, and grand juries, but
found none. He knew better.

What changed in 1995 was that the FDA succeeded in convincing the grand jurors of a new definition of interstate commerce. If you live in New York and order something from a store
in San Francisco, which sends it to you, that store is engaging in

interstate commerce. If you go to San Francisco and buy something in a store and take it home to New York, that store is simply attending a customer and obviously is not engaging in interstate commerce. But for the FDA, it would be. According to the FDA, when someone came from another state, took antineoplaston treatments from Dr. Burzynski and then took the therapy back to their home state, the FDA claimed that Dr. Burzynski was engaging in interstate commerce. This arrangement had been going on for years and the FDA knew it. It wasn't a crime when the FDA convened its first, second, or third grand juries. For the fourth grand jury (which was not told about the first three), Dr. Burzynski's standing procedure suddenly became a crime. It didn't stop there. Based on that argument, the FDA lawyers contended, since Dr. Burzynski was thus breaking the law, he was breaking postal law as well. Here was the infraction; he had sent insurance claims through the U.S. mail without advising the insurance companies that he was breaking the law by engaging in interstate commerce with an unapproved drug. Alice in Wonderland had nothing on such reasoning.

Ironically, while the FDA had indicted Burzynski under its new definition of interstate commerce, by this time he actually was shipping antineoplastons across state lines quite legally as part of the clinical trials which another branch of the FDA had approved.

In January 1996, FDA government lawyers sought to bar Dr. Bursynski from treating any of his patients who did not qualify for the FDA clinical trials. When Dr. Burzynski pointed out that patients would die, the FDA attorney called any resulting harm to patients "irrelevant".

Appalled by the "irrelevant" quote, Texas Congressman Barton called another hearing on FDA Abuses of Authority. Under pressure from Barton, Commissioner Kessler agreed to permit Dr. Burzynski to continue treating current patients and to expand the clinical trials. (FDA clinical trials were a long-standing Burzynski goal.)

In April, the FDA again tried to cut off the flow of new

patients, suggesting that while the treatment was safe for current patients, it would not be safe for new ones. Dr. Burzynski's team felt that this move was an attempt to strangle him financially by cutting off his cash flow. Then, under continuing Congressional pressure, the FDA lifted its clinical "hold" on May 1, 1996.

Not all of the several periods when the FDA cut off patients from access to Dr. Burzynski were at the time of the trial. During one such period, Mary Collins of the IMPRO Co. in Iowa (Chapter 7) suddenly developed breast cancer. A strong supporter of Dr. Burzynski, Mary wasn't worried; she'd just go to Houston and take antineoplastons. But when she called to make arrangements, she learned that the FDA had momentarily shut him down. Antineoplastons weren't available when she needed them, and she died. So in a very real sense, the remarkable Mary Collins may have been an unintended casualty of the FDA. To be sure, antineoplastons might not have stopped her cancer, but she should have had the option to try them.

In regulating Dr. Burzynski's clinical trials, the FDA insisted on some bizarre conditions. Patients with non-Hodgkins lymphoma who did not have a 50% reduction in their tumors within six months would have to stop treatment. One patient, Frances Langham, had happily noted a 44% reduction in her tumor in six months. She was ordered to stop treatment. After bitter protests, again relying on Congressional pressure, the FDA backed off. Virginia Kahn, suffering from breast cancer, had found no relief from Tamoxifen and wanted to start on antineoplastons. The FDA insisted on a three-month waiting period to see if there were any delayed results from Tamoxifen - but cancer does not wait. FDA demanded that treatment be stopped immediately if there were some progression in a brain tumor within the first thirty days. Since some progression in the first month of treatment is a frequent occurrence, this also was an unreasonable demand. Antineoplaston dosage was ramped up gradually and most patients would not have reached the full dose by the end of thirty days. In many of the FDA clinical trials, no patient would be admitted without first having failed one round of orthodox toxic chemotherapy and radiation. For certain types of lymphoma, the FDA demanded that patients must have failed two rounds of chemotherapy before being allowed antineoplastons. Unfortunately, there often is little left of patients after two rounds of chemotherapy, leaving less chance for antineoplastons to do any good.

Krystyna Pataluch and her husband immigrated from Poland to Chicago in 1990. In January, 1996, she discovered that she had colon cancer. After hearing about Dr. Burzynski from other Polish people, she decided she was going to see him, and went to Houston. Then she heard about the FDA. At this point, Dr. Burzynski was under indictment but was allowed to continue his clinic under strict terms that he could only treat people approved by the FDA for its trials. If he treated Krystyna, he would be breaking the conditions of his bail and would go straight to jail. Krystyna told Tom Elias (*op. cit.*), "Who ever heard of stopping a dying person from getting whatever she wants? Not even the Communists did that." Even though her tumor was growing, Krystyna had to wait two weeks, but finally the FDA approved and she started on antineoplastons.

Shawn and Desiree McConnell despaired after seeing their small son Zachary grow desperately ill from chemo and radiation after successful surgery for a brain tumor. Praying for guidance, Shawn felt he had been given a sign when, while washing a woman's windows, he heard her talking on the phone about Burzynski. Soon he was talking to others in the Burzynski patient network. A few days later, he and his wife drove to Houston with Zac. Antineoplastons were started March 19, 1996, and in two months, Zac's MRI was clear. Returning to Houston in May to pick up more medicine, Shawn encountered the FDA. Dr. Robert De Lap, then acting director of the FDA's Division of Oncology Drug Products, had written to Dr. Burzynski on April 26 stating that Zac could only take more antineoplastons after a scan showed that the tumor had returned. De Lap further required a report from a radiation oncologist stating that the tumor could not be treated with radiation. The Burzynski patient network provided the McConnells with medicine to keep Zac going. Meanwhile, the family drove to Washington to testify at a Senate hearing on the FDA, stirring up media attention and letters to congressmen. On July 2, DeLap reversed himself and wrote a letter authorizing Burzynski to renew antineoplaston treatment for Zac. Said Shawn McConnell, "Between those two letters, the only things that happened were political and media pressure. Now we know these FDA decisions aren't based on science or the welfare of the patient. They're based on power and politics". (Elias)

In his July 1996 *Health and Healing* newsletter, Dr. Julian Whitaker wrote about a Burzynski patient, missionary David Smith. Diagnosed with Hodgkins lymphoma, he took four rounds of radiation. This reduced the tumor somewhat, but then it came back. He soon was told that he was at stage IV (terminal) and needed to take chemotherapy. Although sometimes useful in Hodgkins, "chemo" is known to wreck the immune system. David Smith decided against it and went to Dr. Burzynski. After seven weeks of antineoplastons, Smith was greatly improved and most of the metastases had disappeared. About that time, the FDA clamped down, forcing Dr. Burzynski to petition the FDA for a "compassionate use" exemption so that David could continue the treatment. Dr. DeLap refused, directing that David first take chemotherapy before continuing on antineoplastons. Smith refused and sued. However, a federal judge ruled against him, in effect affirming DeLap's right to dictate Smith's cancer treatment. David Smith again refused chemo.

Dr. Whitaker also reported on Dustin Kunnari, who developed a medullablastoma brain tumor at 2 years of age. His parents refused chemotherapy when they learned of the toxic side effects. The oncologist at the University of Minnesota told them that a court order could be used to force them to let their child take the therapy. Instead, they found out about Dr. Burzynski and took Dustin to him. As of 1996, 2 years later, his tumor was entirely gone and Dustin was healthy and robust. As this book goes to print, he is eight years old, healthy, and tumor-free.

Dr. Julian Whitaker, a rising voice in complementary medicine, wrote the following in his February 1996 *Health and Healing* newsletter (which goes to 500,000 subscribers):

Ask yourself what it must feel like to be Dr. Stanislaw Burzynski. You have discovered a powerful nontoxic therapy for cancer. You watch that therapy transform terminally ill patients to full health over a decade. These patients then tell you that their oncologists are angry about their taking the therapy and have told them to stop, even though these same oncologists have never called, even out of curiosity, to find out how it works.

Because you, as Burzynski, are doing something that actually works, you have generated almost unbearable animosity from virtually every part of the cancer industry. Your own government is trying to put you in prison and destroy your discovery. Your offices have been repeatedly raided, and federal agents have lied about you so often that you now expect them to.

Yet the 'victims' of your 'crime' - your patients - are united behind you in fierce opposition to what their government is doing to them. They know that if the government succeeds in getting you, it gets them as well, because without the therapy, they will start to die. Government agents know this, but they don't care.

Everywhere you turn, there is hatred and bigotry, except from those who really know what you're doing - your patients and your staff. The few physicians in the system who understand the value of what you have discovered are now mute because the system would turn on them if they came to your defense. You are very much alone.

The years of persecution have come to a head. Seventy-four indictments have been coerced from the fourth grand jury convened over the last 14 years, with the express task of trying to define your activities as criminal. All of this is on your mind when you walk into an examination room and see the fearful eyes of yet another cancer victim waiting to get started on his or her last chance for survival.

Now ask yourself: If you were Dr. Burzynski, how long could you hold out? I have asked myself that questions hundreds of times, and I am embarrassed at some of the answers it brought forth.

Judge Sim Lake, who would preside over Dr. Burzynski's trial, first stated in December 1995 that he would not close the Burzynski clinic, but then he reversed his decision. When Dr. Whitaker called the judge, his secretary said, "I know that the judge knows that people will die if he shuts off the Burzynski therapy". Many patients told Dr. Whitaker the same thing, "This can't be happening in the United States!" But it did in the 1960's with Krebiozen, and people died then. Judge Lake eventually left the clinic open.

On October 11, 1996, FDA lawyers filed motions to keep all evidence of efficacy out of the upcoming trial set for January 1997. According to the FDA, allowing jurors to see such evidence is a "thinly veiled effort to expose the jury to the specter of Dr. Burzynski in the act of saving lives. Permitting it will certainly infect the jury's consideration of the real issue with irrelevant emotional, prejudicial, and misleading concerns regarding whether antineoplastons work and the unfortunate fate of Dr. Burzynski's patients". If saving lives was irrelevant, what might the real issues be? The FDA was sounding more and more like Detective Javert in *Les Miserables*, to whom justice played a poor second to procedure.

The trial opened in January 1997. Numerous government witnesses were there under coercion; the FDA threatened to prosecute them for aiding and abetting Dr. Burzynski's supposed infractions of interstate commerce laws unless they testified.

They were little help to the prosecution, for not one would speak against Dr. Burzynski. No one denied having frequently picked up medicine at the clinic and then mailing it to patients, and no one believed this was a crime. Most were aware that FDA regulations permit patients returning from Mexico to bring back medical supplies. Why then, they wondered, was it legal to bring home medicine from Mexico but not from Texas?

Outside the courthouse, Dr. Burzynski's patients were demonstrating, chanting "Save the doctor who saves lives!" After the prosecution's coerced witnesses, the defense brought in a parade of patients. Because any mention of efficacy had been ruled out, the patients could not speak of their recovery, but their appearance spoke worlds. Mary Jo Siegel, head of the Burzynski patients defense group, was there when she was not leading demonstrations outside. When Mary Jo was diagnosed with low-grade non-Hodgkins lymphoma, her doctor told her that chemotherapy would have no effect on her cancer. He further declared that there had never been spontaneous remissions in that type of cancer, and therefore she would surely die. When she returned with no tumor after taking antineoplastons, the doctor proclaimed that she had had a spontaneous remission. Pamela Winningham, whose recovery Dr. Prados and his staff had observed, was at the trial. Mrs. Mariann Kunnari was there, pointing to her son, Dustin, recovered from a brain tumor.

The prosecution had a standard question for all the defense witnesses, "Did Dr. Burzynski victimize you?" All replied no, and a few, before being cut off by the prosecutor, managed to state that it was the government who was victimizing them by prosecuting their doctor.

The defense attempted to introduce a report from Dr. Robert Burdick, Seattle oncologist and professor at the University of Washington Medical School. Tom Elias reports that Dr. Burdick's study evaluated seventeen brain tumor patients taking antineoplaston treatment as of April 1996, "'As a rough estimate', Burdick wrote, 'neurosurgeons do well to cure one in every 1,000 brain cancer patients they operate on. Radiation therapy slows the growth of adult tumors, gaining perhaps one month of life, and may result in a cure of only one in 500 - 1,000 patients. Similarly, chemotherapy, despite 30 years of clinical trials, has not resulted in the development of a single drug or drug combination that elicits more than an occasional transient response in primary brain tumors.' Against this dismal background, Burdick said, he reviewed Burzynski's cases. These showed seven complete remissions out of seventeen. There were nine partial remissions of 50% or more, and one case of stable disease. Summarized Burdick, 'I am very impressed with the number of complete and partial responses...compared with the number of responses that I have seen in my personal experience. The responses here are far in excess of any prior series of patients published in the medical literature...the response rate here is an astounding 81%, with an equally astounding 35% complete remission... It is very clear the responses here are due to antineoplaston therapy and are not due to surgery, radiation, or standard chemotherapy.'"

Judge Lake took the Burdick report under advisement for one day and then ruled it irrelevant.

On March 3, 1997, Judge Lake declared a mistrial. The jury was hopelessly deadlocked, 6 to 6, on all counts and could not reach a verdict on anything. The judge overruled the jury and threw out the 34 counts of insurance and mail fraud stating "there is no evidence of insurance or mail fraud in this case". The FDA immediately scheduled another trial for May on the remaining interstate commerce charges.

Reporting the case to his readers, Dr. Whitaker noted that "Robert Spiller, FDA chief enforcement officer, the architect of this charade...took up residence in Houston at the Hyatt Regency at your expense in an attempt to 'get his man'". Whitaker reported that Congressman Richard Burr said that the government's treatment of Dr. Burzynski was "one of the worst abuses of the criminal justice system" he had ever witnessed.

One of the jurors, Darlene Phillips, published a letter in the July 1997 issue of the *Townsend Letter for Doctors and Patients*. In it, she stated that the case should never have been tried in a criminal court. Instead, it should have been returned to the civil court of Judge Gabrielle McDonald, who presided over the civil action of May 24, 1983, which the FDA lost. Ms. Phillips stated that a second reason the case should not have gone to trial was because the FDA had already approved 71 clinical trials in which Dr. Burzynski was given full liberty to ship antineoplastons out of the State of Texas. This was not known to the jurors during the trial, she pointed out. When she learned this, she felt that "I had been involved in… a ridiculous waste of two months of my life. After all, wasn't this a moot point at this time (shipping across state lines)? Surely our government has real 'criminals' to prosecute." She also wrote, "since the prosecution has been working on the case for four years, I expected the exhibits, witnesses, and evidence to be compelling. It was not and they didn't come close to proving their case."

Shortly after the March verdict, Robert Spiller threw out the remaining interstate commerce charges, which were not selling very well to jurors. The remaining charge to be considered at the May trial was contempt of court. In 1983, Judge Gabrielle McDonald had specifically permitted Dr. Burzynski to treat patients in Texas but had forbidden him from engaging in interstate commerce. The FDA charged that since Dr. Burzynski had engaged in interstate commerce by letting people take antineoplastons out of state, he thereby had violated Judge McDonald's order. Therefore, said the FDA, he was in contempt of court, a criminal offense.

Going into the second trial, prosecutor Michael Clark "tried to negotiate a settlement, finally offering to drop all criminal charges if Burzynski would plead guilty to one count of civil contempt of court and pay a $250,000 fine. But Burzynski would have no part of any settlement. 'I don't want to admit to anything that makes it look like I did anything wrong at all', he said. 'I did nothing wrong. I was always very careful to obey every court order.'" (Elias, *op. cit.*)

When jury selection began, one potential juror said, "The FDA is like the Gestapo" and another asked, "why isn't the FDA on trial instead of Dr. Burzynski?" (Elias) Obviously, the prosecution barred the inclusion of these two on the jury.

The trial lasted three days. It took the jury just two hours to acquit Dr. Burzynski.

After the trial, Michael Clark said, "It concerns me as a government employee to see a trend toward government bashing, and this was part of it". (Elias) But the government bashed first. Perhaps a government prosecutor would have a hard time understanding what was expressed by juror Stephanie Shapiro, a Houston attorney, "I found the government behavior offensive. A lot of people felt it was. This was a Big Brother issue." (Elias, *op. cit.*)

The Department of Health's request for a court order to destroy antineoplastons became moot once the FDA approved a number of clinical trials. The case was dropped in December 1997.

The Texas Board of Medical Examiners finally succeeded in having Dr. Burzynski placed on ten years of probation, which started in 1994. During these years, he is permitted to treat only patients admitted to clinical trials by the FDA; this amounts to about six out of every hundred who apply. Since there are a large number of employees in the antineoplaston manufacturing plant and the clinic, these conditions clamped a vise around the doctor's cash flow.

When he and his lawyers were free to focus on things other than his staying out of jail, Dr. Burzynski discovered that on October 21, 1991, Dvorit Samid had filed patent application #779.774 on phenylacetate in the use of cancer, declaring to the U.S. Patent Office in January 1992 that she was the sole inventor of the subject matter of her October 21 application. She told Tom Elias "all these studies came from natural compounds that were developed in my laboratory". However, Dr. Burzynski's files contain a letter from Dvorit Samid dated December 4, 1989, which states, "I will now need to examine the effect of the sodium salts of phenylacetylglutamine and phenylacetic acid (phenylacetate) separately. Could you please provide me with these agents?

(about 10 g of each will do). What is the molecular weight of each of the chemical compounds?" Burzynski sent her the materials she requested. On June 3, 1997, she was issued U.S. Patent #5,635,533 on "Methods for inducing differentiation of a cell using phenylacetic acid and derivatives". On August 5, 1997, she was issued U.S. Patent #5,654,333 on "Methods for prevention of cancer using phenylacetic acid and derivatives thereof". On August 26, 1997, she was issued U.S. Patent #5,661,179 on "Methods for treating neoplastic conditions using phenylacetic acid and derivatives thereof".

Elan Pharmaceutical obtained a "use" patent on phenylacetate which lists Dvorit Samid as the inventor of phenylacetate as a cancer treatment. However, phenylacetate was mentioned, although not claimed as a treatment for cancer, in Dr. Burzyski's first patent in 1984, and in several subsequent ones, all preceding Samid's and Elan's patents. It would have been customary in such circumstances to list Dr. Burzynski as co-inventor.

All of Dvorit Samid's patents are assigned to the U.S. Department of Health and Human Services (HHS), which contains the NIH, which in turn contains the NCI, where she was working when she filed the patent applications in 1991. After her stay at NCI, Dr. Samid, along with her colleague Dr. Alain Thibault, transferred to the University of Virginia Medical School, which, she told Tom Elias (*op. cit.*), has made a major commitment to phenylacetate research.

Burzynski wrote the NCI about their contract with Elan Pharmaceutical. NCI answered him on February 26, 1996, stating that they had a license with Elan Pharmaceutical, NCI License #L-178-94-1, entitled, "Composition and Methods for Therapy and Prevention of Cancer". Since this was presumably the one announced in the NCI journal in 1992, the doctor's lawyers requested a copy. NCI stonewalled them for two years, finally sending the contract in January 1998 only after it was demanded under the Freedom of Information Act.

To no one's surprise, the contract does indeed cover the Samid/NCI patents and the contract arranges for NCI to license the patents to Elan Pharmaceutical. In the contract, the first sentence states, "Dr. Samid made inventions..." which the second sentence states were assigned to NCI, which now owns them.

The NCI-Elan-Samid interactions may represent a long campaign to separate Dr. Burzynski from his discoveries in subtle and sometimes not so subtle ways. There may be some sensitivity within NCI to the appearance of what they have done. An internal NCI memo dated April 29, 1993, states, "Political issues are a real concern. Former Congressman Berkley Bedell is concerned that we are taking the antineoplastons away from Burzynski."

Phenylacetate, then, turned out to be the NCI's own patent medicine. NCI started out to test both phenylacetate and antineoplastons in separate trials, quickly aborting the antineoplaston trial but continuing with phenylacetate. NCI's having obtained patents on phenylacetate (assigned to its parent organization, HHS), puts its favoring of phenylacetate in a particularly poor light.

Even as it continued its go-slow with Dr. Burzynski, in 1997 the FDA approved an Eli Lilly drug called Gemcitabine, which will allow pancreatic cancer patients to live a few weeks longer and in less pain. No one can quarrel with something that lessens pain and extends life even if only for a few weeks. Still, this is hardly the sort of breakthrough in the War on Cancer the public hopes for and expects from the medical/pharmaceutical establishment. And, of course, FDA approved interleukin-2, which patients may have no more than a 15% chance of surviving.

Over the years, Dr. Burzynski has noted that the attitude of the FDA and Official Medicine has swung back and forth like a pendulum, first repressive, then favorable, then back. In June 1998, Dr. Burzynski was invited to speak at a major conference on alternative medicine in Washington where several other presentations on antineoplastons were made. At the end of the conference, Dr. Robert Temple, an FDA official in new drug approval, stated that the time may be coming for the approval of antineoplastons. This was the most favorable comment ever heard from anyone in FDA.

Then the pendulum swung back. In September, 1998, a publication called *The Cancer Letter* put out a collection of observations on antineoplastons in the spirit of the JAMA article of June 1992. There were criticisms on the design of Dr. Burzynski's protocols and complaints about hypernatremia, (excess of salt) following administration of antineoplastons. Dr. Temple gave remarks for the publication indicating that he was nowhere near considering approval of antineoplastons. There was one significant difference from the JAMA article of six years before; unlike JAMA, *The Cancer Letter* printed Dr. Burzynski's rebuttal. He pointed out that excessive salt build-up happens in only a handful of patients and is readily corrected by lowering dosage. As to his protocols, he reminded *The Cancer Letter* that his protocols were designed by Memorial Sloan Kettering.

Dr. Burzynski states that he has developed a considerably improved version of antineoplastons which would immediately put an end to hypernatremia problems. However, the FDA does not let him use it. I.e., government controls are preventing progress in making a relatively non-toxic therapy even less toxic - and more effective. Until his new version is permitted, the therapy is given in large volumes of fluid via a small pump which the patient carries around most of the time.

Requests for antineoplastons occasionally come to Dr. Burzynski from abroad. An American woman married a Mexican doctor and went to live in Mexico. When her husband developed cancer, she got the Mexican government to ask the FDA to release antineoplastons. FDA took three months to give approval; meanwhile, the Mexican doctor died. The Russian Minister of Health requested antineoplastons for the wife of a professor of gynecology. Again, the FDA took three months to give approval; meanwhile, the woman died. But when the Saudi Arabian government requested antineoplastons, it was another matter; the FDA approved the same day.

In October 1998, three-month-old Tori Moreno was diagnosed with a brain stem tumor and given 1-4 weeks to live. Her father, a Los Angeles County deputy sheriff, heard of Dr.

Burzynski, secured a compassionate exemption from the FDA, and started Tori on antineoplastons. An MRI in mid-December showed a 20% decrease in the tumor; another in late February 1999 showed a further 25% decrease. Her doctors told her parents that "there really is no medical explanation why she is alive". But, of course, there is; she took antineoplastons, and the doctors know that. On June 22, 1999, a happy, normal Tori celebrated her first birthday. In mid-March 2000, the tumor was down by over 80%.

Dr. Michael Friedman, who had observed that "human brain tumor responses (to antineoplastons) are real", was transferred to the FDA, where he became a Deputy Commissioner and a colleague of Mary Pendergast, Deputy Commissioner for Litigation and Robert Spiller's boss. On January 5, 1998, Elan Pharmaceutical announced that Mary Pendergast had become its Executive Vice President for Governmental Affairs.

Antineoplastons do not work all the time - nothing does. But there is enough data and case histories to demonstrate conclusively that these medicines do represent a breakthrough. The bottom line is simple; many of those who have cancer are very low in the chemicals Dr. Burzynski identified, the more effective of which he patented. When these chemicals are given to people with cancer, many of them recover, particularly when they are given before a patient has been treated with radiation and chemotherapy. In the February 1999 *Townsend Letter*, Dr. Burzynski explains that "antineoplastons represent a type of gene therapy that targets the signal path of errant ras oncogenes and the p53 tumor suppressor gene. Malfunctions in these (ras) genes are believed responsible for up to 60% of all human cancers." Dr. Burzynski has evidence that the signal of the ras gene is interrupted by antineoplastons.

In 1989, FDA Commissioner Frank Young proclaimed that FDA would approve a new drug if it proved effective in as few as ten patients. Antineoplastons passed that milestone years ago, yet FDA still drags its feet. In 1996, Former Commissioner David Kessler and Vice President Al Gore made a joint appearance stating that henceforth the FDA would move rapidly ahead to approve promising new cancer drugs. Did they mean anything except antineoplastons? Or is there basically just the policy of former FDA official Dr. Crout, who said that he would approve nothing unless it was proposed by a large pharmaceutical company with unlimited resources?

For a time Ric Schiff was the youngest full sergeant on the San Francisco police force. He was decorated for heroism in rescuing people trapped in debris after the earthquake of 1993 and was on the cover of the *Time* magazine issue that reported the event. In 1999, Ric Schiff filed suit against Dr. Michael Prados and the staff of the UC/SF over their treatment of his daughter. California law requires that a doctor tell patients and/or their relatives all "material" information relative to their case and proposed therapies. Germany has a similar law which requires doctors to tell patients about all alternatives, allowing them to choose. Dr. Prados and his staff were well aware of the success of antineoplastons in two cases, yet they told Ric and Paula Schiff that they knew of nothing other than the toxic therapies they recommended. They did not provide all material information to the Schiffs. It will be an interesting case.

During the 2000 Republican presidential debates in Iowa and Los Angeles, at the suggestion of Ambassador Alan Keyes, the video camera picked up four-year old Thomas Navarro and his father in the audience. The Navarros are from Arizona, where Thomas was successfully operated in September 1999 to remove a golfball-size medullablastoma brain tumor. The problem is that this type of tumor invariably returns, usually about 45 weeks after removal. Cancer doctors urged the Navarros to start Thomas on radiation and chemotherapy. Visiting the hospital where treatment was to be given, James Navarro pointed out to his wife, "Donna, this isn't helping those kids, it's killing them...kids with....no hair, veins sticking up all over their heads, ashen, gray, dark, lifeless eyes." (*People's Magazine*, March 20, 2000).

Looking for alternatives, they learned that Dr. Burzynski had successfully treated several children with medullablastoma, among whom is Dustin Kunnari. "Dr. Burzynski was the only doctor who introduced us to his patients", Navarro recalls (*ibid.*). To Jim and Donna Navarro's dismay, Dr. B. sorrowfully told them that the FDA would not allow him to treat Thomas unless Thomas first underwent radiation and chemotherapy. But, they learned, chemo in a child that young generally leaves a child either retarded, deaf, or unable to sit up or stand. Median survival for children treated with chemo is seven years and the oldest survivor of the FDA's recommended protocol is twelve years.

FDA Dr. Dianne Murphy urges the chemo, saying that the child would have a 70% chance of surviving at least five years. Says she, "The risks would be minimal - at the worst, a 10-20 point loss in I.Q." The FDA cites the "St. Jude report" as justification for requiring chemo, St. Jude being the patron saint of the hopelessly ill. Apparently the FDA presumed nobody would read the report, but the Navarros did. The study, on effects of chemo in young children, shows that all children in the study suffered significant brain damage; while the median survival is five years, nobody survived more than twelve. If the Navarros were to follow the FDA's suggestion, lively, intelligent Thomas would very likely end up retarded and before they could plan where he'd go to college, he'd be dead, of a certainty. The Navarros refused this Faustian bargain for their son. Back in Arizona, an oncologist who had seen but not treated Thomas filed charges of medical neglect against the Navarros. Concerned that a court might order treatments they are convinced would damage their child, the Navarros moved to Houston and applied to the FDA for a compassionate exemption for Thomas.

An independent businessman, James Navarro immediately perceived that the situation was political. He sought out Ambassador Alan Keyes, for whom the case was an obvious example of government interference in an area where it doesn't belong. At the Michigan debate, the eloquent Keyes asked his fellow candidates to sign a letter to FDA Commissioner Jane Henney, requesting a compassionate exemption for Thomas Navarro. The FDA did not budge.

Political pressure may yet work for the Navarros, as it did in 1996 when Shawn McConnell and his wife took their son Zach to a Senate hearing in Washington, and generated political and media pressure on the FDA. Sadly, that story did not end well. After the static had died down, the FDA's Dr. DeLap again refused to allow Zach to receive his next batch of antineoplastons, and Zach died shortly afterward.

Dustin Kunnari had a medullablastoma, the same type of tumor as Thomas. At that time, FDA rules were a little more flexible. Dustin never underwent surgery but began antineoplastons soon after the tumor was diagnosed. Within six weeks, his tumor was gone, but antineoplastons were continued for four years, just to be sure. Dustin Kunnari is the longest surviving child with medullablastoma who has never received any conventional therapy - he made medical history. In the year 2000, Dustin is a normal, bright, not retarded 8-year old, and tumor-free.

Michael and Raphaele Horwin wanted the treatment Dustin got for their son Alexander. He was stricken with medullablastoma at age 2, when the tumor was removed in two operations. Learning about Dr. Burzynski, they were horrified to learn that FDA would only allow him to accept children who had taken chemo and radiation and who still had measurable tumors in their brains. Unable to obtain antineoplastons, they were assured by oncologists that the chemo would help Alex. The rationale for chemo is that it can shrink tumors - but Alexander had no tumor.

Furthermore, most chemotherapies are Class 1 carcinogens. The Horwins reluctantly agreed, but the tumor returned while their son was on chemo. Raphaele Horwin wrote in the December 1999 *Townsend Letter*, "Alex died in my arms three months later". Afterwards, the Horwins read over 1,200 abstracts of medical literature and found that chemo for children with medullablastoma is toxic, carcinogenic, unproven, and ineffective. They wrote in the *Townsend Letter*, "After 20 years of this therapy, there was absolutely no credible evidence that it had any value (other than to the doctors prescribing it or the drug companies marketing it)."

The Navarros know what happened to little Alexander Horwin.

Dr. Burzynski has treated twelve children with medullablastoma, one of whom was Dustin Kunnari. Seven did not have chemo or radiation and five did. Of the seven, six are alive, with tumors either completely gone or stabilized - not growing. The five who had chemo or radiation have all died.

To review the facts, antineoplastons have worked on medullablastoma in a way no other therapy has, leaving a child normal and with an expectation of growing up. No child with this disease who was given chemo or radiation has survived more than 12 years, and most who took that protocol became retarded. And why wouldn't they? Almost all the chemos FDA pushes are Class 1 carcinogens. Consider the impact of such a drug on a young child's brain. "It will only lower his I.Q. 10-20 points." Former House Speaker Newt Gingrich may have had his faults, but he was pretty close to the mark when he called the FDA a "Stalinist bureaucracy".

The Navarros arrived at the Burzynski Clinic on November 10, 1999. At that time, a number of children were being treated with antineoplastons. All of them had previously been treated with chemo or radiation, as required by the FDA, and all arrived with prognosis of only a few weeks or months to live. As of mid-April, 2000, all the children who were in treatment when the Navarros arrived have died. Requiring chemo or radiation prior to antineoplastons leaves very few survivors - no more Dustin Kunnaris. At some point, the FDA will announce the results of their tests of antineoplastons in children with medullablastoma. With no mention of the chemotherapy they required, FDA will declare that (X) children were treated and all died; therefore, the FDA will conclude, the antineoplastons failed.

Forty years ago, Governor George Wallace stood in a schoolhouse door, barring access to black children. As this book goes to print, the FDA stands in the door of Dr. Burzynski's clinic, barring access to the only therapy that has had any success in giving normal lives to children with medullablastoma.

In Washington, Congressman Dan Burton has introduced a Thomas Navarro bill (HR 3677) that would restrict FDA's authority to bar access of any patient to any investigational new drug, providing the patient or his/her parent or guardian gives "informed consent", indicating awareness of risks.

In a better world, a freer world, Dr. Burzynski and researchers dealing with non-toxic therapies simply would be let alone to develop their medicines to the maximum - as long as they don't hurt anyone. Hippocrates' first rule - Do No Harm - is still what counts. If this were the case, Dr. Burzynski would be free to offer another improvement he has developed which appears to be one thousand times more potent than his current medicine - and still nontoxic. In lab tests, this product causes cancer cells to revert back to normal and then die at the next normal cell division. To attempt to offer this breakthrough anytime in the near future would mean starting all over again with the FDA. Would they again take six years to approve an IND for this new antineoplaston? Dr. Burzynski does not have the resources to try to push two products through the FDA simultaneously. Meanwhile, one American dies of cancer every minute. It is said that Roman Emperor Nero fiddled while Rome burned. What will history say of the FDA and the NCI?

Are antineoplastons more effective than the Koch treatment? Who knows? How could anyone tell? When there is a free market for all non-toxic therapies, then there can be open competition between antineoplastons, glyoxylide, krebiozen, the Hoxsey treatment, DMSO/hematoxylon, electrical therapies, others presently unknown, and ones to come. In such a free market, we can compare therapies in a new field of study to be called comparative therapeutics. In that free market, radiation and chemotherapy will also compete, and there may well be cases where those harsh therapies are useful and appropriate. Let them all compete on a level field, so a free market can indicate which works best.

Incredibly, against unbelievable odds, the stalwart Stanislaw Burzynski has survived and his therapy continues to help sufferers considered hopeless by conventional medicine. His story is the latest chapter in the war between toxic and nontoxic therapies, in which he has been forced to become a general in a war of attrition. Dr. Victor Penzer wrote of him, "Bright, intelligent, inventive, luckily he is also tough, very tough".

Shontelle Hiron of Mandurah, Australia was chosen to carry the torch into the opening ceremonies of the 2000 Olympic Games in Australia, and Dr. Stanislaw Burzynski was invited to accompany her. In 1993, Shontelle was given three months to live after an inoperable astrocytoma brain tumor was discovered. When her parents learned about Dr. Burzynski, the town of Mandurah helped them raise money to send her to Houston. As soon as antineoplastons were started, the tumor began to shrink and eventually disappeared. So in an emotional and rare moment of public recognition, Dr. Burzynski accompanied the Olympic torch, since he had saved the life of the woman who carried it. (*Health and Healing*, September 2000)

Many who are aware of Dr. Burzynski's struggle do not realize that politics in healing has been discouraging imaginative pioneers for many years, since the same story, in varying details, has been repeated many times. The same institutions (different people) seem determined to do the same thing over and over. It recalls the French Bourbon Dynasty of whom it was said, after they were deposed for the last time, "they forgot nothing and they learned nothing".

The Bourbons have not run France for a long time, but their kissing cousins run Official Medicine in the U.S., which showed no tolerance for nontoxic cancer therapies during the entire 20th century. Will the Thomas Navarro case be the last straw which finally brings down the FDA, the bastille of Official Medicine?

Is Dr. Stanislaw Burzynski's case the fiercest battle of the long war between toxic and nontoxic therapies? If it is, does this mean that the end of the war is near? If so, who will win?

A sad postscript: brave little Thomas Navarro died in October 2001, a casualty of the FDA which, by withholding appropriate treatment, undoubtedly caused his death.

A MATTER OF LIFE AND DEATH

As we enter the new millennium, most Americans are not very inclined to trust government. Even so, it is dismaying to contemplate the losses we have sustained from the public and private institutional malfeasance described in these ten stories. This continuous succession of relentless suppressions during the entire second half of the 20th century represents a cancer on the American healthcare system. We saw how:

The AMA drove the Hoxsey treatment out of the country to Mexico.

The FDA hounded Dr. Koch out of the country, the AMA persecuted the doctors using his treatment, and we lost his science, a new science - we have nothing like it today.

The AMA threatened the medical licenses of the doctors using the Rife instruments, and we lost those.

The AMA and the FDA lied about Krebiozen, persecuted Drs. Ivy and Durovic, and we lost Krebiozen. It's not in Mexico; it's not underground; it's lost.

The FDA persecuted DMSO, which the *New York Times* called the wonder drug of the 1960's, to the point that it has become almost the forgotten drug. As a legal chemical, it can be obtained, but in the face of FDA censorship as to what it can accomplish, few know what it can do. Doctors who might use DMSO intravenously to dissolve a stroke or reverse arthritis would risk losing their licenses.

FDA censorship prevents us from being informed on what targeted colostrums could do for us.

The FDA has Gaston Naessens' 714-X on a watch list at the border, so that people bringing it in legally are often hassled.

FDA censorship and restrictive rules deny us access to or the knowledge of the marvels of electromedicine.

The FDA continues to raid Donna Shuster, distributor of the legal chemical hydrazine sulfate (HS), on a fairly regular basis. FDA censorship prevents more Americans from being informed of the value of this chemical - if, per Dr. Joseph Gold's protocol, one doesn't take barbiturates, sleeping pills, or alcohol, which are incompatible with HS. The NCI gave barbiturates to most of 600 patients during clinical trials with HS from 1989 to 1993. Instead of following the usual pattern of 40-50% improvement seen in four previous HS trials (where the incompatibles were avoided), there were more survivors of the Titanic than of the NCI trials. The NCI may be sued for genocide by family members of those who died in the NCI trials. Most of this information is on the Internet, the great wild card in escaping FDA censorship.

Dr. Burzynski offers a therapy with a demonstrated track record against increasingly prevalent brain tumors. His case is a classic of the pattern of repression; first the Texas Board of Medical Examiners went after Dr. B., and finally managed to put him on a 10-year probation to end in 2004; until then, he is prohibited from taking private patients other than those admitted into FDA trials; FDA accepts about 6 out of every 100 who apply - if they first take chemotherapy. The FDA unsuccessfully tried to put Dr. Burzynski in jail. The NCI diluted his antineoplastons in the small test they carried out, and all patients in the trial died. To add insult to injury, NCI rushed to patent one of the antineoplastons which Dr. B. had not patented. Then NCI spent millions of taxpayers' dollars to test it, only to find out what Dr. Burzynski had said all along; it was not as effective as his other antineoplastons. Is it appropriate that a national institute which is supposed to study cancer therapies objectively should own a product that is in active competition with one of the products it is testing? Or is it a roaring conflict of interest and highly unethical?

These games the medical bureaucrats (or medicrats) play are pretty serious, for after all, they are dealing with matters of life and death.

The U.S. system expects bureaucrats to be watched by elected officials. That doesn't work anymore, since elected officials are too busy raising money for their next campaigns. As to the press, they will tear any elected official limb from limb given the chance. Yet they seem to regard the pronouncements of the med-icrats or any part of Official Medicine as something handed down from Mt. Sinai.

If everything were all right, it wouldn't matter, but everything is not all right. Every minute an American dies of cancer - 10,000 a week, over 500,000 a year, equal to ten times the casualties of the Vietnam War - every year. Clock how many minutes it takes you to read this page - that will be the number of Americans who died from cancer while you were reading. Every four or five min-utes, an American dies of the fourth leading cause of death in the U.S. - drugs approved by the FDA. Those dying in hospitals from this cause number over 100,000 a year. This is roughly 3-5 times the approximately 30,000 dying each year from AIDS, and about 3-5 times the number dying each year from illegal street drugs. In response to the latter, we have a drug czar. When the number dying at home from FDA-approved pharmaceutical drugs is included, the number mounts to around 140,000 a year, according to Centers for Disease Control statistics. All of these drugs are patent medicines, which used to be a pejorative term. The num-ber dying in hospitals each year from legal drugs is about three times the 44,000 who died in 1996 from auto accidents (*Monthly Vital Statistics of 1996*). We have a Wall to commemorate the 50,000 who died in the Vietnam War, but where is the memorial for the approximately three times that number who die each year from FDA-approved drugs? For them, we have only silence and indifference. Since we raise no protest over this calamity, is it considered all right, in our society, to die from prescription drugs but not all right to die from all the rest? Over just the past ten years, this means that between 1,000,000 and 1,400,000 (not counting those who died at home) have died from approved drugs - a veritable drug company-FDA-generated Holocaust. Where is the constituency to protest these deaths? In addition, approved drugs are the fourth leading cause of hospital admissions - around

2,200,000 a year - at a cost estimated in *Business Week* on January 18,1999, of more than $5 billion a year. That number means that every half minute an American is harmed and hospitalized from an FDA-approved pharmaceutical drug.

The situation is not likely to get better very soon. On January 11, 1999, *US News* reported that, "Drug companies lobbied Congress hard against beefing up post-marketing surveillance at the FDA" during the 1998 debates over the FDA Modernization Act. In other words, checking on how a drug performs once it has been approved and is on the market was not a popular idea with the drug companies, who are among the largest contributors to congressional campaigns.

The FDA was set up to make sure that drugs are safe, but, as seen in this book, the FDA seems more concerned at protecting Americans from nontoxic drugs than from toxic ones. Every treatment discussed in this book is or was nontoxic. The question must be; where are the bodies? With nontoxics or harmless devices, there are none by definition; they can't hurt us. With toxic, FDA-approved pharmaceutical drugs, the bodies are all over the floor. A month after Peter Jennings announced the JAMA study about an average 106,000 dying each year from FDA-approved drugs, he returned to the subject. He reported that JAMA had published another article stating that the FDA would never have enough money to monitor toxic drugs (never mind that being their core mission) and would surely need more money. Curiously, a graph of the number of NCI employees compared with the number of Americans dying of cancer would show that the more NCI employees, the more Americans die of cancer. Similarly, the more FDA employees, the more Americans die of FDA-approved drugs.

Official Medicine, of which the FDA, AMA, and NCI are part, has not served the United States very well in the 20th Century. In the 19th Century, there was no Official Medicine, and very little cancer or heart disease. But look how much longer people are living, apologists will say, and that's an interesting point. In the April 1999 issue of *Alternatives*, Dr. David Williams explains, "The U.S. ranks 16th in life span... In this country, the average life span is currently 71.6 years for males and 78.6 years for females. Nor are we living much longer than we used to. In 1900, the average life expectancy in the U.S. was 45 years. At first glance, this 30-year increase in less than a century seems quite impressive - and conventional medicine is quick to take credit for it. But what most people don't realize is that the increase from 45 years to over 70 years is almost entirely due to a reduction of infant mortality. If the reduction in infant mortality is taken out of the equation, life expectancy has only increased 3.7 years over the last 100 years. (*Stat. Bull* 94; July-Sept:11-17). In other words, if one managed to live through childhood in the old days, one's chances of living to a ripe old age were good. Reduction of infant mortality has indeed been a great triumph, but as noted earlier, rates are lower in Cuba than in the U.S., and lower in Shanghai than in New York City. A United Nations World Health Organization (WHO) study issued in June, 2000, measured a new concept; "healthy life expectancy". The WHO found Japan leading the world, with the United States falling behind almost every country in Europe as well as Canada, Australia and Israel. In terms of overall quality, the WHO ranked the U.S. health system #37, largely because of the excessive financial burden it places on its citizens.

Official Medicine in the U.S. cannot cure most cases of cancer, it cannot cure cardiovascular disease, it cannot cure AIDS, it cannot cure a frighteningly large number of new cases of TB, and cannot cure a growing number of bacterial infections. Vancomycin-resistant-enterococcus or VRE is a bacterial infection resistant even to vancomycin, which is considered the antibiotic of last resort. It has been privately reported that 20% or more of the patients in San Francisco hospitals are in this category. When the Muppets' Jim Henson was stricken with such a bacteria, Official Medicine had nothing for him, and he was gone in three days. In central Texas in 1998, eight people were suddenly dead from strep A since there was no medicine that could help them.

Over the past ten years, the Centers for Disease Control (CDC) data has shown that Americans' lymphocyte counts are progressively going down, down, down, *i.e.*, a steady decline in immune systems. In 1981, Dr. H. F. Pross did a study of the Natural Killer (NK) cell count of average Americans; NK cell count is measured in lytic units, or LU. The LU count was 152. In 1991, Dr. R. D. Herberman made a similar study and found the LU count of average Americans had dropped to 135. In 1997, Dr. Gerald See did another NK cell count study and found the LU count of average Americans had dropped to 108, or a 1% drop per annum since Dr. Pross' study. A weakened immune system leads to cancer, or lowered resistance to flu, cold, infections, or the next epidemic. Official Medicine has nothing for a weakened immune system, which you don't get from a lack of antibiotics - but you may from too many of them. Similarly, you don't get cancer from a lack of chemotherapy.

America faces a Health Challenge and is not prepared for it. Meanwhile, a hidebound medical system stuck on toxic therapies - patented poisons - will not change unless shoved. If we do nothing, the dreadful statistics will only continue and get worse.

The solution is remarkably simple, and is contained in the words that brought down the Soviet Union: Freedom, Competition, and Free Markets. These ten stories should have made it very clear that there is no free market in the U.S. in non-toxic therapies, *i.e.*, no competition for often toxic drugs. We regularly hear cries to beware of socialized medicine. But with the FDA, and the NCI, and even the Federal Trade Commission (FTC) interfering to decree what is or is not proper medical treatment, socialized medicine is just what we've got, dictated from the top down. With astronomical costs and poor results, the American version is even worse than we were warned. This is despite the fact that the U.S. spends nearly 12% of its gross domestic product on healthcare, a far larger proportion than any other industrialized country. This situation has the hallmarks of a cartel, where institutions are manipulated to keep prices high and to keep competition down.

When there is real health freedom in the U.S., competition will force the costs of healthcare down so far that universal health coverage for every American will be affordable. The universal health insurance plans that failed of passage in recent years had no plans to provide for competition between toxic and non-toxic treatments. Real Health Freedom means:

1) Yes, the freedom to choose your own doctor but

2) When you find the doctor you want, that doctor must be free to provide you with any therapy you and he/she decide is in your best interest. This would be in line with the Helsinki Declaration, which was adopted in 1964 at an international conference proposed by President Gerald Ford. The Declaration states, *"In the treatment of the sick person, **the doctor must be free to use a new therapeutic measure if in his/her judgment it offers hope of saving life, reestablishing health, or alleviating suffering"***. The Helsinki Declaration was ratified by the U.S. Congress the year after Krebiozen was outlawed. Apparently health officials of the time felt no need to be consistent.

3) Freedom for a doctor to use any provably nontoxic therapy or harmless device without interference from state medical boards - unless, of course, harm is done to the patients.

4) Freedom to place on the market any provably nontoxic therapy or harmless device without interference from government agencies.

5) Freedom to tell consumers the truth about what such a product or device could do for them, without censorship of "health claims" by the FDA or the FTC. If someone lies or makes fraudulent claims, let fraud laws take care of the problem.

6) When a patient obtains a nontoxic treatment of his/her choice, the freedom to have his/her insurance company pay for it.

Of the entire list, the only one Americans enjoy at the beginning of the 21st century is No. 1, and that only within limits because of health maintenance organizations.

This is a sorry picture. These stories of blatant, gross government intrusion into the healing arts has cost thousands, even millions of lives. How could one begin to estimate the lives that would not have been lost if the various therapies described in this book had not been swept away?

In the last decades of the 20th century, we heard a great deal about deregulation, restructuring, and downsizing. The time has come to apply these principles to the FDA. Set up in 1906 to make sure that drugs are safe and food is pure, every day of the week the FDA does a thousand things we want it to do - and quite a few we do not want it to do. Such as approving Viagra in six months while the Burzynski antineoplastons are still in limbo. Such as putting on its staff a Monsanto expert in recombinant bovine growth hormone (rBGH). After FDA approved the Monsanto rBGH product, the expert returned to Monsanto. Because rBGH is now used in almost all American beef cattle, the European Union has put its foot down and refused to import American beef. For Americans, that leaves most people as guinea pigs in an experimental trial to see what will happen, since rBGH is given to most American dairy cattle to boost milk production. Some of what may happen is sadly predictable. Cancer expert Dr. Samuel Epstein wrote in *Politics of Cancer Revisited* that, "Lilly Industries, in its application to the European Community Committee for Veterinary Medicinal Products, has admitted that rBGH milk may contain more than a ten-fold increase in IGF-1 concentrations" (over non-rBGH milk). IGF-1 (insulin-like growth factor) causes cells to divide and proliferate, and this factor increases milk production in cows. (Pasteurization does not disable IGF-1 but rather elevates it, FDA research found in 1990.) **What does this mean for American consumers**? On May 1998, *The Lancet* reported that elevated levels of IGF-1 in milk are associated with a sevenfold increased risk of breast cancer in menopausal women younger than 51. The researchers concluded that there is substantial indirect evidence of a relation between IGF-1 and the risk of breast cancer. Monsanto reported to the FDA that Posilac (commercial name for rBGH) could increase mastitis in cows by up to 79%, which means more antibiotics given to cows, some ending up in the milk. The Monsanto label admits that there may be increased somatic cell counts (SCC's), i.e., pus and bacteria, in the milk from cows given rBGH. British researchers published in *Nature* that rBGH treatment caused a 19% increase in SCC's (again, that's pus and bacteria) in milk compared to controls. This is how the FDA carried out its mandate to keep food pure. The late Carl Schleicher, Ph.D., of Mankind Research Foundation, tried to work with the FDA on several projects, without much success. Someone once asked him, **"Have you ever seen any sign of good faith on the part of the FDA?"** Startled, he paused a moment, and then said, **"No."**

Surgery needs to be performed on the FDA, which is not the Rock of Gibraltar. It was created by Congress and can be changed by Congress - if its members can get past their contributions from the pharmaceutical companies. The principle for restructuring FDA is very simple; Congress needs to remove from the FDA any regulatory authority over anything non-toxic or harmless. If a product is nontoxic or a device harmless, what is the point or need of spending money to have government bureaucrats (FDA, FTC) protect us from it? Instead of processing tons of make-work documents, FDA's role, then, would be to go back to basics and examine products for toxicity or harmfulness, such as rBGH. When Congress prohibits FDA from wasting money, time and personnel protecting us from things that can't hurt us, it will be discovered that the FDA will have all the people it needs to return to its core mission of making sure that food is pure and drugs are safe. In some ways, this would be a return to the status quo before the Kefauver-Harris amendments of 1963, which had the effect of outlawing Krebiozen. Before that legislation, Dr. Ivy notified the FDA that Krebiozen was non-toxic, that he intended to start testing it, and that he would keep them informed. Dr. Jacob did the same with DMSO - until after 1963. Removing FDA regulatory authority over anything nontoxic or harmless resolves another problem; FDA censorship.

In 1990, the FDA made a power grab for regulatory control over nutritional supplements, with the idea of regulating them like drugs. FDA's proposed regulations stimulated the formation of several strong health freedom lobbying groups, notably Citizens for Health and the American Preventive Medical Association. The resulting campaign these groups waged caused Americans to write over one million letters of protest to Congress, even more than had been written during the Vietnam War. Impressed by the size and intensity of the well-informed Vitamin Vote, Congress staved off the FDA and passed the Dietary Supplement and Health Education Act (DSHEA). This was sponsored by Senator Orrin Hatch and then Congressman, now Secretary of Energy Bill Richardson. The law was intended to head in exactly the opposite direction from what the FDA proposed, permitting manufacturers to inform the public about how supplements affect the "structure and function" of the body. This was aimed to expand Americans' knowledge of what nutritional supplements - vitamins, minerals, botanical herbs - could do for them.

It has been well known in scientific circles for almost a decade, and announced by the NIH, that the spinal bifida birth defect can be prevented if a prospective mother takes the inexpensive B vitamin folic acid. FDA would not allow manufacturers to advertise this fact. Finally, Congress told FDA to get the message out to the public. Four years later, FDA put out a statement acknowledging that folic acid prevented spinal bifida, but asserting that enough of the nutrient is obtained from the diet. This is not true, and has been made clear by statements of other government agencies; to get enough folic acid, especially for an expectant mother, supplements are necessary. During the four years FDA dragged its feet before partially obeying the Congressional mandate, how many thousands of babies were born with this defect, at what dreadful cost to the infant, and at what cost in dollars to the parents and the public till? In the

March 1996 issue of *Health and Healing*, Dr. Julian Whitaker stated, "All the FDA had to do was to take its boot off the neck of the nutritional supplement industry and allow manufacturers to put a simple claim on the label, stating that folic acid is necessary to prevent these neural tube defects. But they didn't". The March of Dimes is trying to help spread information on folic acid. Dr. Whitaker added that in a 1995 March of Dimes poll of childbearing age women, only 6% knew the importance of folic acid and 52% of the women had never heard of it.

Such nonsense as this would end once the FDA is forced by Congress to get out of regulating and censoring information on things which by definition can't hurt us. If there were no FDA censorship, manufacturers of grapefruit seed extract could advertise that clinical studies have shown the product superior to antibiotics in defeating some of the worst hospital infections. The label on one bottle states, "to be used by healthcare professions as nutritional support for individuals with certain health problems". The manufacturer is censored from stating that these "certain health problems" include infections. If there were no FDA censorship, manufacturers of DMSO could remind us to keep a bottle in the medicine chest for use at first sign of a stroke. "My people die from lack of knowledge", Russian Czar Peter the Great said, and they still do, everywhere. With the FDA out of censorship, that could change in the U.S.

When the FDA is barred from regulating nontoxic products, how would nontoxicity be determined? One way would be for a manufacturer to supply to the FDA three tests from unrelated, independent testing labs finding a product no more toxic than aspirin (or the Underwriter's Lab certification finding a device harmless). Upon receipt, the FDA would have 90 days to contest these reports; if it did not do so, the product or device would be free to go on the market. If the FDA decided that for some reason the three labs were in error, then it would submit its contrary findings in the form of sworn testimony. Some FDA official, then, would have to face the risk of going to jail for perjury if he/she were the one to submit false sworn testimony. Had this been the law of the land in the 1960's, DMSO would have gone on the market. The FDA would not have been able to prove their assertion of possible lens changes, since there were none in humans. Had the FDA been out of censorship, DMSO's ability to avoid paralysis after spinal cord injury, proven in the work of Drs. Jacob and De La Torre, would have become known. Those doctors who attended Christopher Reeve might have learned of this, and, who knows, perhaps he would never have been paralyzed. Censorship of truthful scientific information is a fearful thing, and can exact a frightful cost from society and its individual members.

Allowing nontoxic products to go on the market unless FDA can prove in sworn testimony that a product is not nontoxic would restore free markets in our health care. Catching the FDA lying about Krebiozen, Senator Paul Douglas said "It's a terrible thing that we cannot really trust the FDA (or the NCI)". Given the FDA's history, sworn testimony is a must. Had that been the law of the land, we'd still have Krebiozen.

With the FDA out of censorship of "health claims", manufacturers would then be able to educate the public about such things, for example, as folic acid. Informing the public of truthful information on a product is an appropriate part of marketing, and so long as the statements are true, it is not the proper function of any level of government to interfere.

But what of the charlatans, some will ask. We have excellent fraud laws, at both the federal and state levels. The fraud laws are quite adequate to take care of the charlatans. Will people occasionally buy something that's harmless - and useless? Of course - but they won't buy it again, and they'll disparage it to their friends.

The law about commercial speech is very clear about lying; it's considered fraud. Generally, one would expect the Federal Trade Commission (FTC) to go after fraud cases. However, the FTC did a number on Dr. Koch 50 years ago after the FDA was unable to convict him. Recently, the FTC has decided to promote itself to become another part of Official Medicine. With no legally assigned responsibilities to pronounce on the values of healing therapies, it has intruded in medical matters again, taking a position as to which therapy is appropriate for treating cardiovascular disease. In chelation therapy, the nontoxic chemical EDTA is administered intravenously with the goal of increasing circulation. With well documented success, used all over the world, and with never a report of harm since the treatment was perfected twenty years ago, chelation is seen as an increasingly attractive alternative to heart bypass surgery, with its 2-5% mortality rate. According to the government's *Monthly Vital Statistics*, in 1996, 40,000 died of cardiac surgery complications, the 9th cause of death in the U.S. Who would not prefer 20-30 albeit tedious but painless sessions of EDTA to having one's chest cut open? Economically, there's no comparison; heart bypass runs $30-40,000, while 20-30 chelation treatments, at $75-$100 a session, is not going to go over $3,000. However, there's a catch. Insurance companies willingly pay for bypass surgery, as recommended by Official Medicine, but drag their feet or refuse to pay for chelation. Chelation is not covered by Medicare; bypass surgery is, and generally is the largest single item in the Medicare budget.

In a free market, chelation is an easy winner, but we do not have a free market in health. State medical boards, always influenced by the AMA, in which cardiac surgeons may have some influence, have been hauling in chelation doctors all over the country, sometimes succeeding in revoking their licenses. In the 1980's, a group of chelation doctors formed the American College for Advancement in Medicine (ACAM) to keep standards high by giving training and board certification to chelation doctors. In 1998, the FTC went after ACAM on the basis of an ACAM brochure which stated that chelation is an effective treatment for cardiovascular disease. While ACAM has plenty of evidence to support that statement, it did not have two double-blind, placebo-controlled studies on chelation, which the FTC demanded. But the FTC imposed a standard on chelation it does not impose on others; few toxic chemotherapies have such studies.

In the absence of double-blind studies, FTC claimed ACAM's brochure was false advertising and asked a court to place ACAM under FTC supervision for twenty years. Congressman Dan Burton was outraged and held hearings on the FTC action.

The campaign against chelation is worth reviewing. First, the FDA went after Dr. Ray Evers (DMSO chapter). Evers fought back and won a historic court ruling that opened the door for doctors legally to use EDTA chelation for circulatory problems. Then the FTC went after ACAM, and we have the spectacle of a federal agency getting a court order to place a respected, non-profit professional organization on probation as though it was a criminal outfit. And the attack continues and gains force. In early 2000, the *Harvard, Berkley,* and *Mayo Clinic* newsletters showed their independence of thought by all taking positions condemning chelation. Had they just noticed something that has been around for twenty years? It doesn't take a psychic to detect a carefully coordinated campaign - and note the extent and degree of the manipulation; the FDA, the FTC, and even prestigious newsletters. Who is pulling the strings?

Moral of the story; it's the FTC's assigned job to go after fraud, but Congress needs to put the FTC on probation to keep it on target.

There will be those who will not want to change anything in the FDA, claiming that it protects us. They should pay attention to what former FDA Commissioner Herbert Ley said of the agency after he left it,

"The thing that bugs me the most is that people think the FDA is protecting them - it isn't. What the FDA is doing and what the public thinks it is doing are as different as day and night." Dr. Ley also complained of "merciless pressure" from the pharmaceutical companies, where an estimated 65% of FDA employees go to work upon retiring from the FDA. Congress might well decide that this "revolving door" is a little too cozy an arrangement. It would do well to bar any employee of any federal agency from going to work in the industry regulated by the agency where he/she worked until at least five years after retire-

ment - a sort of cooling off period. Or a president so inclined could do this by Executive Order, if pharmaceutical contributions had not overly clouded his or her judgment.

Former Commissioner Ley was right; the FDA is not protecting us. The agency has become something of a rogue elephant, even an Evil Empire, ignoring Congress whenever it feels so disposed. In its constitutionally-mandated oversight of the Executive Branch's agencies, Congress is short-handed. It needs the ability to reach deep within a bureaucracy, pick up some errant bureaucrat by the back of the neck, and turn on the spotlight of publicity. The Swedes developed the Ombudsman system to handle such problems. American legislators at both the state and federal levels reject the Swedish system on the grounds that they, the legislators, act as ombudsmen. Fine in theory, but in practice, they don't do it. Congress has the power to impeach elected officials and appointed judges; it needs to arm itself with the power to impeach appointed officials, pointing them out when their bias is obvious, when they are incompetent, or when they refuse to obey the law. It would have to be set up with great care, lest it become runaway partisan, but it could be done - a certain number of legislators from each party and from both houses of Congress needed to move an impeachment motion.

As noted in the first chapter, the U.S. Court of Appeals in the District of Columbia held in January 1999 that FDA censorship of health claims was unconstitutional under the First Amendment governing freedom of speech. Yet on November 30, 1999, the FDA denied the truthful health claim about the saw palmetto herb's ability to shrink the male prostate gland. In May 2000, Dr. Julian Whitaker reported in *Health and Healing* that he'd just returned from an FDA hearing held to "seek input" on whether or not health claims should be allowed on nutritional supplements. Whitaker testified that the question was stupid since the Court of Appeals had already ordered the FDA to do so 14 months earlier.

This puts the FDA not only in contempt of the Court of Appeals for refusing to obey a court order but also in contempt of Congress for ignoring the clear intent of the Dietary Supplement and Health Education Act (DSHEA). In effect, the FDA is thumbing its nose at both Congress and the Court of Appeals.

While Congress at present has no power to impeach bureaucrats, it does have the power to hold them in contempt of Congress, which carries a jail term (just as does contempt of court). It would appear likely that the FDA's illegal activity will continue until Congress holds whoever is the FDA Commissioner at the time in contempt and send that person to jail. Or the Court of Appeals might do so - just as you or I would be sent to jail if we ignored and defied a court order - and limited ourselves to hold discussion sessions to "seek input" on whether or not we should obey the order.

Never before have Americans been better educated, better informed, and better able to make their own decisions. Yet the FDA continues under a policy well articulated by its former commissioner, Dr. David Kessler, who said on the Larry King Live Show in 1992, "The American public does not have the knowledge to make wise health care decisions... FDA is the arbiter of truth... Trust us... We will tell you what's good for you." On June 24, 1992, the *Wall Street Journal* quoted Kessler as saying, "If members of our society were empowered to make their own decisions about the entire range of products for which the FDA has responsibility, the rationale for the agency would cease to exist." Exactly. But not the whole range; how about just the nontoxic and harmless ones?

President Dwight D. Eisenhower had a different understanding of Health Freedom. "The right of the individual to elect freely the manner of his care in illness must be preserved", he stated in a speech to the Brazilian Congress in 1960 (*Susan B. Anthony University Journal*, October 1975). On June 1, 1961, after he had retired, President Eisenhower warned, "We consider it sheer arrogance to believe that people in Government know better for the people than they know for themselves." (Both quotations are derived from Barry Lynes' latest book, *Cancer Solutions*, with his permission.)

After getting the FDA out of protecting us from things that

can't hurt us, the second area for deregulation is freeing doctors to use the non-toxic therapies which, decontrolled, will then become available. This could even include some mentioned in this book. If a state medical board revokes a doctor's license for having used some good nontoxic product, then we won't have made much progress. There must be deregulation for nontoxic products and harmless devices and freedom for doctors to use them. The Helsinki Declaration stated: *the doctor must be free.*

A good place to start is for Congress to pass the Access To Medical Treatment Act. This was conceived by former Congressman Berkley Bedell out of a desire to permit his fellow citizens access to innovative and nontoxic therapies such as the ones he used successfully to recover from Lyme disease (Chapter 7) and to defeat a possible recurrence of prostate cancer (Chapter 8). Since he is well known and highly regarded by congressional leaders of both parties, as of 1999, the legislation has been introduced in both houses of Congress with strong bipartisan support. Offering a simple way around the present obstacle course, the Act provides that a manufacturer may market in interstate commerce a product not approved by the FDA so long as it's clearly marked "Not approved by the FDA". It requires that patients sign a consent form stating that they realize that they are being treated with something not approved by the FDA. It requires doctors to inform the FDA of any adverse reactions produced by such experimental medicines.

As a general principle, the Act states that any person will have the right to be treated by any treatment he/she desires. A memo detailing the provisions of the Access to Medical Treatment Act is in the Appendix on pages 437 and 438.

Hospitalization accreditation boards, organized under the AMA's Joint Commission on Accreditation of Health Care Organizations, are quick to withdraw hospital privileges of doctors using new methods. It would be well if the "Access" Act also contained this additional provision, "Hospital accreditation boards may not revoke or suspend hospital privileges of a doctor solely for the use of therapies not approved by the FDA". Without this, if a patient were suddenly taken to a hospital because of a stroke, his/her doctors might not be able, for instance, to give DMSO intravenously to break up the stroke, and that patient might become paralyzed.

States have been plugging along to liberate doctors following a pattern started in Alaska. Dr. Robert Rowan of Anchorage was one of the first doctors to reverse a stroke in progress by giving DMSO intravenously. When the Alaska Medical Board went after him over his various innovative therapies, Rowan launched a counterattack. He drew up a very simple concept which said that a doctor's license cannot be suspended or revoked solely for the use of unapproved or experimental therapies unless demonstrable physical harm is done to the patient. The AMA fired its Alaska lobbyist the day after Dr. Rowan convinced the Alaska Legislature to pass the bill. Governor Wally Hickel, a bit of a maverick himself, signed the legislation. Then, to the consternation and over the fierce opposition of the AMA, he appointed Rowan to the next vacancy on the State Medical Board.

Each state has a medical board, established by state law, with authority to grant, suspend, or revoke a doctor's license to practice medicine. State medical boards are heavily influenced by state medical societies, from whose recommendations governors are apt to make appointments to the board. State medical societies, in turn, are heavily influenced by the AMA in Chicago, and this is as true in the Year 2000 as it was in the 1920's.

Rowan's "Alaska Law" came down to the "lower 48" and, as of 1999, has passed in various versions, over stern AMA opposition, in seven more states: Washington, North Carolina, New York, Oregon, Oklahoma, Colorado, and Georgia. The Georgia Law, entitled the "Access to Medical Treatment Act", specifically authorizes doctors to use "drugs or medical devices that have not been approved by the Food and Drug Administration", providing patients are informed of this fact, and of the nature of the treatment. Feeling the winds of change, the Texas Board of Medical Examiners adopted as internal regulations the provision of the Colorado law, considered one of the best. However, the

Board defeated a proposal in the 1999 legislative session to cod-
ify these progressive provisions into law, where they could not be
reversed at the next board meeting. When the Board revokes the
ten year suspension it imposed on Dr. Burzynski in 1994, its new
mood can be taken more seriously.

The Minnesota Natural Health Legal Reform Project supporters celebrated on May 11, 2000, when Governor Jesse Ventura
signed their Complementary and Alternative Health Freedom of
Access Act. The bill was sheparded through the Legislature by
Project leaders Diane Miller and Jerri Johnson and field organizer Leo Cashman. Miller was one of the two lawyers who successfully defended the late dairy farmer/healer Herb Saunders,
who passed on in 1999 (Colostrum Chapter). Inspired by the
example of Saunders, who helped so many and hurt no one, the
Minnesota bill protects lay healers such as herbalists, home-
opaths, naturopaths - and those working with colostrum - as unlicensed professionals. Exempting such healers from the authority
of the Minnesota Medical Board, the Act puts them under a new
office in the Minnesota Department of Health, with ample consumer safeguards. The bill originally contained Alaska-Law-type
provisions protecting licensed practioners who use alternatives
but the Medical Board succeeded in having those clauses
removed. The bill passed with overwhelming majorities: 110 to
23 in the House, where it was sponsored by Representative Lynda
Boudreau, Speaker Pro Tem, and by 58 to 1 in the Senate, where
it was sponsored by Senator Twyla Ring. Minnesota, often a
leader in sensible progressive causes, was considerably politicized by the prosecution of two popular alternative doctors as
well as Herb Saunders by then Attorney General Hubert ("Skip")
Humphrey III. Political analysts consider that the backlash to his
actions contributed to his defeat by Jesse Ventura in the 1998
governor's race.

By protecting the wide and growing range of unlicensed alternative health practitioners from over-zealous prosecutors, the
Minnesota Act takes the lead in providing the medical freedom
called for by Founding Father Dr. Benjamin Rush. Dr. Rush

wrote that all laws which "restrict the art of healing to one class of men are un-American and despotic". Benjamin Rush would be happy with the Minnesota Law but would urge the Natural Health Group, while flush with victory, to keep going and win the right to practice alternative medicine for the licensed professionals.

Fifty years ago, most doctors belonged to the AMA as a matter of course, but at the beginning of the 21st century, the number is falling toward 30%. Doctors, handcuffed by the restrictions addressed by the "Alaska laws", find their patients voting with their pocketbooks for alternative treatments. Indeed, many visits to allopathic (orthodox) doctors are motivated solely by the fact that most insurance companies will only pay for conventional treatments. In 1993, the *New England Journal of Medicine* shocked the medical world by publishing a study by Harvard's Dr. David Eisenberg reporting that 40% of Americans were using "alternative" treatments; by the end of the decade, he estimated the number was over 50% and climbing. This included treatments by chiropractors, a profession the AMA once conspired to stamp out. On February 7, 1990, the Supreme Court upheld the AMA's conviction under the Sherman Anti-Trust Act of conspiring to eliminate the entire chiropractic profession. In the new millennium, fresh AMA leadership may well find it sensible to take stock, undo some of the damage of the past, and change the organization's posture as a likely way to increase membership. The AMA would do well to loosen up its overly close relationship with pharmaceutical companies, whose products it has pushed to the exclusion of other forms of medicine since the days of Dr. Morris Fishbein. Flipping through any issue of JAMA, one finds nothing but drug company ads from front to back. A Congressional committee - or some good investigative journalists - would do well to ask the AMA to disclose any holdings it may have in pharmaceutical stocks - which ones and how many. Americans were forcibly reminded in 1999 that the AMA has a keen eye for a buck when the AMA president contracted to sell its seal of approval for some Sunbeam medical devices. AMA retreated under a storm of protest only to face a lawsuit from Sunbeam for breach of contract. The AMA would do well to be more objective and professional, less commercial, and to recognize that there are effective medicines other than pharmaceutical drugs.

With the rigidity of yesteryear out of favor, the AMA should take the lead in freeing up doctors by supporting legislation more in keeping with the times. For instance, why wouldn't the AMA reverse its position and urge passage of the Access to Medical Treatment Act? It is eventually going to pass. Likewise, the Alaska Law concept is going to pass, state by state, whether the AMA likes it or not, until doctors throughout the U.S. are free to use any effective treatment, so long as they do no harm.

Several years before he conceived of the Access to Medical Treatment Act, Congressman Bedell persuaded his friend Senator Tom Harkin, also from Iowa, to sponsor the creation of an Office of Alternative Medicine (OAM) within the National Institutes of Health (NIH) to "investigate and validate" unapproved or experimental therapies that sounded promising. At that time serving as chair of the Health Sub-Committee of the Senate Appropriations Committee, Senator Harkin put $2,000,000 into the 1992 budget to start the OAM. Rarely has such a modest appropriation caused such a stir. Wide press coverage and considerable excitement gave a clear indication that the people, who are usually far ahead of the politicians, hoped that the OAM would stir Official Medicine to move in new directions. However, the NIH never asked for the OAM, didn't want it, and bound it with straitjackets. In 1998, Congress upgraded the OAM to a National Center for Complementary and Alternative medicine (NCCAM), gave it $50,000,000, but left it in the NIH, a situation set up to fail.

Given the overall health situation that we have reviewed, Congress should free up the NCCAM to be a catalyst for change. This would involve taking the NCCAM entirely out of the NIH, and having it report directly to Congress as an autonomous office like the General Accounting Office or the Congressional Budget Office. Accompanying that transfer, Congress should totally exempt the NCCAM from the FDA and offer Alaska-law-type protection from state medical boards to doctors working in

NCCAM research.

Frustrated and disgusted by NIH's smothering of the OAM-now-NCCAM, Berkley Bedell has organized the National Foundation for Alternative Medicine (NFAM), with headquarters at 1155 Connecticut Ave. NW, Suite 400, Washington, DC 20036. Its mission is to "investigate and validate" breakthrough therapies, both in the U.S. and abroad, as he had expected the original OAM would do. "The job's got to be done," he says, "so if the government won't do it, we'll just have to do it privately." In its first years of life, 1998 and 1999, his foundation's teams have investigated two German hospitals which were reported to be achieving an 80% success rate in all types of cancer. Berk and Elinor Bedell jumpstarted the NFAM with their own money, but he is seeking contributions since "we can't do the whole thing". NFAM is organized as a tax exempt non-profit, so contributions are tax deductible.

When the FDA is removed from regulation of things that can't hurt us - nontoxics - and with doctors free to use them, American hospitals could then offer the healing treatments those two German hospitals use. And some of the therapies described in this book will rise from the ashes, like the phoenix. Doctors who are pioneers will be free to see if they can do a better job. How many will take advantage of the opening? If 25% of our doctors and of the American population want to go in a new direction and are free to do so, this will open the gates to a new paradigm of health. As people recover from illnesses more quickly, stay healthier, and live longer in good health, the example will be set and attitudes will change. It will take awhile, but it will happen, for ingrained concepts don't change overnight. John Maynard Keynes once said, "whenever there is progress, the difficulty lies not in the new ideas, but in escaping from the old ones."

While FDA's authority over nontoxic or harmless products needs to be removed, there are still things we want the FDA to do:

1) we want the FDA to continue to inspect factories

    where nontoxic or harmless products are made to make sure they are made in a clean environment, and

2) FDA will continue to make sure that labels are accurate, and that packages contain what they say they contain; if the label says there is a pound of product, then there must be a pound of product.

However, civil penalties should be adequate to take care of any infractions of labeling regulations or factory problems. Congress needs to strip away FDA's powers to press any criminal charges regarding products that are nontoxic or harmless. Criminal charges are appropriate where people die from the effects of FDA-approved drugs, but there are no reports of FDA activity along such lines.

At the turn of the millennium, many Americans are becoming wealthy, but wealth cannot prevent anyone from becoming one of the one-in-three Americans expected to be struck by cancer. With their prosperity, they may assume that they have access to the "best medicine". If they get cancer, and take chemotherapy, they will probably not be told that most chemotherapeutic drugs are listed with the FDA as Class 1 carcinogens - *i.e.*, they cause cancer. They will probably not be told that the chemo will kill many of those who take it, and that its overall success rate is about 2-3%. In the *Scientific American* of November 1985, Dr. John Cairns of the Harvard School of Public Health wrote, "Chemotherapy treatments now avert perhaps 2-3% of the deaths from cancer that occur each year in the U.S. Those who organize cancer centers and supervise the many clinical trials look for ways to circumvent these relentless statistics". In other words, chemotherapy fails to prolong survival 97-98% of the time. Oncologists judge cancer therapies by the standard of whether or not a tumor shrinks. While chemo frequently does indeed shrink tumors, a patient will probably not be told that it will also destroy their bone marrow which, when intact, produces their immune system. It is also unlikely that they will be told that cancer arises from a polluted swamp, to use the analogy in the Naessens chapter, and that unless the swamp is drained, and the conditions which gave rise to the cancer in the first place are taken care of, the cancer may return. And if it returns, the immune system, having been destroyed by the chemotherapy, will not be around to protect them. Then such persons, for all their wealth, will become cancer statistics. Perversely, since their tumors may indeed have shrunk, they may be listed as successes of chemotherapy - even though they died. What is puzzling is why it is taking so many people - opinion-makers, leaders of business and industry - so long to catch on that something is wrong. Would they buy stock in a company whose product failed 97-98% of the time? Or a car that failed 97-98% of the time it was driven? Informed on their investments but not on matters affecting their very lives, they follow the "accepted" therapies route as if following the Pied Piper.

In 1989, Ulrich Abel, a German statistician, wrote a study called *Chemotherapy of Advanced Epithelial Cancer* after working ten years in clinical oncology. He confirmed seeing, "incontestable, sometimes dramatic success of chemotherapy" in what are called the **non-epithelial** cancers: leukemia, Hodgkins disease and non-Hodgkins lymphoma. However, he found little evidence of success in **epithelial** cancers, which are all the rest: breast, colon, lung, prostate, brain cancer, etc. Since there are far more of the latter, success in the non-epithelial cancers is what provides chemotherapy with whatever success rate it can boast, about 2-3% overall. (Since Dr. Abel's study, chemotherapy has been found effective in testicular cancer.) Abel wrote that, "there is no direct evidence that chemotherapy prolongs survival in patients with advanced epithelial malignancies". He noted that most cancer publications "equate the effect of chemotherapy with response irrespective of survival. Response is the question of whether the tumor shrinks. If it shrinks, this is counted as a success, regardless of whether the patient survives or not". Dr. Abel states that, "The thesis of the efficacy of chemotherapy assumes the character of a dogma, which…is hardly compatible with the requirement of science." Abel states, "oncology has been unable to provide a solid scientific foundation for cytotoxic therapy in the present form".

Why would oncologists give cancer patients carcinogenic chemo for the epithelial cancers? Perhaps it's because of a fundamental misunderstanding. Official Medicine has pronounced that all alternative cancer treatments are quackery for so long that many cancer professionals have ended up believing it. Accepting what they've been told, they conclude that since (in their view) there are no viable alternatives, the patient is, of course, going to die. Therefore, they use surgery, radiation, and chemotherapy, as they're expected to do. Chemo, they reason, might shrink a tumor and give the patient a few more months.

One who stepped off that bandwagon is Dr. Vincent Speckhart of Norfolk, Virginia, former U.S. Air Force flight surgeon, medical missionary in Africa, and for 13 years a conventional oncologist. As he puts it, around 1990, **"I got tired of signing death certificates."** Reviewing his files, he found he had signed 1,700 in ten years, an average of 170 per year or three a week. At a hearing of Congressman Dan Burton's committee, Dr. Speckhart testified:

> *After 13 years of using FDA-approved chemotherapy protocols, I concluded that such therapies were extremely toxic, poorly tolerated, and not effective in prolonging survival in most solid tumors of adults. In 1983, my patients began to request therapies other than chemotherapy. I agreed, and without even knowing it, I became an 'alternative practitioner' and was red-flagged by opponents of this form of therapy.*

There are no hard figures on how many people die of chemotherapy rather than from cancer; obviously, oncologists are not going to write "chemo" as the cause of death on a death certificate. Informal estimates have reported 25%, but this may be low in view of Dr. Speckhart's cases, since the 1,700 who died were mostly chemotherapy patients. In retrospect, he presumes that those who survived must have been doing something else and preferred not to tell him. The late Senator Hubert Humphrey, who died of cancer, was not far off when he called chemotherapy "death in a bottle".

As long as his patients were dying as expected, nobody protested. However, once he changed to non-toxic therapies and his patients began to recover, complaints were filed with the Virginia Medical Board, and not by his patients. The Board hauled him in on charges of using "unapproved" therapies; the fact that they worked was beside the point. The Board placed him on probation, but Dr. Speckhart fought back. "For five years", he says, "I didn't know whether or not I'd have an office to go to the next day". He was greeted sympathetically several times at hearings of Congressman Dan Burton's committee. The Richmond press reported extensively on these appearances, and this helped him. Finally, after spending $300,000 to defend himself, his license was restored without restrictions. When enacted, the Access to Medical Treatment Act should protect doctors from such harassment. Dr. Speckhart reports (personal communication) that his nontoxic methods are producing a response rate of about 80% - tumors shrink and go away, without poisoning the patient, and with about 50%+ recovery in terminal patients.

The National Cancer Institute (NCI) seems wedded to toxic chemotherapy. It never tested Koch's glyoxylide, refused to test the Hoxsey treatment, refused to test Krebiozen, decided the Rife Ray couldn't work without looking at it, and cheated on trials of hydrazine sulfate and antineoplastons. Senator Douglas spoke of not being able to trust the NCI. With the cancer scourge rising inexorably and steadily, **perhaps it's time for Congress to pass a "Sunset" law on the NCI**; give it ten years to find some cures for cancer - or go out of business. It used to be said that the knowledge that one was going to be hanged in the morning had a remarkable ability to clear the mind. Someone in the NCI once boasted to noted English radiotherapist Dr. Alice Stewart that the NCI has someone on the board of every medical journal and could stop the publication of any article. So NCI, as well as FDA, is into censorship. Who needs this? The late legendary Dr. Hans Nieper of Hannover, Germany, told a conference of the

Foundation for Advancement in Innovative Medicine (FAIM) in New York City that he regularly received as patients high officials (and their relatives) of the NCI (and the FDA and the AMA) who came to take treatments they do not allow in the U.S. Who needs such hypocrisy? The NCI may be sued for genocide because of its handling of the hydrazine sulfate trials. We do not need this sort of organization. Why did the NCI get Congress to pass a law making secret the names of people dying in NCI trials? - and the numbers? Until that law is repealed, we cannot know the number who die in NCI trials. And in the case of Dr. Burzynski's antineoplastons, have the people in the NCI never heard of ethics? A government agency charged with evaluating cancer therapies has no business owning any of them. The U.S. does not need such an organization. While it is notoriously well known that many avoidable pesticides are known to be carcinogenic, NCI pays no attention to alerting the public to this danger. Noted cancer authority Dr. Samuel Epstein, professor of Occupational and Environmental medicine at the School of Public Health, University of Illinois Medical Center in Chicago, states in *The Politics of Cancer Revisited* that most cancers are preventable, and indicts the NCI for ignoring this fact.

It is not even clear that prevention or finding a cure is accepted as a mission. Dr. Epstein (*op. cit.*) quotes Dr. Harold Varmus, director of the National Institutes of Health (NIH), which contains the NCI, as saying, in relation to NCI/NIH genetic research, "I have no idea when we'll know enough to develop anything clinically applicable, and I don't know who's going to do it. It's not a high priority in my thinking... Talking about cures is absolutely offensive to me. In our work, we never think about such things even for a second. You can't do experiments to see what causes cancer... It's not the sort of things scientists can afford to do." It may be offensive to most Americans that the head of the NIH does not want to think about cures while a cancer epidemic is raging. Do we want to spend our money on such medicrats? The May 1998 issue of *The Lancet* contained an article on "the promise of a good death" by Dr. E. J. Emanuel of the

NCI and Dr. L. L. Emanuel of the AMA. They wrote, "In 1998, we have the capacity to make a good death the standard of care in developed countries. Increasingly, society is focused on ensuring a good death; physicians have more powerful medications and other interventions to alleviate pain than ever before..." How many people thought that our society is increasingly "focused on ensuring a good death?" It's more likely that most Americans thought, or at least hoped, that NCI and AMA were focusing on ways to keep us alive instead of helping us to die 'a good death'. But maybe they aren't.

There is an old saying, "lead, follow, or get out of the way". Has the NCI become irrelevant, or should it be downsized until it gets real? Congress should give the NCI ten years to mend its ways or go out of business, reducing NCI's budget 10% each year. We might see some results once it was understood that the NCI would no longer be a career bureaucracy where one could study cancer forever, with no concern for cures. Freed of career considerations, NCI bureaucrats should be encouraged to form teams to investigate and validate anything that works, whether or not they understand how it works. Special arrangements would be made for such teams to report directly to designated committees of Congress, so that any bright ideas lurking around NCI would no longer get lost in its byzantine bureaucracy. Such teams would in effect be encouraged to work themselves out of a job. Therefore, their rewards should be great. For teams that come up with solutions, not studies, Congress should provide "golden parachutes" equivalent to what business executives arrange for themselves. This would enable successful teams, who demonstrate cures, to retire in considerable comfort as a reward from a grateful nation. If they do nothing more than bring back the therapies written about in this book, it would be a great victory. Since NCI has rigorously refused to look at nontoxic therapies that work, and remains fixated on toxic therapies with an overall 2% success rate, who needs it?

For those half dead from strokes, it is shameful that Dr. Dan Kirsch, restrained by FDA censorship, cannot shout from the rooftops that microcurrents have restored victims of strokes in a few cases - so let's have a look and try the technique in, say, a thousand cases. And it's shameful that it isn't household knowledge that DMSO can stop strokes in their early stages, so that people could demand that their doctors use it when dreaded strokes occur - the third U.S. cause of death.

It's shameful that Official Medicine still has its clamps into Dr. Burzynski, preventing him from going forward with his science, forcing him to leave on the shelf a breakthrough which, in the lab, appears thousands of times more powerful than his already effective medicine.

The Control Mechanisms which push patented, often toxic pharmaceuticals over nontoxic alternatives are:

1) FDA control over things that can't hurt us and
2) the tendency of AMA-influenced state medical boards to discipline doctors using nontoxic, non-pharmaceutical therapies.

These two mechanisms are fundamental flaws in the American healthcare system and will continue to distort it unless Congress takes action. Until then, nothing will change. If the Koch, Hoxsey, Rife treatments or Krebiozen were again to be offered, they would be stamped out as ruthlessly as before, as ruthlessly as Official Medicine has tried to stamp out Dr. Burzynski's antineoplastons. Not only is the War on Cancer being lost, but the unnoticed War between Toxic and Nontoxic Therapies is being lost to the toxics. Chemotherapy reigns supreme while one out of three Americans will be struck by cancer, and one out of four will die. Breakthroughs waiting in the wings will stay there as long as the present repressive climate continues.

The stories in this book may seem to suggest a puppet show being manipulated behind the scenes. However, when the Control Mechanisms are cut, then whatever puppeteers there may be will find themselves with a lot of loose strings in their hands, and will lose the ability to obstruct competition in a free and uncensored market. If the pharmaceutical companies are the puppeteers, then the very simple solution is to eliminate the FDA's authority to keep nontoxic alternatives off the market, which is how FDA protects pharmaceuticals from competition. The pharmaceutical companies constitute the richest industry in the world, even richer than the oil industry. If pharmaceuticals subscribe to the belief that competitive free enterprise is the most efficient system, then competition will be good for them. As the movement grows to strip the FDA of regulatory authority over anything nontoxic, it will be interesting to hear what arguments will be offered against the eminently sensible concept that we don't need government protection from things that can't hurt us. Perhaps the pharmaceuticals will say "Unfair competition! We have to spend millions of dollars to get FDA approval of our products and the nontoxics should do the same". But there's the rub; pharmaceutical products are often toxic and should be controlled; indeed, should be controlled much better. It's hardly the same business if someone wants to market something harmless.

A draft of the Health Freedom of Choice Act, which would prohibit FDA regulation of anything nontoxic or harmless, is in the Appendix on page 439. Both it and the Access to Medical Treatment Act (also in the Appendix, page 437) can be passed, but only after heavy insistent and persistent citizen pressure. The right thing can be made to happen - with pressure; only on the rarest of occasions would the right thing happen in a legislature without pressure. To help build that pressure, write your Congressperson! The draft of a suggested letter is in the Appendix on page 448. Legislators pay far more attention to handwritten letters than to form letters.

Once the Control Mechanisms are cut, the stage is set for free and open competition between toxic and nontoxic therapies. This was almost unknown in the U.S. during the 20th Century, the Century of authoritative Official Medicine, with decisions dictated from the top down, just as in the worst forms of socialized medicine. This was the century where it never occurred to most people that medicine could be other than a drug, and most likely a patented and usually expensive drug. This was the Century of the AIDS epidemic, the Century of the Cancer epidemic, the Century of the Heart Disease epidemic, and now the Century of the epidemic of deaths from FDA-approved pharmaceutical drugs. Frighteningly, it is now the Century of a conceivable epidemic from antibiotic-resistant infections. This was the century when Official Medicine's insistence on toxic, patent medicine has been accompanied by skyrocketing health costs. And this was the century when Official Medicine carried out an abominable, unconscionable suppression of medical breakthroughs in order to protect increasingly expensive patent medicine against competition from inexpensive, effective, non-toxic therapies such as the ones described in this book. And this was the century when the FDA came into being as a progressive triumph and then moved out from its role of making sure drugs are safe into a role of determining how doctors practice medicine, a role never assigned to it by Congress. The 20th Century is a good one to leave behind, moving on to a better approach.

If the proposed reforms had been the law of the land during the 20th Century, this book would not have been written. These stories that should not have happened would not have happened. When the Control Mechanisms are cut, competition will cause health costs to plummet. This will be of major significance not only to individuals, but also to businesses and state and federal budgets, thus leading to lower taxes.

One of the old truisms in politics is that people get the government they deserve. Does that hold true in healthcare? If people let their vigilance down, special interests move into positions of power and set directions. Finally, since nothing has the inertia of an adopted policy, no one even questions the situation.

We can market almost anything in the U.S. - hideous violence, gore, certainly pornography, protected, we learn, by the First Amendment guaranteeing free speech. But at the dawn of a new century and a new millennium, we have not secured the right freely to market nontoxic therapies, and the freedom to tell people what they will do. The results of this lack of competition are seen in the health statistics and costs.

Well-known cancer researcher and author Dr. William Regelson (*The Melatonin Miracle*) says, "In America, we all go to different churches; it's our choice. It's not the government's business what we say or pray once we get there. Health should be the same; It's not the government's business whether we go to an M.D., a chiropractor, a homeopath, or a naturopath. And it's not government's business what medicine we take when we get to (whichever). All we need from government is to make sure the medicine isn't poisonous. From there on, it's our choice."

Some readers may consider that most of these stories in this book happened in the past, and that surely things must be better as we enter the new Millennium. However, as this book is published, the FDA is still trying to make hydrazine sulfate illegal and still restricts access to Dr. Burzynski's treatment, even for four-year-olds. This is enough to demonstrate that the FDA policy of repression continues in full force. But there is more.

Late-Breaking Developments

Allen Hoffman, Baltimore health researcher, could not have predicted in 1994 that something simple, natural, wonderfully effective, and published in the medical literature, could be illegal. Coming across some five-year old medical journals, he read an article on how concentrated aloe vera could elevate lymphocyte counts enough to effectively treat AIDS. It can't be true, he thought, or else everyone would know about it. Still, as a researcher, he was curious, so he arranged for a lab to make an aloe vera saturated solution; this is a solution so concentrated that it cannot hold another molecule of the substance being concentrated. The FDA approved the use of aloe vera as an adjunct in AIDS treatment in 1994, and aloe vera is on the FDA's GRAS list - "generally regarded as safe." In addition, it is a traditional botanical used in healing for millennia. At the suggestion of Aristotle, his tutor, Alexander the Great conquered an island in the Red Sea in order to secure a supply of aloe vera for his troops;

Julius Caesar carried aloe into battle to treat his soldiers' wounds, and so did Genghis Khan. How could anyone get in trouble over aloe vera?

Yet Alexander's aloe vera plant landed Allen Hoffman in federal court on criminal charges of distributing an unlicensed drug. The charges were brought by the Justice Department at the request of the FDA. Hoffman adds absolutely nothing to the aloe vera, so the only difference from the aloe that Alexander's physicians used is that Hoffman concentrates it.

After preparing the concentrated aloe vera solution, Hoffman sought out indigent AIDS patients and donated it to them to be taken orally. In exchange, he asked permission to monitor their immune systems. To his amazement, he found that lymphocytes doubled every three weeks. The lymphocytes then pulled up the T-cell count, which characteristically drops in AIDS. In a few months, the "opportunistic infections" were gone and viral load dropped. Then, in four months, AIDS-related tumors began decreasing and disappearing as well. In addition, Hoffman reports that after 18 months, about half the AIDS victims "seroconverted" - their AIDS tests went back to HIV negative. AZT won't do that.

Hoffman calls his concentrated aloe vera solution "T-PLUS", and finds that one teaspoon of it contains 500 mg of mucopolysaccharides and 500 mg of polypeptides. He discovered that when the concentration is less, even at 400 mg of each, nothing happens, but at 500 mg, it's like turning on a switch. As the lymphocytes increase, they cause the body to produce cytokines. These are interleukin, interferon, and Tumor Necrosis Factor (TNF). As its name implies, TNF kills tumors - the body's own chemotherapy. Official Medicine, playing the Patent Game, has tried to synthesize and patent the cytokines. Results are poor, since the body sees them as toxic when used individually and in far larger quantities than the body makes for itself. Dr. Steven Rosenberg (one of the co-authors of Dr. DeVita's cancer textbook mentioned in the hydrazine sulfate chapter) used interleukin in a study of 25 cancer patients, curing one. The other 24 died, but

Official Medicine trumpeted Rosenberg's 4% success rate as a breakthrough. In contrast, when one works with nature, stimulating the body with a natural product to make its own cytokines, they work like a charm. Medical science knows that interleukin and interferon kill viruses and bacteria, and that TNF shrinks tumors, so there's nothing mystic about how the aloe vera solution accomplishes its results.

Hoffman founded a company, began to distribute T-PLUS and to give lectures, especially to doctors. Hoffman knew about the FDA, but like so many, thought it was there to protect us. He also was aware of the Dietary Supplement and Health Education Act (DSHEA) and firmly believed that it was intended to facilitate exactly what he was doing, and that it allowed him to inform the public of how his T-PLUS affected the "structure and function" of the body. So he told about how the lymphocytes increased, and how they increased the cytokines, and how the cytokines killed viruses and bacteria, and how the TNF killed tumors. Hoffman arranged for the product to be given intravenously in Mexico, and to be injected directly into accessible tumors. In one case, a woman's breast tumor was thus injected and soon disappeared. One of Hoffman's lectures was taped and soon 100,000 copies of the cassette were distributed all over the country. Business boomed, and, more importantly, people were getting well.

Wanting to concentrate on research, he sought a business partner and found one in successful Baltimore businessman Neal Deoul. Things went very well for a couple of years. Deoul, also interested in alternative medicine, asked Allen Hoffman what he knew about cesium; Deoul had read that it too was useful in treating cancer. Hoffman quickly found studies on cesium by Dr. Keith Brewer, and they were staggering. Later, Neal Deoul owed his health to them.

Dr. Keith Brewer (1893-1986) published his research on cesium in 1984. It is well known that cancer cells are acidic and that theoretically, if you could alkalyze them, they would die. However, nobody knew how to do this without also alkalyzing the blood, which would kill the patient. The body's normal cell pH is 7.35-7.4. The pH scale goes from 0-14; 7 is neutral; above 7 is alkaline and below 7 is acid. Cancer is 6.5-7. In a Nobel Prize-type discovery, Dr. Brewer found how to change the pH of the cell and not of the blood. Cesium is one of the most alkaline of the elements, No. 55 in the Periodic Table. Dr. Brewer found that cesium goes directly into a cancer cell when taken with Vitamin C (4 grams a day, one gram with each meal and once whenever) and zinc (50 mg a day). Brewer also found patients should take 800 mg of potassium and 800 mg of lithium a day. Vitamin C and zinc helped cesium to cross the membrane of the cancer cell. Once cesium was in the cell, it raised the cancer cell pH to 8 in a matter of hours, effectively killing it, while leaving the pH of the blood unaffected. In a study published in *Pharmacology, Biochemistry & Behavior*, Vol. 21, Suppl. 1, pp 1-5, 1984 (see Appendix), Dr. Brewer wrote on the High pH therapy for Cancer, as he called the cesium, treatment. He reported that, *"tests have been carried out in over 30 patients. In each case, the tumor masses disappeared* (italics added). Also all pains and effects associated with cancer disappeared within 12-36 hours." Brewer found that small quantities of cesium could do more harm than good, and that the ideal dose is 3-6 grams a day. Since something that alkaline could upset the normally acidic environment of the stomach, he discovered that taking one gram in the middle of each of three full meals caused the least problems. In these quantities, cesium is non-toxic, and is toxic at 135 grams. Note that what Brewer used in cancer treatment is cesium chloride, its natural form, exactly as it comes out of the ground.

In some far-reaching research, Dr. Brewer found that in certain areas of the world where cancer is rare to non-existent, the inhabitants ingest cesium in their food or their water. In the Vilcabamba Valley in Ecuador, which the ancient Incas called the Sacred Valley, the concentration of cesium in the soil is 140 parts per million. In Hunza in northern Pakistan, where the Hunzakuts regularly live to 125 years with no disease, cesium is in the water, but the concentrations are not known.

Knowing that cesium makes a beeline for cancer cells, oncologists, in order to trace chemotherapy, regularly attach it to cesium to which radioactive isotopes have been added. But they do not use cesium for its alkaline properties. Cesium is considered safe by the FDA. It is not a rare element, nor is it expensive.

So Hoffman and Deoul added one-gram capsules of cesium to their product line. To date, about 2,000 people have taken cesium for cancer. It has been found very effective in liver cancer, and cancer pains generally vanish within 12-24 hours of starting the treatment. It has not been used in brain tumors, because cesium does not pass the blood-brain barrier without help. DMSO crosses that barrier, but if anyone has yet tried combining cesium with DMSO, it is not known. Cesium also has not been effective in pancreatic cancer, but for a different reason; this type of cancer is usually discovered only when the pancreas is mostly destroyed. At that point, killing cancer cells would very likely be too little, too late.

The classic pattern of persecution started when the Maryland Medical Board called in Allen Hoffman on charges of practicing medicine without a license. But he was selling nutrients, not practicing medicine, so they dropped the investigation. Next to take up the case was the Maryland Attorney General (AG). In 1998, he pressed charges of consumer fraud against Hoffman and Deoul under the Maryland Consumer Protection Act, although no consumers had complained. The "administrative law" court judge before whom they were brought works for the Consumer Protection Board. The Board is part of the Attorney General's Department of Justice; therefore, in effect the judge worked for the AG, their prosecutor. Deoul and Hoffman found themselves in a trial with no jury, with no rules of evidence, and where they could not cross-examine witnesses testifying against them. The judge accepted anything the AG offered as evidence and rejected anything Deoul and Hoffman offered. Convicted, they are appealing but the Maryland Consumer Protection Board prevents them from getting the case to a venue where they can exercise their right to a trial by jury, as guaranteed by the U.S. Constitution.

Under the stress of the "trial", Neal Deoul came down with prostate cancer, Refusing surgery or any conventional treatment, he decided to take his own medicine. After three weeks of one gram of cesium three times a day during meals, he went to Mexico and took both cesium and aloe vera intravenously for one week. He returned to Baltimore cancer-free. He has put up a website to tell his remarkable story at www.cancer-coverup.com.

The science behind cesium has the elegance of a really simple solution, good, hard science, and simple enough that anyone can understand it. Like the concentrated aloe vera, there's nothing mystic about how cesium works. Just as negative attracts positive, acid attracts alkaline. When alkaline cesium gets into the body, it looks for acidic conditions and thus is attracted straight to acidic cancer cells. Levi Rabinowitz, an associate of Hoffman and Deoul, wonders if cesium is the bromoseltzer of cancer. Just as bromoseltzer alkalyzes an acid stomach, cesium alkalyzes acidic cancer cells, thereby killing them.

One particular lead in the cesium story points a way to putting an end to the scourge of cancer. Instead of putting fluoride in our water supplies, which can cause cancer, how much better it would be to put cesium, which very likely could prevent it.

Before Hoffman and Deoul had much time to savor the latter's triumph over prostate cancer, the second arm of the persecution struck. The FDA indicted Hoffman for selling an unapproved drug; (his concentrated aloe vera), as well as for wire fraud (he had talked about aloe on the phone) and for mail fraud (he had sent out literature on it). They did not or could not indict Neal Deoul. Anyone can obtain aloe vera in various forms in any health food store. But if you concentrate it, even if you add absolutely nothing at all, which is the case with Hoffman's T-PLUS, that seems to turn it into a drug as far as the FDA is concerned, even if it is a botanical and thus covered by the DSHEA. Above all, apparently, if the concentration successfully treats AIDS, for sure it's a drug. The FDA does not contest that Hoffman's T-PLUS works, but rather that he didn't follow the rules and file for a new drug. Unpatentable, aloe vera would have as much luck as saw palmetto. Since aloe vera is a venerable, age-old botanical, the FDA's stance appears to be in open defiance of the intent of DSHEA, thus placing the FDA, in effect, in the position of being in contempt of Congress.

As in the Burzyski trial, the FDA asked the court to bar testimony from anyone helped or cured by T-PLUS. The only question, said the FDA, was whether or not Hoffman broke FDA rules - which would make him a criminal. Unlike in the Burzynski trial, the federal judge did not agree. "Since you have presented people to testify against him", he told the FDA, "he can bring in people to testify in his defense". Over the past three years of their investigation, the FDA interviewed 5,000 people who had used T-PLUS. Hoffman had long maintained a policy of refunding money to anyone requesting it. Some did, since T-PLUS sometimes causes diarrhea before the body gets accustomed to it. Despite that, only seven out of the 5,000 came forward to complain at the trial. All seven of the complaints related to an I.V. treatment done by doctors in Virginia, which was not done by Allen Hoffman. On May 1, 2000, a renowned oncologist appeared for the FDA, testifying that the immune system had nothing to do with cancer. Hoffman's lawyer displayed to the eminent doctor two respected textbooks (including Dr. DeVita's). When shown that the books contradicted him, the doctor declared "Sometimes the books are wrong, but I am right". The jury laughed.

The FDA usually doesn't do too well before juries, and this case was no exception. After deliberating two weeks, the jury sent the judge a question, "If we find Hoffman acted in good faith, what should we do?" The judge replied, "Then you should vote to acquit." The prosecutor audibly uttered an "expletive deleted" four letter word. On June 22, 2000, the jury announced its decisions on the FDA's 20 counts; acquitted on one and hopelessly hung on the rest. Allen Hoffman intends to go on doing just what he has been doing, but outside the U.S. With invitations from several countries, he may go to the Caribbean. (Unlike the case of Dr. Koch, he is free to leave the country.) The cost of his legal defense will keep him in debt for years. And the FDA has already set a date for a second trial on April 16, 2001. So the onslaught goes on.

Brilliant, articulate, and anxious to help people, Allen Hoffman wonders whether people will ever wake up and demand the changes needed to take politics (government) out of cancer. Once cancer happened to somebody else, but in recent years, it comes closer and closer; hardly anyone has not lost a friend or relative to cancer. Hoffman wonders if anyone cares if cancer and AIDS cures are snuffed out by the FDA. He quotes Germany's Pastor Niemoller, who in the 1930's wrote of the Nazis, *"First they came for the Communists, but I was not a Communist and I did nothing. Then they came for the trade unionists, but I was not a trade unionist, so I did nothing. Then they came for the Jews, but I was not a Jew, and I did nothing. Then they came for me, but by then there was nobody left to stand up for me."*

Philosopher George Santayana once wrote that people who do not learn from history are doomed to repeat it. Will we learn from the history of the tragic truth about politics in healing? Will we demand that the needed changes be made before Americans die of cancer even more rapidly than one every minute? In almost every field, we judge things objectively; if they work, we use them - but not in healthcare, and especially not in cancer.

The U.S. has decontrolled nearly every aspect of its economy, which has caused it to be the most vibrant in the world. But we haven't decontrolled healthcare, and our health statistics show it; No. 1 in degenerative disease in the world - in spite of spending more money per capita on healthcare than any other country in the world.

The United States has changed itself and the world in the last part of the 20th century by preaching the virtues of open competition and free markets. "Let the market work its magic", Ronald Reagan used to say, and it has - except in healthcare. Business magazines regularly extol how the New Economy thrives on free markets. If the U.S. economy were regulated like the nontoxic products described in this book, it would have looked like the Soviet system. If IBM had had an FDA to defend its interests, we'd still be using punch cards. In *US News* of June 8, 1998, Mortimer Zuckerman wrote, "Our open-ended....system has proved... adaptable to revolutions in technology and logistics that are simply too dynamic and too complex for any top-down centralized system to exploit." In the December 7, 1998 issue of *Business Week*, a revolutionary breakthrough in fiber optics was described; wave-length division multiplying, or WDM. This multiplies "bandwidth", a previous constraint. This will permit an almost unlimited number of channels for broadcasting, and is "advancing swiftly". In this field, there's no bureaucratically administered system but a free market where breakthroughs can "advance swiftly". Speaking at Harvard's 1999 commencement, Federal Reserve Chairman Alan Greenspan recalled the late Professor Joseph Schumpeter's concept of "creative destruction". In a free economy, taught Schumpeter, a new technology (such as WDM) pushes out old ones in a continuous churning of economic creativity and renewal. Given the Control Mechanisms, this is impossible in healthcare. Until they're cut, neither cesium nor aloe vera, nor anything else in this book has any chance to push aside chemotherapy. Where there is freedom in the U.S. economy, the system works great. But when freedom is restricted, then there is trouble, as indicated by the cancer statistics.

These principles of free markets and open competition need to be applied to healthcare, with a complete lack of government interference where therapies are nontoxic or harmless, with the encouragement of a free flow of uncensored information, and with doctors free to use what works - so long as they do no harm.

That was Hippocrates' First Rule, and it's an excellent basis for reforming our health system.

As the new millennium dawns, consciousness of health issues is unquestionably rising. At some point will Americans decide to take the politics out of cancer and healing? Or are we going to leave things just the way they are - the same old stuff? Will we learn from history? Is there an awakening, a critical mass large enough to turn a page in healthcare and make the needed changes happen? Or has this one-time country of rugged individualists become a supine, follow-the-leader society? A large segment of America wants to become more self-reliant, to take better care of themselves, to stay healthy, and wants the government to stay out of the way of things that will help them to do so. But can they stay focused on this? There are still so many distractions; baseball, football, basketball, hockey, television, or where one will go on the next vacation. However, one thing is certain; when there's as much interest in having a cancer cure as in who will win the World Series or the Super Bowl, we'll have a cancer cure, in fact a variety of them. But this will only happen after people require that the government get out of the way. President George H.W. Bush once said, "If you don't like the way things are, don't sit on the sidelines". It may take nothing short of a cataclysm to stir people enough to demand the changes proposed in this book, but when they do, things will change, and quickly.

The late Margaret Mead once said, "Never doubt that a small group of thoughtful citizens can change the world. Indeed, it's the only thing that ever has."

It's really a very simple agenda: Freedom. If freedom is good for the economy, it will be good for healthcare. Let the market work its magic!

After all, it *is* a Matter of Life and Death.

APPENDIX

On Dr William F. Koch: www.williamfkoch.com

On Hoxsey: cmain@alaska.net
www.afinerview.com
www.wellmedia.com
The Hoxsey Clinic
Centro Biomédico
Tijuana, Mexico
Tel. 011 52 66 84 9011

On Rife: www.kalamark.com
www.keelynet.com/rife
www.rife.org

On DMSO: www.PHARMA21.net
www.dmso.org
PHARMA 21
1363 Shinly, Suite 100
Escondido, CA 92026

On Naessens: www.cerbe.com
www.cose.com
Centre Experimental de Recherches
Biologiques de l'Estrie
5260 Mills St., Rock Forest, Quebec, J1N 3B6
Canada
Tel.: (819) 564-2195
Email: naessens@cerbe.com

On Hydrazine Sulfate: www.ngen.com/hs-cancer

On Electromedicine: www.alpha-stim.com

On Burzynski: www.cancermed.com
www.burzynskipatientgroup.org
S. R. Burzynski Clinic
9432 Old Katy Road, Houston, TX 77055
Tel. (713) 335-5697

On Cesium: www.cancer-coverup.com
www.cureamerica.net/med
www.mwt.net/~drbrewer

VIDEOS: *The Hoxsey Story - Quacks Who Cure Cancer*,
                 by Ken Ausabel. Can be ordered from Winstar -
                 (800) 283--6374

                 Hoxsey's Bio-Medical Center - The Experience.
                 Can be ordered from Carol Main, P.O. Box 152,
                 Soldotna, Alaska 99669

Both videos, as well as *You Don't Have to Die*, by Harry Hoxsey, can be
ordered from Centro Biomédico, Tijuana, Mexico; tel: 011-52-66-84-9011.

American Preventative Medical Association: www.apma.net
P.O. Box 458   Great Falls, Virginia   22066
Tel. 800-230-2762   Fax   703-759-6711

Citizens for Health: www.citizens.org

California Citizens for Health   www.citizenshealth.org

The Alpha-Stim 100 may be purchased from:

    Electromedical Products International, Inc.
    2201 Garrett Morris Parkway, Mineral Wells, TX 76067-9484
    Tel. (800) FOR-PAIN (367-7246), (940) 328-0788
    Fax (940) 328-0888, email: alpha-stim@epii.com
    Web Site: www.alpha-stim.com

The legal chemical hydrazine sulfate may be purchased from most "compounding" pharmacies (ask your pharmacist for the location of one or consult
the internet).

The mineral cesium, which is found in the human body, is for sale to
licensed health professionals by:

    Bio-Tech
    Box 1992
    Fayetteville, AR 72702
    Tel. (800) 345-1199

    It can also be obtained from some compounding pharmacies.

Meg Patterson drug addiction treatment center: Ken Small (619) 421-5610.

ACCESS TO MEDICAL TREATMENT ACT (AMTA)

During the 2000 session of Congress, this bill was S-1955 in the Senate and HR-2635 in the House of Representatives. During the 2001 session, the bill will have to be reintroduced, so the numbers will change, and perhaps some provisions, but the name and objectives will remain the same.

What is the Access to Medical Treatment Act?

This is a Health Freedom bill. It will create a federal statutory right for consumers to use unapproved drugs and devices, so long as they follow the safety provisions in the bill. It will free practitioners from the fear of censorship, harassment, or worse for using unconventional therapies. It will guarantee your right to access the medical treatments of your choice, without the need of FDA approval. It will give Americans the ability to use therapies that are available to millions of people worldwide, and eliminate the need for Americans to go to Canada, Germany, Mexico, and elsewhere for therapies that are still considered illegal here in the U.S.

Would this bill open the door to dangerous quackery?

NO. Consumer protections are an essential element of the bill. The AMTA was conceived as a patients' rights bill, to ensure that all Americans have access to the full range of therapies. Practitioners need to be protected from those who want to censure them or even to eliminate unconventional treatments.

This is a freedom of choice bill. It gives Americans access to therapies that are being used safely and effectively in other countries, but which are not available here because FDA has not approved them.

Freedom of choice is one of the bedrock principles upon which our nation rests. Asserting the right to use alternative treatments, provided that patients are not misled or misinformed, extends freedom of choice to the realm of medicine. This legislation stems from the conviction that an individual, suffering from a disease for which conventional medicine offers limited or no hope, should not be denied access to a nonconventional treatment if there is reason to

believe that it might be beneficial. It also recognizes that not everyone is willing to suffer the side effects of conventional therapies
when less toxic remedies are available.

What specific safeguards are there for consumers?

The legislation requires that unapproved treatments must be
administered by licensed or otherwise authorized health care
providers. It does not permit them to exceed their normal scope of
practice. The products may not be advertised or promoted, which
would prevent unscrupulous individuals from profiting from the sale
of unapproved drugs. In addition, practitioners would be prohibited
from charging more than an amount necessary to recover their costs.
This restraint, coupled with other consumer protections in the bill, is
meant to limit the use of unapproved drugs and devices to practitioners and manufacturers who have the best interests of the patients
in mind.

Don't we need the FDA to approve these substances to ensure that they are safe and effective?

The FDA is not in the business of regulating the practice of medicine, yet it has tried to insert itself into the process through its ham-
merlock on the dissemination of scientific information, its attempts
to classify natural substances as drugs, and its delay in approving
therapies that have been used successfully in other countries for
decades. If Americans are to achieve the best health care in the
world, the present system of regulation must be altered.

Why don't companies simply get their therapies approved by the FDA?

The present system doesn't work for therapies that are
unpatentable (because they incorporate natural substances). It costs
upwards of $300 million and takes a decade or more to obtain FDA
approval of drugs today. Without patent protection, a manufacturer
could not recoup that expense. In addition, many foreign companies
are unwilling to commit that time and expense for products already
approved for use overseas.

Health Freedom of Choice Act

1) Regardless of the definition of a drug used by the Food and Drug Administration (FDA), as of the effective date of this Act, FDA is prohibited from exercising jurisdiction over products which are nontoxic or devices which are harmless.

2) Nontoxicity is defined as any substance less toxic than aspirin and is established when a manufacturer submits to the FDA tests from three independent, unrelated, and unconnected testing laboratories certifying that the product which the manufacturer proposes to place in interstate commerce is no more toxic than aspirin.

3) Harmlessness is established when the Underwriters Laboratory certifies as harmless a device which a manufacturer proposes to place into interstate commerce.

4) The FDA may contest such findings of nontoxicity or harmlessness, if it chooses, but it is required to do so within 90 days (as it routinely did before 1963), and must do so in sworn testimony made available to the manufacturer and to the public.

5) In the failure of the FDA to contest certification of nontoxicity or harmlessness in sworn testimony, the manufacturer is free to place the product in question in interstate commerce.

6) FDA officials up to and including the Commissioner will be guilty of committing a felony if they fail to observe the 90-day deadline. Manufacturers subjected to delays beyond the 90-day deadline are hereby authorized to press both criminal and/or civil charges against such FDA officials as seek to delay introduction of a product into interstate commerce, after the 90-day deadline has passed, without the presenta-

tion of sworn testimony establishing that the product is more toxic than aspirin or that it is harmful despite certification of its harmlessness by the Underwriters Laboratory.

7) Once a product is placed into interstate commerce, the FDA is expressly forbidden from seeking an injunction to prohibit such introduction into interstate commerce. Any FDA official will be guilty of a felony who seeks such an injunction, or seeks in any way to delay the introduction into interstate commerce of a product certified as nontoxic or harmless in the manner above stipulated.

8) From the effective date of this Act, FDA's authorization to press criminal charges is restricted to products which are toxic, and FDA is prohibited from pressing criminal charges in any regulatory action when products have been certified as nontoxic and harmless in the manner stipulated. Similarly, the FDA is prohibited from confiscating such products as have been certified as nontoxic and harmless.

9) Employees of the FDA, upon their departure from the FDA, are hereby prohibited for ten years from working in any capacity, either as an employee, consultant, or member of a board, for any company subject to regulation by the FDA.

10) Employees of the Federal Trade Commission (FTC) upon their departure from the FTC, are hereby prohibited for ten years from working in any capacity, either as an employee, consultant, or member of a board, for any company subject to regulation by the FDA.

11) The General Accounting Office (GAO) will carry out a study to determine which and how many FDA employees will be rendered superfluous when the FDA is prohibited from regulating nontoxic substances or harmless devices, after the effective date of this law.

12) When the said GAO study is completed, and when the said number of FDA employees to be rendered superfluous is determined, the FDA is then required to put such superfluous employees to work in "post-marketing surveillance". Post-marketing surveillance is the regulatory inspection of substances already approved by the FDA as prescription drugs. Since such drugs, used in the indicated way, have become one of the top causes of death in the U.S., extensive and intensive additional regulatory supervision is needed. FDA was created to make sure that drugs are safe and needs to return to that focus. The American public has no need of protection against products certified as nontoxic or harmless, which have no place under FDA jurisdiction. Relieved of unnecessary regulation over products certified as nontoxic and harmless, the FDA will then be free to return to its basic duty of protecting the American public from toxic drugs, a duty at which it has failed in recent years. Thus FDA regulatory efforts will be focused and concentrated upon products which can do harm rather than dissipated in examination of products which cannot do harm.

The Fitzgerald Report

The following is excerpted from the report made in 1953 by Benedict Fitzgerald of the U.S. Department of Justice, to the Senate Interstate Commerce Committee on the Need for Investigation of Cancer Research Organizations. The report was requested by Senator Charles Tobey of New Hampshire, Chairman of the Committee, who soon thereafter died suddenly. Senator John Bricker of Ohio, Senator Tobey's successor as committee chairman, refused to see Fitzgerald or to accept his report. At the request of Senator Tobey's son, Senator William Langer of North Dakota inserted the report into the Congressional Record, where it can be found dated **August 3, 1953**, on page A5350 of the Congressional Record Appendix.

FROM: Benedict F. Fitzgerald, Jr., special counsel to the Committee on Interstate and Foreign Commerce

TO: Hon. John W. Bricker and members of the Interstate and Foreign Commerce Committee of the United States Senate

SUBJECT: Progress report on study requested by the late Senator Charles W. Tobey, chairman, Senate Interstate and Foreign Commerce Committee

The undersigned, as special counsel to the Senate Interstate and Foreign Commerce Committee, was directed to supervise a study of the following:

The facts involving the interstate conspiracy, if any, engaged in by any individuals, organizations, corporations, associations, and combines of any kind whatsoever, to hinder, suppress, or restrict the free flow or transmission of **Krebiozen, glyoxylide**, and/or mucorhicin, and other drugs, preparations, and remedies, and information, researches, investigations, experiments, and demonstrations relating to the cause, prevention, and methods of diagnosis and treatment of the disease cancer.

The undersigned traveled to Illinois to investigate the so-called **Krebiozen controversy**... The controversy is involved and requires further research and development. **There is reason to believe that the American Medical Association (AMA) has been hasty, capricious, arbitrary, and outright dishonest**, and of course, if the doctrine of "respondeat superior" is to be observed, the alleged machinations of Dr. J. J. Moore (for the past 10 years the treasurer of the AMA) could involve the AMA and others in an interstate conspiracy of alarming proportions. The principal witnesses who tell of Dr. Moore's rascality are Alberto Barreira, Argentine cabinet minister, and his secretary, Anna D. Schmidt.

Being vitally interested and having tried to listen and observe closely, it is my profound conviction that this substance **Krebiozen** is one of the most promising materials yet isolated for the management of cancer. It is biologically active. I have gone over the records of 530 cases, most of them conducted at a distance from Chicago, by unbiased cancer experts and clinics. In researching my conclusions, I have of course discounted my own lay observations and relied mostly on the opinions of qualified cancer research workers and ordinary experienced physicians.

I have concluded that in the value of present cancer research, this substance and the theory behind it deserves the most full and complete and scientific study. Its value in the management of the cancer patient has been demonstrated in a sufficient number and percentage of cases to demand further work.

Behind and over all this is the weirdest conglomeration of corrupt motives, intrigue, selfishness, jealousy, obstruction, and conspiracy that I have ever seen.

Dr. Andrew C. Ivy, who has been conducting research upon this drug, is absolutely honest intellectually, scientifically, and in every other way. Moreover, he appears to be one of the most competent and unbiased cancer experts that I have ever come in contact with, having served on the board of the American Cancer Society and the American Medical Association and in that capacity having been called upon to evaluate various types of cancer therapy. Dr George O. Stoddard, president of the University of Illinois, is assisting in the cessation of Dr. Ivy's research at the

University of Illinois, and in recommending the abolishment of the latter's post as vice president of that institution, has, in my opinion, shown attributes of intolerance for scientific research in general...

Now, passing on to another institution, I have very carefully studied the court records of three cases tried in the Federal and State courts of Dallas, Texas. A running fight has been going on between officials, especially Dr. Morris Fishbein, of the American Medical Association, through the journal of that organization, and the **Hoxsey Cancer Clinic**. Dr. Fishbein contended that the medicines employed by the Hoxsey Cancer Clinic had no therapeutic value; that it was run by a quack and a charlatan. (This clinic is manned by a staff of over 30 employees, including nurses and physicians.) Reprints and circulation of several million copies of articles so prepared (by Fishbein) resulted in litigation. The Government thereafter intervened and sought an injunction to prevent the transmission in interstate commerce of certain medicines. It is interesting to note that in the trial court, before Judge Atwell, who had an opportunity to hear the witnesses in two different trials, it was held that the so-called Hoxsey method of treating cancer was in some respects superior to that of X-ray, radium, and surgery and did have therapeutic value. The Circuit Court of Appeals of the Fifth Circuit decided otherwise. This decision was handed down during the trial of a libel suit in the District Court of Dallas, Texas, by Hoxsey against **Morris Fishbein**, who **admitted that he had never practiced medicine one day in his life and had never had a private patient**, which resulted in a verdict for Hoxsey and against Morris Fishbein. **The defense admitted that Hoxsey could cure external cancer** but contended that his medicines for internal cancer had no therapeutic value. The jury, after listening to leading pathologists, radiologists, physicians, surgeons, and scores of witnesses, a great number of whom had never been treated by any physician or surgeon except the treatment received at the Hoxsey Cancer Clinic, concluded that Dr. Fishbein was wrong; that his published statements were false, and that the Hoxsey method of treating cancer did have therapeutic value. In this litigation, the Government of the United States, as well as Dr Fishbein, brought to the court leading medical scientists, including pathologists and others skilled in the treatment of cancer. They came from all parts of the country. It is significant to note that a great number of these doctors admitted that X-ray therapy could cause cancer. This view is supported by medical publications, including the magazine entitled *Cancer*, published by the American Cancer Society, May issue of 1948.

Report of Dr. George Miley, medical director of Gotham hospital, New York, of a survey made by Dr. Stanley Reimann (in charge of tumor research and pathology, Gotham Hospital). Dr. Reimann's report on cancer cases in Pennsylvania over a long period of time showed that **those who received no treatment lived a longer period than those who received surgery**, radium, **or X-ray**. The exceptions were those patients who had received electrosurgery. The survey also showed that **following the use of** radium and **X-ray, much more harm than good was done to the average cancer patient.**

Doctors Warned to be Wary in Use of X-Rays in Disease Treatment, by Howard W. Blakeslee, Associated Press Science Editor.

New York, July 6, 1948. X-rays and gamma rays can cause bone cancer, is a warning issued in *Cancer*, a new medical journal started by the American Cancer Society... One of the most dangerous things about this kind of bone cancer, the report states, is the very long delay between the use of the rays and the appearance of the cancer. The delay time in the 11 cases (reported) ranged from 6 to 22 years. Dr. Herman Joseph Muller, Nobel Prize winner, a world-renowned scientist, has stated **the medical profession is permanently damaging** the American life stream through the unwise use of X-rays. There is no dosage of X-rays so low as to be without risk of producing harmful mutations.

The attention of the Committee is invited to the request made by Senator Elmer Thomas following an investigation made by the Senator of the **Hoxsey Clinic** under date of February 25, 1947, and addressed to the Surgeon General, Public Health Department, Washington, DC, wherein he sought to enlist the support of the

Federal Government to make an investigation and report. No such investigation was made. In fact, every effort was made to avoid and evade the investigation by the Surgeon General's office. The record will reveal that this (Hoxsey) Clinic did furnish 62 complete case histories, including pathology, names of hospitals, physicians, etc., in 1945. Again, in June 1950, 77 case histories, which included the names of the patients, pathological reports in many instances, and in the absence thereof, the names of the pathologists, hospitals, and physicians who had treated these patients before being treated at the Hoxsey Cancer Clinic. The Council of the National Cancer institute, without investigation, in October 1950, refused to order an investigation. The record in the Federal court discloses that this agency of the Federal Government (NCI) <u>took sides and sought in every way to hinder, suppress, and restrict this institution in their treatment of cancer</u> (See testimony of Dr. Gilcin Meadors, pp. 1125-1139, transcript of record, Case No. 13645, U.S.C.A.)

Accordingly, we should determine whether existing agencies, both public and private, are engaged in and have pursued a policy of harassment, ridicule, slander, and libelous attacks on others sincerely engaged in stamping out cancer, this curse of mankind. Have medical associations, through their officers, agents, servants, and employees engaged in this practice? **My investigation to date should convince this committee that a <u>conspiracy does exist</u> to stop the free flow and use of drugs in interstate commerce which allegedly have solid therapeutic value. Public and private funds have been thrown around like confetti at a county fair to close up and destroy clinics, hospitals, and scientific research laboratories which do not conform to the viewpoint of medical associations.**

Respectfully submitted,
Benedict F. Fitzgerald
Special Counsel

Suggested Items to Include in a Letter to Your Senator or Congressman:

American medicine is too tilted toward toxic drugs. We urgently ask you to pass the Access to Medical Treatment Act (bill #) and the Health Freedom of Choice Act (bill #).

We don't need to pay bureaucrats to protect us from things that can't hurt us; the government has no business regulating non-toxic medicines or harmless devices. We need a Free Market in such therapies, with no FDA controls.

One American dies of cancer every minute. Pass the Access to Medical Treatment Act and the Health Freedom of Choice Act so that we can have access to effective nontoxic therapies now only available outside the United States. We're tired of having to go to Mexico or abroad to obtain nontoxic medications. We want the freedom to have these here in the U.S. These medicines would provide stiff competition to the pharmaceutical toxic therapies.

Of all the special interests, pharmaceutical companies are the biggest contributors to Congressional campaigns. We ask you to refuse to accept contributions from the drug companies, and we ask you to vote for the Health Freedom of Choice Act, which will open the doors to real competition.

Do you know how much less it costs to buy almost any drug in Canada or Mexico? It's a bundle! Give the drug companies some stiff competition by passing the Access to Medical Treatment Act and the Health Freedom of Choice Act so as to create a free market in nontoxic therapies. This will permit significant competition for the drug companies. Competition will make their prices come way, way down, in the way that only a free market can do. This is a much better idea than taking taxpayers' money to pay for drugs; that's a handout to the drug companies. What you need to do is to give them real competition which will drive their inflated prices way down. This will happen when you pass these two pieces of legislation.

Do you know that some estimates report that 65% of FDA employees take cushy jobs at the drug companies when they retire from FDA? We want you to vote to prohibit that, by voting for the Health Freedom of Choice Act.

A list of all Senators and Representatives can be obtained by calling the Congress (202) 224-3121, or by consulting the Internet. The house website is www.house.gov; it links with the Senate website.

THE HIGH pH THERAPY FOR CANCER
TESTS ON MICE AND HUMANS
A. Keith Brewer

A. Keith Brewer Science Library, Richland Center, WI 53581

BREWER, A. K. The high pH therapy for cancer: tests on mice and humans.
PHARMACOL BIOCHEM BEHAV 21: Suppl. 1, 1-5. 1984. --- Mass spectrograph
ic and isotope studies have shown that potassium, rubidium, and especially cesium are
most efficiently taken up by cancer cells. This uptake was enhanced by Vitamins A and
C as well as salts of zinc and selenium. The quantity of cesium taken up was sufficient
to raise the cell to the 8 pH range. Where cell mitosis ceases and the life of the cell is
short. Tests on mice fed cesium and rubidium showed marked shrinkage in the tumor
masses within 2 weeks. In addition, the mice showed none of the side effects of cancer. Tests have been carried out on over 30 humans. In each case the tumor masses
disappeared. Also all pains and effects associated with cancer disappeared within 12 to
36 hr; the more chemotherapy and morphine the patient had taken, the longer the withdrawal period. Studies of the food intake in areas where the incidences of cancer are
very low showed that it met the requirements for the high pH therapy.

Cancer therapy   Cesium   High pH   Pain   Potassium   Rubidium   Tumor   Vitamins

The High pH Therapy for cancer was arrived at from an
extensive series of physical experiments. These involved the isotope effect across membranes of many types, normal plant and
animal, embryonic, cancer, and synthetic. It also involved mass
spectrographic analyses of membranes and cells, as well as fluorescence and phosphorescence decay studies of many types of
cells and parts thereof. It is the thesis of this paper that the results
obtained throw a direct light upon the mechanism of carcinogenesis, and also indicate a therapy. Tests on both mice and humans
substantiate this theoretical approach [1-8].

BACKGROUND

The isotope effect throws a very direct light on the mechanism of carcinogenesis. In this study it was shown that the
$^{39}K/^{41}K$ ratio in ocean water down to 6000 ft was 14,20000 [9-11].

In normal matured cells, both plant and animal, the ratio varied from 14.25 to 14.21. Embryonic and cancer cells all gave a ratio of 14.35. In the case of all synthetic cells across which there was a potential gradient, the ratio was 14.35. From these values it will be seen that the ratio in normal living cells indicates that as many isotopes leave the cell as enter.

In the case of potassium for embryonic and cancer cells as well as synthetic type cells with all types of membranes even including liquid mercury films the observed isotope ratio was given by equation 1.

$$\left(^{39}K/^{41}K\right)_O = \left(^{39}K/^{41}K\right)_n (41 + m / 39 + m) \, \tfrac{1}{2} \qquad (1)$$

where n refers to the normal ratio, o to the observed ratio, and m is the associated mass for the ions.

All cations in solution are associated. The attached mass for Cs^+ is 3 molecules of water, for Rb^+ it is 5 molecules, for K^+ is 7 molecules. For cations below potassium in the Electromotive Series all ions are highly associated. This is to be expected from their position in the Hoffmeister Series. In the case of Ca^{++} the association is 30 molecules, while Na^+ is 16. Equation (1) holds for all cations tested from H^+ to U^+. The value of m however will vary when polar molecules are present in the solution. For example, K^+ can also attach glucose. In contrast, Ca^{++} can attach a wide variety of molecules; it is this cation that transports peroxides into the cell, as well as metabolic products out of the cell.

The results given in equation (1) are most significant in that they show that transport is dependent entirely upon the frequency with which the ions strike the membrane surface. It is not a matter of capillary action, but one on which the ion and its associated mass pass directly through the bonding space between molecules which comprise the membrane. That the associated molecules are not lost in this transport is due to the fact that the attraction between the molecules and the ion is far greater than their attraction by the material of the membrane.

In the case of potassium an exact similarity exists between embryonic and cancer cells. The isotope ratio indicates that the

K^+ ions are taken up by the most efficient process possible. The same held true for Cs^+ and Rb^+.

In contrast to the above, a vast difference exists for cations below potassium in the EMS. In the case of embryonic cells all cations tested obeyed equation (1). In the case of cancer cells cations below potassium were taken up sparingly, if at all. For example the amount of calcium in cancer cells is only about one percent of that in normal cells [18].

The above isotope effect for potassium which transports glucose into the cell, and for calcium which transports oxygen are most significant with respect to cancer. They mean that glucose can readily enter cancer cells but that oxygen cannot enter. This accounts for the anaerobic state of cancer cells pointed out by Warburg as early as 1925 [26].

The mechanism responsible for the similarity in the isotope effect for potassium and rubidium in cancer and embryonic cells and for their marked difference in case of calcium was investigated in some detail using mass spectrographic analyses, and also fluorescence and phosphorescence decay patterns.

The phosphorescence decay patterns were found to be peculiar to and specific for all cell types or parts thereof [12-15]. It should be mentioned that the decay spectra is due entirely to the light emitted from the energized double bonds. All double bonds are capable of being raised to the energized state. While the fluorescence spectra and the phosphorescence decay patterns are both specific for each double bond they can be influenced by adjacent strong polar radicals. Again, both can be completely depressed by molecules absorbed over the surface; thus morphine, as well as attached polycyclic type molecules, will completely depress the excitation of the P=O radicals which characterize all cell membrane surfaces.

It was observed that the membranes tested gave a phosphorescence decay pattern due almost entirely to the P=O radicals which are composed of phospholipids. These radicals are specifically oriented over each type of membrane. This is most significant from the point of view of membrane action, since the P=O radicals are moderately strong electron donors in the ground state and strong to powerful donors in the energized state. This is due to the fact that the ionization potentials, 1st to 5th, are appreciably higher for the 0 than the P atom. This means that the 4 bonding electron orbitals will be displaced nearer the 0 atom thus surrounding this atom with a pronounced negative field. The P atom is thus positive in nature.

The above results are most important with respect to membrane action. They show that the strong electron acceptors Cs^+, Rb^+, and K^+ can be attracted into the membrane so that they will enter the negative potential gradient which exists across all living membranes. In contrast to these cations, the highly associated cations farther down in the EMS are not sufficiently strong electron acceptors to be drawn into this gradient except when the $P=O$ radicals are in the energized state. This means that K^+ cations which transport glucose into the cell can readily enter cancer cells, but that Ca^{++} ions which transport oxygen into the cell cannot enter. In the normal cell the glucose, upon entering the cell, reacts with the oxygen in the cell and is burned to carbon dioxide and water with the liberation of heat. This heat in turn is absorbed on the membrane surface and raises the $P=O$ radicals to an energized state which permits them to attach more Ca^{++} ions. Thus it will be seen that the amount of oxygen entering the cell is determined by oxidation within the cell, primarily that of glucose. This action is responsible for the pH control mechanism of the cell which maintains a value near 7.35.

The reactivity of the double bond has been studied in some detail using both light absorption and electron impact. It was found that energy states of the order of those produced by metabolic processes were not reactive. In contrast, high energy states such as those that are induced by radioactivity. are very reactive. Intermediate energy states in the ultra violet range were not reactive. Intermediate energy states in the ultra violet range were not reactive by electron impact, but slightly with light quanta. Here however the reactivity increased with a high power of the energy intensity per unit area [16]. This suggests that the reactivity may be due to the multiple absorption of light quanta, thus raising the energy of the bond to the sum of the quanta absorbed (see Table

1).

TABLE 1

THE RELATIONSHIP BETWEEN REACTIVITY DOUBLE BOND
REACTIVITY, INTERMEDIATE ENERGY STATES, WAVE LENGTH
AND RADIATION

Volts Ve=h $\times 1.235 \times 10^x$	Wave Length Å	Radiation	Reactivity
10^{-4}	1 cm	Rotation Spectra	
			Zero
10^{-3}	10^7 Å	Infra Red	
10^{-2}	10^6 Å		
10^{-1}	10^5 Å	Solar	Zero
1	10^4 Å	Ultra Violet	
10	10^3 Å		Low
10^2	10^2 Å	X-Rays	High
10^3	10 Å		
10^4	1 Å	Gamma	High
10^5	0.1 Å		
10^6	0.01 Å		

THE MECHANISM OF CARCINOGENESIS

The experimental information presented in the previous section involving the isotope effect, mass spectrographic analyses, and fluorescence and phosphorescence decay, combined with the pH data supplied by Von Ardenne [23-25], makes it possible to define the mechanism involved in carcinogenesis. This mechanism is very different from the accepted one of carcinogens entering the cell and becoming attached to the DNA. This mechanism will not explain any of the experimental data outlined briefly herein.

The proposed mechanism can be outlined in four steps.

Step 1

The attachment of carcinogenic type molecules to the membrane surface. This involves two factors: (a) the presence of carcinogenic-type molecules primarily of the polycyclic type, and (b) an energized state of the membrane, which may result from prolonged irritation. When these molecules are attached to the membrane glucose can still enter the cell, but oxygen cannot. The cell thus becomes anaerobic.

Step 2

In the absence of oxygen, the glucose undergoes fermentation to lactic acid. The cell pH then drops to 7 and finally down to 6.5.

Step 3

In the acid medium the DNA loses its positive and negative radical sequence. In addition, the amino acids entering the cell are changed. As a consequence, the RNA is changed and the cell completely loses its control mechanism. Chromosomal aberrations may occur.

Step 4

In the acid medium the various cell enzymes are completely changed. Von Ardenne has shown that lysosomal enzymes are changed into very toxic compounds. These toxins kill the cells in the main body of the tumor mass. A tumor therefore consists of a thin layer of rapidly growing cells surrounding the dead mass [3]. The acid toxins leak out from the tumor mass and poison the host. They thus give rise to the pains generally associated with cancer. They can also act as carcinogens.

HIGH AND LOW pH THERAPYS

Only two therapys will be mentioned here. Both are apparently effective. These are the Low pH therapy devised by Von Ardenne *et al.* [23-25] and the High pH therapy developed by the writer.

The Low pH Therapy

In this therapy devised by Von Ardenne, glucose is injected into the blood stream. As a consequence, the cancer cell pH will drop eventually to the 5.5 range. The patient is then placed in a furnace heated to 104°F for a matter of hr [23-25]. The older the patient, the fewer the number of hours. The patient is allowed to breathe cold air. Diathermy is also applied over the tumor area which, in the absence of a blood supply, will cause the temperature of the mass to rise to something over 106°F. At these high temperatures and in the acid medium, the life of cancer cells is very short. The only drawback to the therapy is that a case of severe toxemia may result from the out-leakage of the acid toxins within the tumor masses [23-25].

The High pH Therapy

The ready uptake of cesium and rubidium by the cancer cells lead the writer to the High pH therapy. This consists of feeding the patient close to 6 g of CsCl or RbCl per day in conjunction with the administration of ascorbic and retionic acids, Vitamins C and A, which being weak acids, upon absorption by the tumor cells will enhance the negative potential gradient across the membrane, and also zinc and selenium salts which, when absorbed on the membrane surface, will act as broad and moderately strong electron donors. Both types of compounds have been shown in mice to drastically enhance the pickup for cesium and rubidium ions.

The toxic dose for CsCl is 135 g. The administration of 6 g per day therefore has no toxic effects. It is sufficient however to give rise to the pH in the cancer cells, bringing them up in a few days to the 8 or above where the life of the cell is short. In addition, the presence of Cs and Rb salts in the body fluids neutralizes the acid toxins leaking out of the tumor mass and renders them nontoxic.

TESTS OF THE HIGH pH THERAPY ON MICE AND HUMANS

The therapy has been tested and the results will be discussed briefly below.

Tests on Mice

The High pH therapy was first tested at American University in Washington, DC using mice. In these tests, 2 mm cubes of mammary tumors were implanted in the abdomens of mice and allowed to grow for 8 days. The mice were then divided into two groups. Both groups were continued on mouse chow, but the test group was given 1.11 g of rubidium carbonate by mouth per day in aqueous solution. After 13 more days the controls were starting to die so all mice were sacrificed and the tumors removed and weighed. The tumors in the test animals weighed only one eleventh of those in the controls. In addition, the test animals were showing none of the adverse effects of having cancer [3].

Results similar to those mentioned above were obtained at Platteville, WI using CsCl. More recently, Platteville has studied intraperitoneal injection of cesium carbonate for mice with abdominal tumor implants with 97% curative effect.

Tests using intraperitoneal injections of CsCl were carried out by Messiha et al. [21]. The results were most successful and showed a drastic shrinkage in the tumor masses.

Tests on Man

Many tests on humans have been carried out by H. Nieper in Hannover, Germany and by H. Sartori in Washington, DC as well as by a number of other physicians. On the whole, the results have been very satisfactory. It has been observed that all pains associated with cancer disappear within 12 to 24 hr, except in a very few cases where there was a morphine withdrawal problem that required a few more hours. In these tests 2 g doses of CsCl were administered three times per day after eating. In most cases

5 to 10 g of Vitamin C and 100,000 units of Vitamin A, along with 50 to 100 mg of zinc, were also administered. Both Nieper and Sartori were also administering nitrilosides in the form of laetrile. There are good reasons to believe that the laetrile may be more effective than the vitamins in enhancing the pickup of cesium by the cells.

In addition to the loss of pains, the physical results are a rapid shrinkage of the tumor masses. The material comprising the tumors is secreted as uric acid in the urine; the uric acid content of the urine increases many fold. About 50% of the patients were pronounced terminal, and were not able to work. Of these, a majority have gone back to work.

Two side effects have been observed in some of the patients. These are first nausea, and the second diarrhea. Both depend upon the general condition of the digestive tract. Nieper feels that nausea can be prevented by administering the cesium in a solution of sorbitol. The diarrhea may, to some extent, be affected by the Vitamin C.

Only one case history will be presented here. A woman with 2 hard tumor masses 8 to 10 cm in diameter, one on her thyroid and one on her chest, was given 3 to 6 months to live. She had been subjected to chemotherapy, but was discontinued because it weakened her. She was taking laetrile on her own. She was given a 50 g bottle of CsCl and was told to take 4 g per day. She reported her case a year later. Being very frightened she took the entire 50 g in one week. At the end of that time the tumor masses were very soft, so she obtained another 50 g of CsCl and took it in another week. By the end of that time she could not find the tumors, and two years later there was no sign of their return.

LOW INCIDENCE CANCER AREAS

There are a number of areas where the incidences of cancer are very low. Unfortunately, the food composition in these areas has never been analyzed. At the 1978 Stockholm Conference on Food and Cancer it was concluded that there is definitely a connection between the two, but since the relationship was not understood, no conclusions could be drawn [22]. The food intake has been studied by the author as far as possible from the high pH point of view. The results found will be discussed for a number of low incidence areas.

The Hopi Indians of Arizona

The incidence of cancer among the Hopi Indians is 1 in 1000 as compared to 1 in 4 for the USA as a whole. Fortunately their food has been analyzed from the standpoint of nutritional values [17]. In this study it was shown that the Hopi food runs higher in all the essential minerals than conventional foods. It is very high in potassium and exceptionally high in rubidium. Since the soil is volcanic it must also be very rich in cesium. These Indians live primarily on desert grown calico corn products. Instead of using baking soda they use the ash of chamisa leaves, a desert grown plant. The analyses of this ash showed it to be very rich in rubidium. The Indians also eat many fruits, especially apricots, per day. They always eat the kernels. The results indicate clearly that the Hopi food meets the requirements for the High pH therapy.

The Pueblo Indians of Arizona

Some 20 years ago the incidence of cancer among the Pueblo Indians was the same as that for the Hopi Indians, since their food was essentially the same. But unlike the Hopi, these Indians have accrued certain items from outside their environment, hence supermarkets were installed in the area. Today the incidence of cancer among the Pueblos is 1 in 4, the same as the U.S. It is reported that there is a regular epidemic of cancer among them. It must be emphasized here that the high incidence of cancer is not due to what is in the supermarket foods, hut rather to what is not in it. It is essentially lacking rubidium and cesium and low in potassium.

The Hunza of North Pakistan

Cancer is essentially unknown among the Hunza, but unfortunately their food has never been analyzed. Talks with Hunza themselves and with Hindu professors who have spent some time in the area, have thrown sufficient light upon the food intake to show that it meets the requirements of the High pH therapy. They are essentially vegetarians, and are great fruit eaters, eating ordinarily 40 apricots per day; they always eat the kernels, either directly or as a meal. They drink at least 4 liters of mineral spring waters which abound in the area. Fortunately this water has been analyzed and found to be very rich in cesium. Since the soil is volcanic in nature, it must be concluded that it will be rich in Cs and Rb, as well as K.

Central and South America

The Indians who live in Central America and on the highland of Peru and Equador have very low incidences of cancer. The soil in these areas is volcanic. Fruit from the areas has been obtained and analyzed for rubidium and cesium and found to run very high in both elements. Cases have been reliably reported where people with advance inoperable cancer have gone to live with these Indians, and found that all tumor masses disappear within a very few months. Clearly the food there meets the high pH requirements.

In conclusion, the High pH therapy, as has been pointed out, was arrived at from physical experiments carried out on cancer and normal cells. It has been tested and found effective on cancers in both mice and humans. There can be no question that Cs and Rb salts, when present in the adjacent fluids, the pH of cancer cells will rise to the point where the life of the cell is short, and that they will also neutralize the acid toxins formed in the tumor mass and render them nontoxic.

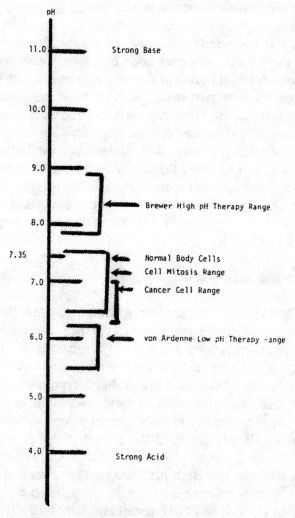

FIG. 1. The relationship between pH of cancer cells and cancer progression: the high and low pH therapies.

Cesium Dosage and Side Effects

Several problems have arisen in the therapy which require further study. One of these is to determine the minimal dosage of CsCl that will kill cancer cells. Would cesium carbonate be better? Related to this are the effectiveness of intravenous injections, and, in certain cases, intraperitoneal injections. Both have been found to be effective in mice, but they have not yet been tested on humans.

The minimal dosage for curative action has not been determined. It has been observed by several physicians that the administration of 0.5 g per day of CsCl will actually enhance the rate of tumor growth. This is to be expected, since this low amount is sufficient only to raise the cell pH into the high mitosis range (see Chart 1). The data so far reveal that any quantity of 3.0 g or above will be effective.

A side effect which occurs in some cases, especially those who have had stomach ulcers, is nausea. This is far smaller for 3.0 g per day than for 6 to 10 g. The nausea can be minimized by administering cesium salt in a sorbitol solution as mentioned earlier. Further studies are necessary.

A limited number of patients have experienced diarrhea. Since cesium is a nerve stimulant [19], this can be expected. The effect is enhanced by taking large doses of Vitamin C, but it apparently is lowered by laetrile.

A further study is being made to determine the amount of cesium, rubidium or possible potassium in the diet that is sufficient to prevent cancer. Some data is available on the food composition in areas of the world where cancer is very low, but it is difficult to quantify, since the amount eaten varies greatly between individuals.

The effectiveness of potassium salts is yet to be determined. Tests to date have not been made on leukemia patients.

CESIUM BIOLOGICAL USES

In addition to the cancer therapy outlined in this paper, a [19] U.S. Patent has been issued on the use of cesium chloride as a nerve stimulant. Cesium salts are very effective in regulating heart arrhythmia. In areas of the world where cesium in the food intake is high, it has been noted that longevity of well over 100 years is not at all uncommon. Based on experimental data available [21] Cs salts may be useful in the treatment of manic-depressives.

REFERENCES

1. Brewer, A. K. The mechanism of carcinogenesis: Comments on therapy. *J Int Acad Prev Med* 5: 29-53, 1979.
2. Brewer, A. K. Cancer: Comments on the physics involved. *Am Lab* 5: 12-23. 1973.
3. Brewer, A. K., B. J. Clarke, M. Greenberg and N. Rothkopf. The effects of rubidium on mammary tumor growth in C57BL K/6J mice. *Cytobios* 24: 99-101, 1979.
4. Brewer, A. K. and R. Passwater. Physics of the cell membrane. I. The role of the double bond energy states. *Am Lab* 6: 59-72, 1974,
5. Brewer, A. K. and R. Passwater. Physics of the cell membrane. II. Fluorescence and phosphorescence in cell analysis. *Am Lab* 6: 19-29, 1974.
6. Brewer, A. K. and R. Passwater. Physics of the cell membrane. III. The mechanism of nerve action. *Am Lab* 6: 49-62, 1974.
7. Brewer, A. K. and R. Passwater. Physics of the cell membrane. IV. Further comments on the role of the double-bond. *Am Lab* 7: 41-50, 1975.
8. Brewer, A. K. and R. Passwater. Physics of the cell membrane. V. Mechanisms involved in cancer. *Am Lab* 8: 37-45, 1976.
9. Brewer, J. Isotopes of potassium. *Ind Chem Eng* 30: 893, 1938.
10. Brewer, J. Abundance of the isotopes of potassium in mineral and plant sources. *J Am Chem Soc* 58: 365-369, 1936.
11. Brewer, A. K. Man spectrographic analysis of the constancy of the atomic weight of potassium in ocean water. *J Am Chem Soc* 58: 370-375, 1936.
12. Brewer, A. K. Excitation of the hydrocarbon double bond. *Am Sci* 56: 259, 1968.
13. Brewer, A. K., S. Adelman, H. Hoerman and W. Sanborn. Differential identification of biological entities by phosphorescence decay. *Nature* 213: 718-719, 1976.
14. Brewer, A. K. and S. Adelman. Method for analysis and identification of biological entities by phosphorescence decay. U.S. Patent 3, 470, 373, 1969.
15. Brewer, A. K. Methods and means for the detection of microorganisms in the air. U.S. Patent 3, 566, 114, 1970.
16. Brewer, A. K. Chemical action in low volt arc. *Physiol Rev* 42: 785, 1932.

17. Calloway, D. R., R. D. Giaque and F. N. Costa. The superior mineral content of some American Indian food, in comparison to Federal donated counterpart commodities. *Ecol Food Nutr* 3: 203-210, 1974.

18. Editorial. *Lancet* 1: 1204, 1964.

19. Masco. H. L. U.S. Patent 3, 614, 242, 1972.

20. Messiha, F. S. The antidepressant action of cesium chloride and ethanol preference in rodents. In: *Alcoholism: A Perspective.* edited by F. S. Messiha and B. S. Tyner. New York: PJD Pub., 1980, pp. 247-259.

21. Messiha, F. S., A. El-Domeiri and H. F. Sproat. Effects of lithium and cesium salts on sarcoma-I implants in the mouse. *Neurobehav Toxicol* 1: 27-31, 1979.

22. Special report. Food and cancer. *Nutr Rev* 36: 313-314, 1978.

23. Von Ardenne M., P. G. Reitnauer and D. Schmidt. Theoretische Grundlagen und in vivo Messungen zur Optimierung der selekiven übersäurung von Krebsgewebe. *Acta Biol Med Germ* 22: 35-60, 1969.

24. Von Ardenne, M. Selective multiphase cancer therapy: Conceptual aspects and experimental basis. *Adv Pharmacol Chemother* 10: 339-380, 1972.

25. Von Ardenne, M. and A. Von Ardenne. Berechnung des pH-Profile im Interkapillarraum der Krebsgewebe für die Faelle mit und ohne Langzeit-Glucose-Infusion. *Res Exp Med* 171: 177-189, 1977.

26. Von Warburg, O. Metabolism of human tumor cells. *Klin Wohnschr* 4: 2396-2397, 1925.

Note: In later writing, Dr. Brewer wrote: "The goal of high pH therapy is the transport of large quantities of Cs^+, Rb^+ and glucose-free K^+ across the membranes of cancer cells. During high pH therapy Dr. H. Nieper observed a loss of potassium which should be replaced." Two booklets discussing Dr. Brewer's theories about cesium are available from the Brewer Science Library: "High pH Cancer Therapy With Cesium," by A. Keith Brewer, Ph.D. and "Cancer Its Nature and A Proposed Treatment." For information, contact the Brewer Science Library by phone (608) 647-6513, by fax (608) 647-6797, by e-mail drbrewer@mwt.net, or by mail: 325 N. Central Ave., Richland Center, WI 53581. The library web site is: http//:www.mwt.net/~drbrewer.

The Brewer Science Library offers Dr. Brewer's writings for information purposes only and will assume no responsibility or liability for the use of any of the information in his writings.

This study, as it appeared in *Pharmacology, biochemistry & Behavior*, Vol 21, Suppl 1, 1-5, is reprinted by special arrangement with Elsevier Science, holder of the copyright.

Neal Deoul (pp 428-9, www.cancer-coverup.com) caused his prostate cancer to go into remission using Dr. Brewer's cesium protocol. Working closely with his doctor as he started taking cesium, Deoul found that his PSA count (indicator of prostate cancer) was climbing considerably. Although his doctor warned him to stop the cesium, Neal Deoul persisted and after several months, his PSA started to drop, eventually returning to normal. Deoul learned that this same phenomenon could occur with another cancer marker, the CA count, as dead cancer cells are dumped into the blood. Having studied chemistry, Neal Deoul knew that cesium could leach out of his body minerals that were below cesium on the Periodic Table of Elements, and these included postasium, magnesium, and lithium. Since a deficiencey of potassium and magnesium could lead to a heart attack, he took these supplements.

ABOUT THE AUTHOR

Daniel Haley served in the New York State Assembly from 1970 to 1976 representing St. Lawrence County. To date he is the only Democrat ever elected to the Assembly from that district in the history of the state.

In the Assembly, he chaired the Legislature's Joint Commission on Energy, emphasizing the need to develop alternative energy resources. He authored the Safe Energy Act of 1975; this established the NYS Energy Research and Development Authority, which is directed by statute to focus on renewable energy resources.

Before entering politics, Haley was an international businessman in Brazil. After managing the Mosler Safe Co.'s Brazilian subsidiary, he assembled the beach real estate project which became the Rio de Janeiro Sheraton. This followed service in the U.S. Air Force as an intelligence officer in Korea, the Philippines, and Japan. He graduated from Harvard College cum laude.

Haley spent four years, 1997-1999 inclusive, writing *Politics in Healing*, and a good deal of the previous ten researching for it.

BIBLIOGRAPHY

Arnott, D. H., MD. Proceedings of the Ontario Cancer Commission regarding Koch Treatment, with commentary, www.williamkoch.com

Bailey, Herbert. *A Matter of Life and Death*, G.P. Putnam's Sons, New York, NY

Becker, Robert O., MD. *Body Electric*, Quill, William Morrow & Co., New York, NY

Becker, Robert O., MD. *Cross Currents*, Jeremy P. Tarcher, Inc., Los Angeles, CA

Bird, Christopher. *Gastons Naessens, Galileo of the Microscope*, Les Presses de l'Université de la Persone, St. Lambert, Quebec, Canada

Bird, Christopher. *The Trial and Persecution of Gaston Naessens*, H.J. Kramer, Tiburon, CA

Bird, Christopher. "What Became of the Rife Microscope?" (*East-West Magazine*)

Borderland Sciences. *The Rife Report*, Borderland Sciences, Garberville, CA

Brown, Raymond Keith, MD. *AIDS, Cancer, and the Medical Establishment*, Robert Speller Publishers, New York, NY

Cantwell, Alan, MD. *The Cancer Microbe*, Aries Rising Press, Los Angeles, CA

Congressional Record of December 6, 1963 on Krebiozen.

Crane, John. *Polarity Research Manual*; collection of papers of Royal Rife, out of print

Elias, Thomas. *Burzynski Breakthrough*, General Publishing Group, 1997

Epstein, Samuel, MD. *The Politics of Cancer Revisited*, East Ridge Press, Fremont Center, NY

Gould, Jay, MD. *Deadly Deceit*, Four Walls Publisher, 1990

Hoxsey, Harry. *You Don't Have to Die*, Centro Médico, Tijuana, Mexico (see other resources)

Ivy, Andrew, MD. *Observations on Krebiozen in the Management of Cancer*, Regnery, Chicago, IL

Kirsch, Daniel L., PhD. *The Science Behind Cranial Electrotherapy Stimulation (CES)*, Medical Scope Publishing Corporation, Edmonton, Alberta, Canada

Koch, William F., MD. *Natural Immunity*, www.williamkoch.com

Koch, William F., MD. *Psychosomatic Judgment*, www.williamkoch.com

Koch, William F., MD. *Survival Factor in Neoplastic and Viral Diseases*, www.williamkoch.com

Lang, Avis. On the Public Record: *Cancer Patients Take the U.S. Government to Court*

Lynes, Barry. *The Cancer Cure That Worked*, Marcus Books, Queensville, Ontario, Canada

Lynes, Barry. *Cancer Solutions*, Marcus Books, Queensville, Ontario, Canada

Lynes, Barry. *The Healing of Cancer*, Marcus Books, Queensville, Ontario, Canada

McGrady, Patrick. *DMSO, The Persecuted Drug*, Doubleday & Co., New York, NY

Moss, Ralph, PhD. *The Cancer Industry*, Paragon House, New York, NY

Natenberg, Maurice. *The Cancer Blackout*, Cancer Control Society, Los Angeles, CA

Natenberg, Maurice. *The Legacy of Dr. Harvey Wiley*, Regent House, Chicago, IL

Pelton, Ross, PhD, and Overholser, Lee, PhD. *Alternatives in Cancer Therapy*, Fireside, Simon & Schuster, New York, NY

Simpson, Mark. *The Rife Way*, out of print

Walker, Morton, DPM. *DMSO, Nature's Healer*, Avery, Garden City Park, New York, NY and Freelance Communications, 484 High Ridge Road, Stamford, CT 06904-3095

Wahl, Albert, MD, Rehwinkel, Bessie L., MD, and Reilly, Lawrence, DD *Birth of a Science*, www.williamkoch.com

Wahl, Albert, MD. *The Least Common Denominator*, www.williamkoch.com

Wiley, Harvey W., MD. *History of a Crime*, Lee Foundation, Milwaukee, WI

Winrod, Gerald, D.D. *Koch Treatment Relieves Suffering*, www.williamkoch.com

INDEX TO POLITICS AND HEALING